Reading and Mental Health

"This volume constitutes a landmark in health humanities research. Many people assume there must be a positive correlation between literary reading and mental well-being but remarkably few studies have looked at the relationship systematically. This volume is a compendium of the most up-to-date and comprehensive evidence, bringing together a diverse range of researchers, practitioners and policy-makers, to shine a light on this fascinating and tricky area. Josie Billington and her fellow contributors have produced a collection that will be required reading for health humanists, practitioners, psychologists and literary readers."

—Neil Vickers, *Professor, Centre for the Humanities and Health, King's College London*

"The power of literature to enhance well being and mental health has been increasingly recognized in recent years. This definitive study brings together the relevant practice and research, with contributions from GPs and neurologists as well as literary scholars, and with hard evidence of the benefits of bibliotherapy for those in prisons, hospitals and care homes. Rich both in historical insights and in pointers to how 'shared reading' can be developed to alleviate disadvantage and distress, it is a comprehensive and invaluable book."

—Blake Morrison, *Poet, Author and Professor of Creative and Life Writing, Goldsmiths, University of London*

"This is an excellent and long overdue book. It brings together into one volume the full range of thinking - from psychology, medicine, psychoanalysis, literature and neuroscience - on why reading matters to human flourishing. As well as the most recent compelling evidence of the value of reading in clinic and care home, community and secure mental health settings, the book offers persuasive testimony from health professionals and service users who have first-hand knowledge of the transformative power of literary reading. Above all, this book brings shared literary reading powerfully to life. It is an essential read for those new to the shared reading phenomenon and to all who have been part of the journey. This book bears witness to how far we have come."

—Jane Davis, *Founder and Director of The Reader*

Josie Billington
Editor

Reading and Mental Health

palgrave
macmillan

Editor
Josie Billington
Centre for Research into Reading,
Literature and Society
University of Liverpool
Liverpool, UK

ISBN 978-3-030-21761-7 ISBN 978-3-030-21762-4 (eBook)
https://doi.org/10.1007/978-3-030-21762-4

This Palgrave Macmillan imprint is published by the registered company Springer Nature Switzerland AG
The registered company address is: Gewerbestrasse 11, 6330 Cham, Switzerland

Contents

Notes on Contributors

Nick Benefield is a former Advisor to the Department of Health Personality Disorder and Offender Personality Disorder Programme and retired Head of the Department of Health/National Offender Management Service. He established in criminal justice settings the environmental model of living, management and care known as PIPES—Psychologically Informed Planned Environments.

Josie Billington is Reader in English and Deputy Director of the Centre for Research into Reading, Literature and Society at the University of Liverpool. She has published extensively on the power of literary reading to influence health, including *Is Literature Healthy?* (Oxford UP, 2016).

Gavin Brookes is a Senior Research Associate in the ESRC Centre for Corpus Approaches to Social Science within the Department of Linguistics and English Language at Lancaster University, with research interests in corpus linguistics and health communication.

Melissa Chapple holds an Economic and Social Research Council Ph.D. studentship in the Department of Psychology at the University of Liverpool and is working with autism organisations to study reading habits and impacts in respect of people living with autism. She was diagnosed with autism at the age of eighteen.

Charlotte Christiansen is a Ph.D. student in the Department of Anthropology in the School of Culture and Society at Aarhus University, Denmark.

Gillian Claridge is based in the School of Language and Culture, Institute of the Pacific United, New Zealand, and Lead Applied Linguist and Research Fellow on the Reading and Dementia Programme at the University of Otago, Wellington.

Katie Clark is a Reader Leader at The Reader, UK, and, since 2008, has pioneered the reading aloud of poetry in residential care groups for people living with dementia.

Helen Cook is a National Health Service-user living with chronic pain, who has been attending a reading group at her pain clinic for several years, and has recently completed a volunteer training course to become a group leader herself.

Rhiannon Corcoran is Professor of Psychology and Public Mental Health at the University of Liverpool, concerned with the psychological, social and environmental mechanisms that underpin mental distress and wellbeing, and leads the Community Wellbeing Evidence Programme of the UK's What Works Centre for Wellbeing.

Anne Line Dalsgård is Associate Professor, and Director of the Ph.D. programme in Anthropology, Global Studies, and the Study of Religion at Aarhus University, Denmark.

Charles Darby-Villis was a Reader in Residence at HMP Low Newton, Durham, and a project worker with The Reader for five years.

Philip Davis is Emeritus Professor and former Director, Centre for Research into Reading, Literature and Society at the University of Liverpool. He is author of *Reading and the Reader* (OUP, 2013) and has published on literature and brain-imaging. He is launching a series with Anthem Press on Bibliotherapy and Wellbeing.

Christophe de Bezenac is a researcher in cognitive neuroscience with a particular interest in the dynamics of social interaction in relation to mental health/illness. His Ph.D. research examined the neural correlates of ambiguity in self-other attribution—an interest stemming from his background in improvised music-making (he has performed widely as a saxophonist on the European jazz scene).

Tom Dening is the Head of the Centre for Dementia in the Institute of Mental Health at the University of Nottingham, and former Medical Director for Cambridgeshire and Peterborough NHS Partnership Trust. He is currently an Honorary Consultant in Old Age Psychiatry with Nottinghamshire Healthcare NHS Trust.

Christopher Dowrick is Professor of Primary Care at the University of Liverpool and General Practitioner at Aintree Group Practice, Liverpool, Merseyside, UK. He is author of *Beyond Depression* (Oxford: Oxford University Press, 2009 [2nd ed]) and Chair of the Working Party for the Mental Health World Organisation of Family Doctors (WONCA).

Clare Ellis is a Learning and Quality Leader at The Reader, Liverpool, UK. She completed her Ph.D. at the University of Liverpool where she was post-doctoral research assistant on studies of reading for depression and dementia.

Grace Farrington (Frame) is a Learning and Quality Leader at UK charity, The Reader. She completed her Ph.D. thesis in the Centre for Research into Reading, Literature and Society (CRILS) at the University of Liverpool and was a post-doctoral researcher on a range of CRILS' reading and mental health studies.

David Fearnley is Medical Director of Mersey Care NHS Mental Health Trust and Associate National Clinical Director for Secure Mental Health, England. In his capacity as forensic psychiatrist at Ashworth Hospital, he ran a reading group for several years on a secure psychiatric ward.

Ellie Gray is a Clinical Psychologist in a community-based adult mental health service in Cumbria, UK. She completed her doctoral studies in clinical psychology at the University of Liverpool.

Kelda Green recently completed a Ph.D. study at the University of Liverpool, entitled 'When literature comes to our aid: investigations into psychological understanding in the writing of Seneca and Montaigne, Wordsworth and George Eliot'.

Kevin Harvey is Associate Professor in Sociolinguistics in the School of English at the University of Nottingham with special research interests in interdisciplinary approaches to health communication.

Nusrat Husain is Professor of Psychiatry and Director of Research for Global Mental Health in the Division of Psychology and Mental Health at the University of Manchester. He is also Honorary Consultant Psychiatrist and Lead for Lancashire Care NHS Foundation Trust's Culture & International Mental Health Research Group.

Andrew Jones is a pain medicine consultant at Royal Liverpool and Broadgreen University Hospitals NHS Trust, Liverpool, UK.

David Kidd is a postdoctoral fellow at the Harvard Graduate School of Education and assistant research director of Project Zero's Humanities and Liberal Arts Assessment (HULA) project. David received a Ph.D. in Social Psychology from the New School for Social Research in 2015.

Gundi Kiemle is the academic director of the Doctorate in Clinical Psychology training programme at the University of Liverpool. A clinical psychologist and psychotherapist, she has worked in UK NHS clinical services for over 30 years with research interests in mental health, trauma and post-traumatic growth.

Kremena Koleva (University of York) has research interests in non-literal language processing and meaning access, selection and retrieval in ambiguous situations.

Don Kuiken is Professor Emeritus in the Department of Psychology at the University of Alberta, specialising in the study of literary reading, dreams, and phenomenology. His current research examines shifts in the sense of self that occur through literary reading and impactful dreams.

Nicolai Ladegaard is a clinical psychologist at Aarhus University Hospital, Denmark, and senior researcher in the Department of Depression and Anxiety, School of Clinical Medicine at Aarhus University.

Sofia Lampropoulou is Senior Lecturer in English Language at the University of Liverpool with principal research interests lie in the areas of Interactional Sociolinguistics and (Critical) Discourse Analysis.

James Ledson is a pain medicine consultant at Royal Liverpool and Broadgreen University Hospitals NHS Trust, Liverpool, UK.

Fiona Magee is a researcher at the Centre for Research into Reading, Literature and Society and a project worker for The Reader, delivering Shared Reading in prisons.

Eleanor McCann is a project worker at The Reader, Liverpool, UK, and was Reader in Residence at Mersey Care NHS Trust for a period of two years.

Kate McDonnell is Head of Reading Excellence at The Reader, UK from 2001–2018, and has run a Shared Reading group for people living with chronic pain at the weekly pain clinic of a city hospital for six years.

Susan McLaine co-ordinates State Library Victoria's Book Well program, a collaborative initiative of the State Library of Victoria, the Public Libraries Victoria Network and VicHealth, Australia. Currently, she is a Ph.D. candidate at RMIT University.

Alexis McNay co-ordinated the 'Read and Relax' programme at HMP Walton, Liverpool, UK, as a Project Worker for The Reader, UK.

Kathryn Naylor is an associate specialist in forensic psychiatry at Ashworth, one of the three high-security psychiatric hospitals in England, alongside Rampton and Broadmoor, with special interest in personality disorder, suicide and self-harm and holistic approaches to treatment and recovery. Dr. Naylor runs a Shared Reading group with her patients.

Keith Oatley is Professor Emeritus in the Department of Applied Psychology and Human Development at the University of Toronto. He is a cognitive psychologist whose research has included studies of mental health, emotions, and the reading and writing of fiction. His most recent book is *Our Minds, Our Selves: A Brief History of Psychology*.

Martin Orrell is Director of the Institute of Mental Health at the University of Nottingham and former Professor of Ageing and Mental Health at University College London. He is Chair of the Memory Services National Accreditation Panel and a member of the Prime Minister's Challenge on Dementia Research Group.

Adam Phillips is a practising psychoanalyst and visiting professor in English, University of York. He is the author of numerous works of psychoanalysis and literary criticism, including (*Side Effects* and *Unforbidden Pleasures*), General Editor of the *Penguin Modern Freud*, and Fellow of the Royal Society of Literature.

Sally Rimkeit is a Medical Specialist in Psychogeriatrics at the University of Otago & Capital and Coast District Health Board, Wellington, New Zealand and Senior Research Fellow and Lead Clinical Investigator of the Reading and Dementia Programme.

Jude Robinson is a social anthropologist and Professor of Health and Wellbeing at the University of Glasgow. Her collaboratively and interdisciplinary research focuses on gendered health inequalities and on the development of participatory research methods in different settings.

Rick Rylance is Dean and Chief Executive of the School of Advanced Study and Pro Vice-Chancellor for Research at the University of London. Formerly Chief Executive of the Arts and Humanities Research Council (AHRC), Professor Rylance's chief research interests are 19th- and 20th-century literature with a particular focus on the history of psychology, the psychology of the reading process and the public value of literature.

Dalice Sim is Biostatistician and Senior Research Fellow at the University of Otago, Wellington, New Zealand and Principal Investigator of the Reading and Dementia Programme.

Mette Steenberg is a researcher at Aarhus University, Interacting Minds Center and Director of The Danish Reading Society (Laeseforeningen), a sister organisation to The Reader, UK, which has been promoting Shared Reading in Denmark.

Thor Magnus Tangeraas is Associate Professor of Communication at Westerdals Department of Communication and Design, Kristiania University College, Oslo. He recently completed his Ph.D. thesis, '"How Literature Changed my Life": A Hermeneutically Oriented Narrative Inquiry into Transformative Experiences of Reading Imaginative Literature' at Oslo-Met University.

Ann Walmsley is an author and journalist. Her book, *The Prison Book Club* (Oneworld, 2015), recounts her experience of monthly book discussion groups inside secure federal men's institutions in Canada.

Megan Watkins holds a Mersey Care NHS Trust funded Ph.D. studentship in the Department of Psychology at the University of Liverpool and is studying the effects of reading in relation to self-harm in collaboration with Mersey Care secure and community health services and UK charity The Reader.

Charlotte Weber is a Reader Leader with The Reader, UK, and delivered reading groups for a reading and dementia study conducted by the Centre for Research into Reading, Literature and Society, University of Liverpool.

Adam Zeman is Professor of Cognitive and Behavioural Neurology at the University of Exeter, with research interests in the science and philosophy of consciousness and the relationship between neurology and psychiatry, mind and brain. He is former Chair of the British Neuropsychiatry Association.

List of Figures

List of Tables

1

Introduction

Josie Billington

Over the last two decades, the vital importance of reading to human flourishing and whole-life fulfilment has attracted strong and public notice. Reports from influential international and governmental bodies have shown recreational reading to have a more powerful effect on cognitive development, educational achievement and social mobility than socio-economic status.[1] During the same period, there has been unprecedented attention to the relationship between *literary* reading—specifically the reading of literary fiction and poetry—and mental health and wellbeing.[2] The impetus for this interest has been threefold, influenced by: the increase in third sector organisations and governmental bodies promoting reading; the urgent need of health providers to find economical and humane solutions to health problems; the successful growth of the arts in health and medical humanities movements. This wide constituency of interest has led to research and practice in this area crossing diverse groups and disciplines—reading charities and arts organisations; academic psychologists, neurologists and human scientists; literary academics, writers and philosophers; medical researchers and practitioners. Research alone embraces a wide range of approaches—theoretical, empirical, experimental—and while some such 'applied' studies are specifically related to health outcomes, there is a growing body of 'pure' research with key, and as yet under-mobilised, implications for health and wellbeing.

J. Billington (✉)
Centre for Research into Reading, Literature and Society,
University of Liverpool, Liverpool, UK
e-mail: jbilling@liverpool.ac.uk

J. Billington (ed.), *Reading and Mental Health*,
https://doi.org/10.1007/978-3-030-21762-4_1

'Reading and mental health' is thus a recognisable and burgeoning field of enquiry. What the field currently lacks, however, is a comprehensive recognition of its findings and a core consolidation of its insights: it lacks a '**centre**'. The key priority of this book is to begin to carry out this vital task of consolidation. The volume thus brings into one place some of the best practice and best evidence currently available in the field, together with the diverse and complementary perspectives of practitioners and beneficiaries, pioneers and researchers, commissioners and policy-makers. By gathering and distilling these findings into centralised coherence, the book seeks significantly to advance knowledge of why literary reading matters for mental health. It also provides a foundational text for future practitioners and researchers and a guide to health professionals and policy-makers in relation to embedding reading practices in health care.

The book is divided into five parts. Part I, **Reading and Health: Medicine to Literature; Literature to Therapy**, offers an introductory awareness of the rich cross-boundary and in-between ground which the reading and health field occupies. In the first chapter of Part I, Christopher Dowrick, a professor of primary care and world-leading expert in depression, who is also a general practitioner (GP) in an inner-city surgery in the UK, argues that the general practitioner's essential obligation to patients is the recognition of suffering and the offering of hope. Dowrick considers how GPs who are daily faced with the pressure of patient distress in their consulting rooms might gain from engagement with literature. Three writers who have mattered personally to the author, and who are themselves at the boundary of philosophy and literature and the spiritual and the sick—Robert Burton, Gerard Manley Hopkins and John Paul Sartre—provide rich insights for the modern understanding and management of depression and the interaction of suffering and hope. As Chapter 2 is an example of a medical mind turning towards literature, so Chapters 3 and 4 are written by literature scholars crossing, quite literally in their case, over to medicine. Josie Billington and Philip Davis are co-founders of the Centre for Research into Reading, Literature and Society (CRILS), the first such centre to take academics from a School of English Literature into a Faculty of Health and Life Sciences in order to bring literary reading into closer relation with health and wellbeing. This collaborative enterprise is the inspiration for this book and, as we shall see, supplies much, though by no means all, of the material it comprises. In the second and third chapters of Part I, therefore, these literary people explore what motivated that turn towards health from within their own scholarly backgrounds: namely, the existing grounds for, and origins of, reading as 'therapy' which are to be found within the English literary tradition. In 'The Sonnet "Cure": Renaissance Poetics to Romantic Prosaics', Grace Farrington and Philip Davis trace the therapeutic value of literature to Renaissance poetics. Samuel Daniel's *Defence of Rhyme* (1602) held that the poet made form out of human chaos through the creation of structured rhythmic patterns, a holdfast against disorder. George Puttenham in his *Art of English Poesy* (1589), drew a direct analogy between poet and physician: a poem offers, cathartically, he said, 'one short sorrowing' as 'the remedy of a long and grievous sorrow'. These concerns were re-introduced into the modern lyric tradition, the authors suggest, through the work of Romantic poet, William Wordsworth, for whom 'the turnings intricate of verse' effected 'sorrow that is not sorrow/… to hear of'. In the final chapter of this section, 'The Victorian Novel: Laying the Foundations for Bibliotherapy', Farrington and Davis, together with Josie Billington, take up, historically, from the preceding chapter. Wordsworth's Preface to *Lyrical Ballads*, as has long been acknowledged, offered a blueprint for the nineteenth-century novel's principal literary achievement, realism, which committed literature to ordinary experience during an era when (with the spread of education, literacy and written material) reading itself was becoming democratised. The authors' contention here, however, is that Victorian realism's mission was not simply to represent real life for its own sake, but to reach *into* the real life of the reader, transformatively. Literary realism, as it developed from Charles Dickens to George Eliot, it is argued, offers a model and rationale for modern-day reading therapies.

Part II, **Practices**, turns to contemporary reading practices and modern-day real readers who are engaging, often for the first time, with literature from earlier times. Clare Ellis and Eleanor McCann recount their experiences of taking Shakespeare's sonnets and plays—the Renaissance literature regarded as foundational to reading therapy in Chapter 2—into both community and hospital contexts as part of mental health provision. Katie Clark and Charlotte Weber demonstrate the power of Wordsworth's poetry to trigger spontaneous access to core autobiographical experience, in dementia (residential and day) care. The geographical reach of such practices is shown in Anne Line Dalsgård's report on public librarians' delivery of reading groups to psychologically vulnerable people in Denmark as part of a collaboration between third sector, psychiatric and municipal organisations, and by Susan McLaine's account of a state library's reading programme for older people in Victoria, Australia, in partnership with public health promotion. At such times Part II anticipates the focus on implementation of literary reading within health provision which will come in Part V, by featuring some 'on-the-ground', practical lessons learned by pioneering practitioners and researchers. This is true, too, of Alexis McNay's and Charles Darby Villis's illustration of the unique challenges and rewards of setting up the protected 'thinking space' of reading groups in male and female prisons in the UK. Their experience is contrasted and complemented by an interview with Canadian author and journalist Ann Walmsley on her acclaimed book, *The Prison Book Club*, in which she compares her experience of reading groups in high and medium secure prisons in Ontario, Canada, with her continuing participation in a women's book club in Toronto. The Practices section concludes with Grace Farrington's and Kate McDonnell's accounts of reading with people suffering from long-term and often severe health conditions (personality disorder, psychosis, chronic pain) in clinical (in-patient and out-patient) contexts. The final testimony comes from Helen Cook, an NHS service-user living with chronic pain, who recounts her journey from reading group member to reading group leader.

Many, though not all, of the practices represented in this section are based around UK charity The Reader, with whom CRILS has enjoyed a research partnership since its foundation. The Reader's mission is to 'bring about a reading revolution so that everyone can experience and enjoy great literature which we believe is a tool for helping people survive and live well'.[3] Its distinctive model of Shared Reading is one of the most widely used arts in health interventions in this country and internationally (there are related organisations and partnerships in Denmark, Belgium, Sweden, Norway, Germany, Australia and New Zealand), and, as this volume will show, there is now a strong body of evidence demonstrating the model's success in promoting mental health. Shared Reading groups are distinct from conventional book clubs.[4] The material is not read in advance nor confined to contemporary works. Nor is the material chosen for its targeted relevance as in self-help bibliotherapy[5] or in reading interventions which seek to treat particular cases, conditions or moods.[6] Rather, poems, short stories and novels from the literary heritage down the ages are read aloud, together, live, and the reading is regularly interrupted for group members to share thoughts and responses. One great advantage of this model from the point of view of reading research is that readers have the chance to show some of what is usually private or silent in reading. While admittedly a different experience from reading on one's own, Shared Reading aloud is the nearest we have for research into private acts of thinking made live during reading, not least because, as we shall see, the private emerges within a group made unusually intimate by the presence of the poem or book. A second key reason for basing the Practices section of this book on The Reader model is the sheer amount of (reproducible) examples of practice made available by (ethically approved) research in relation to it. Those who, in Part II, are writing about their experience as reading practitioners have access to the primary research data they themselves collaborated in producing (audio-video recordings, transcripts, diaries, logs), which enables them to recreate and bring to life the reading experience at near first-hand, and give themselves as well as the readers whom they reach a voice in this book. It was an axiom of this volume from the first that practitioners and beneficiaries of literary reading should be heard equally alongside researchers, academics and professionals. It was also important that these voices were heard before the book becomes absorbed by research methodologies and theories in relation to reading and health, for two reasons. First, it is essential that this volume does not lose sight of the human trouble and need, expressed within the literature as well as by those who read it, which is at the heart of this book's endeavour. Second, the methodologies and theories represented later in the book have often emerged *from* the subject they treat, as well as being applied *to* it.

This two-way interaction is reflected in the division of chapters in Part III, **Research Methodologies**. Chapter 9 demonstrates the application of established qualitative methods in reading research. Jude Robinson and Josie Billington illustrate how ethnographic inquiry can be used effectively in the specific (and highly controlled) reading context of prison life. Ellie Gray and Gundi Kiemle demonstrate the appropriateness of Interpretative Phenomenological Analysis in relation to reading and community mental health, while Melissa Chapple shows the application of Framework Analysis in relation to readers living with autism. Chapter 10 turns to innovative qualitative methods which have sought to capture the lived experience of reading at its live, minute by minute, source. Philip Davis, Josie Billington, Grace Farrington, and Fiona Magee show the potential for accessing individual, subjective responses to literary reading—and specifically breakthrough moments where readers are palpably released from default habits of thought—using video-recorded data of reading group sessions and video-assisted interviews; while Mette Steenberg demonstrates her use of the micro-phenomenological interview to elicit the 'felt sense' and cognitive processes of reading. Thor Magnus Tangeraas, in his investigation of life-changing encounters with literary works, has developed an interview method, inspired by narrative inquiry and the dialogic method of Shared Reading, which he calls 'intimate reading'; and, likewise concerned with the individual reader, Kelda Green has evolved a method of tracing the effects on emotional and psychological health of private reading over time, which combines personal diaries with face to face interviews. The value of combining these methods with linguistic (qualitative *and* quantitative) approaches is the focus of Chapter 11 in which Sofia Lampropoulou, Kevin Harvey, Gavin Brookes and Kremena Koleva apply their linguistic expertise to the primary data used by researchers in Chapters 9 and 10, including practical demonstration of a 'worked' transcript. This chapter closes with an attempt to recreate the kind of open, collaborative thinking that can emerge when academics from different disciplines work together on the same material, and illustrate why those disciplines need one another, especially in relation to a phenomenon as multilevelled and multifaceted as reading.

The emphasis on multidisciplinary and multidimensional methods is strong in the final two chapters of Part III also, despite their focus on more measurable aspects of the literary reading encounter. The first two sections of Chapter 12 are concerned with identifying quantitative tools for capturing the complex benefits of reading which have potential to gain currency with policy-makers and health-care providers. Rhiannon Corcoran, Josie Billington and Megan Watkins explain the processes (both experimental and hypothesis-driven) by which they have discriminated clinical outcome measures and indicators of psychological health appropriate to those engaging with literary reading who are experiencing mental health difficulties, including self-harm. Mette Steenberg, Charlotte Christiansen and Nicolai Ladegaard then recount their experience of trying to replicate the use of some of these measures in their research study of the Danish reading programme 'Time to Read', which features in Part II (Practices). The challenges they faced are a salutary reminder of how research in this area is still in its early stages and the process of standardising 'reading for health' might always prove intractable. In the final section of this chapter, Donald Kuiken explicates the objectives of empirical phenomenology: to bring to clarity and coherence—as systematically as possible and with all the nuance language will allow—the full complexity of categories of lived experience. Kuiken offers a rationale for numeric formalisation of phenomenological procedures that facilitate the identification and articulation of types of reading experience with a precision not normally associated with qualitative studies of literary reading. This section uses a specific exemplary study to review the distinctive contributions of numerically aided phenomenological methods in understanding the reading experience, with particular attention to design factors (such as suspension of concern with explanation) that facilitate fresh revelation and clarification of different 'species' of reading experience.

The final chapter of Part III, 'Brain, Mind and Body', brings a biological dimension to the study of reading. In the first section Philip Davis and Rhiannon Corcoran outline their groundbreaking experiments on reading and the brain, which have suggested that the inner neural processing of literary language has the potential to galvanise existing brain pathways and to influence emotion networks and thinking modes, by diverting from ineffective channels towards more diverse reasoning options. Together with Rick Rylance and Adam Zeman—whose own study of the reading brain showed that reading of literary prose and poetry activated regions of the brain previously identified with emotional response to music and with introspection—the authors point to how fMRI studies can help triangulate or complicate findings emerging in social psychology in relation to reading's power to re-orient or 're-wire' perspective. This is the focus of David Kidd's contribution, in which he describes recent studies of how reading literary fiction (as opposed to popular fiction or non-fiction) can foster 'Theory of Mind' (ToM)—the human capacity to comprehend others' mental states and understand that other people hold beliefs and desires distinct from one's own. His findings link the temporary enhancement of ToM to literary fiction's affective simulation of characters' inner lives and the reader's immersed engagement therewith and suggest that exposure to quality literary fiction over a lifetime improves cognitive empathy. Finally, Christophe de Bezenac describes his current cutting-edge work in using physiological measures of emotional processing—such as heart rate variability, skin conductance response, eye movement, facial expression, and vocal features—to offer insight into otherwise hidden aspects of brain and body function during literary reading. Investigation of these implicit processes, de Bezenac argues, can be powerfully combined with both computational linguistics (sentiment analysis) and a range of qualitative methods to provide holistic understanding of the lived cognitive and emotional experiences of readers.

Part IV, **Towards a Theoretical Understanding of Reading and Health**, draws in part upon the makings or foundations of a theory of reading for mental health provided by the rich findings presented in Part III. But this part of the book is principally concerned with how extant theories (established or developing) in the therapeutic disciplines (psychiatry, psychology, psychoanalysis) resonate with emergent thinking and theory in the rest of this volume. In Chapter 14, 'Reading and Psychiatric Practices', David Fearnley (Medical Director of Mersey Care NHS Mental Health Trust and Associate National Clinical Director for Secure Mental Health) draws on his experience as a forensic psychiatrist at a high secure hospital where he ran a Shared Reading group for several years. Together with Grace Farrington, whose own role in secure settings is described in Chapter 8, the chapter considers what it is about the reading of literature that distinguishes this activity from formal therapy and its consequent value in psychiatric contexts. Central is literature's capacity to connect readers both with the experience of men and women across time via (what Jung called) 'historical antecedents' and with their own early experiences, those which pre-date trauma. Literature's non-targeted approach allows connections which may be more primary and more personally relevant than formal treatment could locate, with the potential for deeper-level recovery as a result. Keith Oatley's and Rhiannon Corcoran's chapter, 'Reading Minds: Fiction and its Relation to the Mental World of Others', turns to consider the landmark studies in Psychology (including Kidd's above) which have demonstrated connections between the habit of fiction-reading and enhanced capacity for social interaction and cooperation, and for stronger social understanding and empathy, as well as for longer life. Positing a sense of purpose as more valuable to mental health and wellbeing than the pursuit of pleasure or happiness, the authors survey the evidence for reading as a life-sustaining activity in part because of its emphasis on meaning-of-life issues. They consider fiction's power to make people more socially adaptable by extending emotional and cognitive openness or creativity, as well as the value of group reading or 'reading communities' in engendering and sustaining these benefits as part of a public mental health agenda. The ensuing chapter offers a further theoretical perspective on reading and health from the discipline of Psychology, now intensely focused on the interiority of the individual reader. In 'Metaphoricity, Inexpressible Realizations, and Expressive Enactment', Don Kuiken articulates a theory of expression, informed by phenomenology, which explains how literary reading facilitates the movement towards words or phrases that 'fit' the feelings (being moved, sublime disquietude) elicited by the text. During literary reading, the expression of existential feeling *becomes possible* when textual metaphoric 'fusions' elicit the 'dreamy metaphoric fusions' of the reader's existential feelings. The transition from passive elicitation to reflective explication *begins* here, when the literary text produces an evocative intimation, an *inexpressible realization* where the reader becomes '…conscious of having an emotion but not conscious of what that emotion is'. 'Within the silence of a feeling, finding what might be but has not been said involves listening, not in active search for particular words or phrases, rather in receptive openness to the coming and going of words that seem to "come from" the feeling'. The more effectively silence is realised, the more potential there is for subsequent (and potentially expressive) explication of the intimation. This interest in what is 'there' but 'not said' resonates, across disciplinary bounds, with the psychoanalytical thinking which Adam Phillips introduces in the final chapter of Part IV. In interview with Philip Davis,

Phillips talks across the breadth of his own reading and writing, about the 'overlapping and incommensurate' relation of life to literature, and literature to psychoanalysis. Starting from the position that 'bafflement is integral to a post-religious life or world—we don't know what we are doing and nobody can tell us', Phillips contends that literature offers the reader the chance to think the strangeness of his or her own thoughts, without becoming, as psychoanalysis is prone to do, an 'intelligibility project', privileging understanding at the expense of 'live surprise'. He also considers how literature can help create possible futures by offering 're-describings of life' enabling the reader to do or imagine something else. 'Anything you cannot re-describe is akin to a trauma, and therefore art is to free one's capacity for re-description.' The purpose of Part IV is by no means to offer conclusive theories. None are yet possible and perhaps may never be. Literature's gift after all (to use Adam Phillips words) is 'inspiration' not 'set knowledge or conclusive understanding'. The key task is to engender and mobilise lively intellectual discourse across disciplines in the effort to understand why literature matters for mental health.

For literature to matter to people in trouble, it has to be accessible to them. Part V, therefore, **Reading and Health: Implementation—Barriers and Enablers**, is concerned with what will foster and what will hinder the acceptance of a reading agenda and reading provision within mental health care, particularly the mental health contexts already represented in Parts Two and Three (depression, dementia, prisons and secure contexts, clinical settings). Chapter 18 offers three distinct perspectives on the value of—and potential obstacles to— embedding Shared Reading within the treatment options of health professions and services. Ellie Gray surveys a wide range of reading or book-based interventions recently or currently in use in mental health contexts and considers their implications for clinical practice. Grace Farrington articulates the value of a literature-based intervention from the perspective of occupational therapists working with mental health patients in hospital. Mette Steenberg reports on (and assesses the criteria for success of) a collaborative venture of Danish health services, libraries and local government in which people living at risk of mental health issues are referred to reading groups. Chapter 19 brings together perspectives, problems and solutions from expert academics and practitioners working in the field of old age mental health and dementia. Martin Orrell and Tom Dening make a case for reading in dementia care based on both the evidence base and health economics considerations, and explain the requirement for the scientifically robust research study which a Randomised Controlled Trial would provide. Nusrat Husain outlines the special case for Shared Reading among the BME population (specifically older British South Asians) who are more vulnerable than other groups to the twin mental health difficulties of dementia and depression, and considers the barriers that will need to be overcome to make reading provision viable. Finally, Sally Rimkeit, Gillian Claridge and Dalice Sim, working on a reading and dementia programme in New Zealand, begin to answer some of the issues raised by their UK colleagues in outlining their current three-stage programme (feasibility, pilot, RCT) for a robust study which can help to mainstream reading in old age care. This detailed explication offers a potential model for researchers across the breadth of the reading and health—and arts in health—spectrum. The final two chapters of the volume take the form of interviews. Chapter 20 offers two complementary perspectives on the practice of shared group reading in two distinctive secure contexts. Talking to Fiona Magee (who herself runs reading groups in prisons), psychotherapist and policy-maker, Nick Benefield, former lead of the National Personality Disorder Team, recounts his successful introduction of Shared Reading groups within the criminal justice system—specifically as part of the environmental model of living, management and care known as PIPES, Psychologically Informed Planned Environments. Kathryn Naylor, a forensic psychiatrist at Ashworth (high-secure) Hospital, talks of her experience of running a Shared Reading group with patients who, because of what they have 'missed' or 'lost', present a grave danger to themselves or others. She speaks of reading's special power to help patients find what 'they do still have' as an alternative to habitual self-harm as a reflex of inarticulate pain. Finally, in the concluding chapter of the volume, Andrew Jones and James Ledson, pain medicine consultants at an inner-city hospital, are interviewed by Kate McDonnell, who has lived with pain for forty years having been diagnosed with rheumatoid arthritis as a teenager and who has been running a reading group in the consultants' pain clinic (see Chapter 8). Jones and Ledson talk about why they have (successfully) fought to commission the reading group for eight consecutive years, how it complements and enhances the effect of existing treatments and therapies they offer, and how it enriches the lives of their 'suffering' patients.

The interviews which conclude this volume give an indication of the quality of dialogue—humane, intelligent, fortifying—which has occurred across the range of stakeholders within reading and health who are represented in this book. I was advised to describe this volume as a compendium, which is what it is certainly designed to be, housing useful examples of endeavour at levels of practice, research and thought. But I prefer to think of it as an expanded and invigorating 'conversation' across conventional disciplinary divisions which will, I hope, inspire others to join it.

Notes

1. See Organisation for Economic Cooperation and Development (OECD), Reading for Change, 2006; Alison Sullivan and Matt Brown, *Social Inequalities in Cognitive Scores at Age 16: The Role of Reading* (London: Institute of Education, 2013); and 'Research Evidence on Reading for Pleasure', Education Standards Research Team, Department of Education, 2012.
2. This body of literature is represented throughout the volume but see: Philip Davis, *Reading and the Reader* (Oxford: Oxford University Press, 2013); Ella Berthoud and Susan Elderkin, *The Novel Cure: An A–Z of Literary Remedies* (Edinburgh: Canongate, 2013); Josie Billington, *Is Literature Healthy* (Oxford: Oxford University Press, 2016); and Jonathan Bate, Paula Byrne, and Sophie Ratcliffe (eds.), *Stressed/Unstressed* (London: William Collins, 2016).
3. See https://www.thereader.org.uk; Jane Davis, Introduction to *A Little Aloud: An Anthology of Prose and Poetry for Reading Aloud to People You Care For*, ed. by Angela Macmillan (London: Random House, 2010), pp. 7–19; Jane Davis, 'The Reading Revolution', in *Stop What You're Doing and Read This!* (London: Vintage Books, 2011), pp. 115–36.
4. Jenny Hartley, *The Reading Groups Book* (Oxford: Oxford University Press, 2002).
5. Debbie Hicks, 'An Audit of Bibliotherapy/Books on Prescription Activity in England' (Arts Council England and the Museums Libraries and Archives Council, 2006).
6. See Berthoud and Elderkin (2013) and Bate et al. (2016).

Part I

Reading and Health: Medicine to Literature, Literature to Therapy

2

Comfort in a Whirlwind: Literature and Distress in General Practice

Christopher Dowrick

I believe we can distill general practitioners' obligations to our distressed patients to two essential elements: the acknowledgement of suffering and the offer of hope. Eric Cassel reminds us that the duty of physicians to relieve human suffering stretches back to antiquity.[1] Ian McWhinney understands medicine as complex, context-dependent, poignant, a reflection of the human condition. He invites us to be open in the face of suffering, and to follow the wisdom traditions with their emphasis on listening. We are too often 'tempted to shy away from suffering', he wrote. 'It is this lack of openness in the face of suffering which closes off compassion and stops us from being healers'.[2] In similar vein, Ronald Epstein recommends that we turn towards suffering: actively seek to recognise it, become curious about the patient's experience and intentionally become more present and engaged.[3] Our commitment to encouraging hope is a fundamental element of overcoming any illness. Hope itself is a therapeutic tool, one of the most powerful aspects of the doctor–patient relationship,[4] especially if it is based on a genuine understanding of the patient's concerns and expectations, and linked with the best evidence-based practice.[5]

C. Dowrick (✉)
University of Liverpool, Liverpool, UK
e-mail: cfd@liverpool.ac.uk

J. Billington (ed.), *Reading and Mental Health*,
https://doi.org/10.1007/978-3-030-21762-4_2

But how on earth are we to practise this in our overwhelmingly busy consulting rooms, faced with the myriad pressures of patients' problems and professional protocols?

Mentors, peer support and supervision are all helpful. Formal training in empathy,[6] mindful communication,[7, 8] and mindfulness-based stress reduction, have been shown to be effective.[9] So too is maintaining a balance between our clinical commitment and our life as a whole.[10]

In this chapter I take a different direction, and consider what benefits general practitioners might gain from engagement with literature. I focus on three writers who mean a great deal to me personally, Robert Burton, Gerard Manley Hopkins and Jean Paul Sartre. Burton (1577–1640), Fellow of Christ Church College, Oxford and vicar of parishes in Oxford and Leicestershire, is best known for his monumental treatise *The Anatomy of Melancholy*. His combined role as scholar and cleric was, in its historical context, remarkably similar to that of the modern academic general practitioner. Hopkins (1844–1889) was an English poet and Jesuit priest who, posthumously, gained a reputation as one of the leading Victorian poets. Between 1870 and 1881, he worked as a parish priest in Liverpool, just a few hundred yards from my university office. Jean Paul Sartre (1905–1980) was a key figure in the philosophy of existentialism and in French literary studies. I was introduced to his *Roads to Freedom* trilogy while studying French A-Level as an angst-ridden teenager.

Sitting as they do on the borders between literature and philosophy, between spirituality and sickness, and encompassing highly divergent world views, these writers provide a rich variety of insights into interactions between suffering and hope. For Burton, melancholy is both a disease and the essence of the human condition, while for Hopkins and Sartre, distress is a consequence of alienation, whether from God or from a tension between social expectations and one's authentic self. Burton and Sartre find hope in possibilities of change, in sociality and activity, though expressed in very different ways. Hopkins' sense of hope is more provisional, more complex, but perhaps also more compelling, involving comfort of the self, the mutual benefits of pastoral care and the ecstasy of God in nature.

Building on ideas I have previously set out in my book *Beyond Depression*,[11] I base my reflections on Burton's *Anatomy*,[12] six of Hopkins' poems[13] and two of Sartre's novels,[14, 15] and intersperse them with remarks on how they influence my own clinical practice.

My Mistris Melancholy

Burton provides us with vivid descriptions of melancholy. He defines it as 'an Epidemicall disease, that so often, so much crucifies the body and minde; .... A kind of dotage without a fever, having, for his ordinary companions, fear and sadness, without any apparent occasion.... suspicion, jealousie, discontent, solitariness, irksomeness, continual cogitations, restless thoughts, vain imaginations &c' (Faulkner et al., vol. 1, pp. 110, 162; vol. 3, p. 297). He is careful to distinguish between melancholy as disease or habit and melancholy as 'Character of Mortalitie' from which 'no man is living free'... 'but more or less some time or other, he feels the smarte of it' (Faulkner et al., vol. 1, p. 136).

Burton is writing not only as a spiritual physician but also as a fellow melancholic: he is 'not a little offended with this maladie, shall I say my Mistris Melancholy' (Faulkner et al., vol. 1, p. 7). Hopkins and Sartre, in much stronger vein, provide us with highly personalised poetic and literary insights into the depths of their own distress.

Hopkins combines personal and spiritual perspectives in harrowing ways, especially in his 'Terrible Sonnets'. Created during a deeply unhappy period of his life while working as a classics professor at University College Dublin, these poems arise from 'a languishment of body and mind'.[16] They explore his deadly sense of terrible evil or ferocity ('the fell of dark'), of unending, unremitting bleak times:

> I wake and feel the fell of dark, not day.
> What hours, O what black hoürs we have spent
> This night! what sights you, heart, saw; the ways you went!
> And more must, in yet longer light's delay.
> With witness I speak this! But where I say
> Hours I mean years, mean life. (Gardner, p. 62)

His anguish is intense, his description of it almost unbearable to read:

> No worst, there is none. Pitched past pitch of grief,
> More pangs will, schooled at forepangs, wilder ring.....
> My cries heave, herds-long; huddle in a main, a chief-
> Woe, wórld-sorrow; on an áge old anvil wince and sing -
> Then lull, then leave off. Fury has shrieked 'No ling-
> ering! Let me be fell: force I must be brief'.

> O the mind, mind has mountains; cliffs of fall
> Frightful, sheer, no-man-fathomed. Hold them cheap
> May who ne'er hung there. (Gardner, p. 61)

Sartre's most vivid description of suffering is his portrayal of 30-year-old Antoine Roquentin, the central character in his novel *Nausea*. Roquentin is staying in a French seaport, completing his research on the life of an eighteenth-century political figure. But during the winter of 1932 a sweetish sickness he calls nausea begins to affect everything he does: his research project, the company of the self-taught man who is reading all the books in the library, a pleasant physical relationship with a cafe owner named Francoise, his memories of Anny, an English girl he once loved, even his own hands and the beauty of nature. He is engulfed by desolation and despair:

> I live alone, entirely alone. I never speak to anyone, never; I receive nothing, I give nothing… When you live alone you no longer know what it is to tell something: the plausible disappears at the same time as the fiends. You let events flow past; suddenly you see people pop up who speak and who go away, you plunge into stories without beginning or end: you make a terrible witness. … I tear myself from the window and stumble across the room; I glue myself against the looking glass. I stare at myself, I disgust myself: one more eternity. Finally, I flee from my image and fall on the bed. I watch the ceiling. I'd like to sleep. (Alexander, p. 46)

Irascible Imagination

Burton's approach to the causes of melancholic suffering has much in common with modern diagnostic practices, apart from his understandable emphasis on supernatural—'from god, the devil or … by magicians, witches' (Faulkner et al., vol. 1, p. 119)—as well as natural causes. Natural causes can be primary e.g. old age, temperament, parents, 'outward or adventitious' (Faulkner et al., vol. 1, p. 203), in the same way that psychiatrists may distinguish between endogenous and reactive depression. Outward causes may be remote, involving terrors, calumnies, imprisonment, poverty and want, 'an heap of other accidents, death of friends, loss &c' (Faulkner et al., vol. 1, p. 356); or what we would now describe as life events and difficulties. Outward causes may also be contingent, inward, antecedent 'in which the body works on the mind and this malady is caused by precedent diseases as agues, pox &c … or by particular parts distempered, as brain, heart, spleen, liver, mesentery, pylorus, stomach &c' (Faulkner et al., vol. 1, p. 119); or what we would now describe as psychosomatic conditions.

For these factors to lead to melancholy, Burton specifies six necessary causes: diet offending in substance, quality or quantity; retention and evacuation; air: 'hot, cold, tempestuous, dark, thick, foggy, moorish &c' (Faulkner et al., vol. 1, p. 235); exercise—excessive or defective; sleep and waking; and passions and perturbations of the mind, including 'irascible or concupiscible' (Faulkner et al., vol. 1, p. 255) imagination. Jennifer Radden notes that Burton's account 'so neatly fits present-day cognitivism' and psychiatry,[17] including network models of depression and the part played by rumination and mind wandering in engendering affective disorders.

Hopkins' distress is grounded in his intense sense of loss, of separation or alienation. Hilary Pearson suggests his move to Dublin in 1884 led to a threefold sense of alienation: from his family, through his conversion to Catholicism; from his country, which had failed to follow his religious beliefs; and now a physical separation to a country whose preference for Home Rule was antithetical to his own patriotic views.[18] To these I would add two further senses of alienation: from his friends and, particularly, from God.

In the second half of 'I wake and feel the fell of dark', Hopkins writes 'And my lament/ Is cries countless, cried like dead letters sent/ To dearest him that lives alas! away' (Gardner, p. 62). This could be a reference to his geographical separation from his close friend Robert Bridges, or perhaps the loss of Digby Dolben whose physical beauty and tragic early death both fascinated and distressed him.[19] However in the wider context of this poem, his lament most powerfully expresses his sense of enforced severance from his Lord. In the subsequent lines we find 'God's most deep decree/Bitter would have me taste' and the poem ends with an empathic vision of the experience of hell: 'I see/The lost are like this, and their scourge to be/As I am mine, their sweating selves; but worse' (Gardner, p. 62). In 'No worse there is none', he cries out for help from above, 'Comforter, where, where is your comforting?/Mary, mother of us, where is your relief?'. But no help is forthcoming; 'all/Life death does end and each day dies with sleep' (Gardner, p. 61).

The crucial difference between Burton and Hopkins on the one hand, and Sartre on the other, is that for the latter there is no God and hence no ultimate source of meaning. There is no recourse, no point of reference with the divine, whether external or internal. It is not a matter of man's separation from God: but of man finding himself to be a thinking, feeling, conscious being faced with the appalling awareness of his place within an essentially hostile and pointless universe.

Roquentin faces the disturbingly provisional and limited nature of existence. He tries to make sense of all the things that had filled his life up to that point, but finds himself face to face with a world and an existence without meaning.

> The essential thing is contingency. I mean that one cannot define existence as a necessity. To exist is simply to be there; those who exist let themselves be encountered, but you can never deduce anything from them. I believe that there are people who have understood this. Only they tried to overcome this contingency by inventing a necessary, causal being. But no necessary being can explain existence: contingency is not a delusion, a probability, which can be dissipated; it is the absolute, consequently, the perfect free gift. All is free, this park, this city, and myself. (Alexander, p. 176)

According to Sartre, inauthenticity occurs when human beings, under pressure from social forces, adopt false values and disown their innate freedom.[20] Bad faith (*mauvaise foi*) involves deceiving myself into thinking I don't have freedom to make choices. It is a kind of self-deception, in which I take myself to be a certain kind of person while all along I am—and know myself to be—actually a different kind of person. Thus, the person who thinks she is a coward 'just as a matter of fact' is excluding from view the ability to transform her existence through changed ways of behaving. But bad faith may be the easier option, as authenticity comes at a price: of being true to the inescapable tension at the core of the human self.

> Authenticity, it is almost needless to say, consists in having a true and lucid consciousness of the situation, in assuming the responsibilities and risks it involves, in accepting it … sometimes in horror and hate.[21]

The Pane of Sorrow

In her wonderful essay on grief in modern China, Vera Schwarcz reminds us that

> To suffer is to be shut in, to be locked up by grief in a world without light. A pane opens when sorrow is somehow voiced, shared, spewn out of the closed world of the individual in pain. When others respond to the voice of

the sufferer … with truthful attentiveness – the window of insight becomes broader still.[22]

Expressing pain in literary form allows the writer a degree of detachment. Moving a step away from the rawness of immediate reality, the pain or distress is observed, modulated and re-expressed (by Hopkins) in highly intricate and innovative technical poetic forms. Further distancing can also be noted within the poems themselves. In 'I wake and feel the fell of dark', he finds company for himself in the form of his heart: 'O what black hoürs we have spent/ This night! what sights you, heart, saw; the ways you went!' with the subtle change from 'we' to 'you' suggesting detachment as time passes.

Sartre argues that although melancholy people sometimes say that they want to be alone with their sorrow, the actual cherishing of passive sadness is in fact rather rare. This wish for a private refuge comes from the fact that 'the entire universe is bleak, and it is precisely in order to protect ourselves from its frightful, illimitable monotony that we make some place or other into a "shelter". That is the one differentiating factor in the absolute monotony of the world: a bleak wall, a little darkness to screen us from that bleak immensity'.[23] Here is resonance with the lines in Hopkins' 'No worse there is none': 'Here! Creep/Wretch, under a comfort serves in a whirlwind' (Gardner, p. 61), which bring to mind an image of huddling under a blanket as storms rage above and around, finding a momentary sense of relief.

For the suffering reader, such deep, clearly articulated expressions of distress offer the sense that we are not alone, that others have been there too, and share the experience. With this in mind, in a recent consultation with Frances, an older, socially isolated Catholic woman who suffers from long term depression, I tentatively suggest she read some of Hopkins' poems. When I next see her she brings with her a copy of his selected poems and tells me how much they mean to her. 'It's like finding a friend. I felt like he was sitting next to me, reading to me. It brings a closeness'. She also finds it brings legitimacy to her own distress, something she often doubts: 'It's allowed' she says, 'you're entitled to feel that depth'.

There are similarities too with the practice of mindful meditation. Mindfulness involves attending to relevant aspects of experience in a non-judgmental manner. The essence of this state is to 'be' fully in the present moment, without judging or evaluating it, without reflecting backwards on past memories, without looking forward to anticipate the future, as in anxious worry, and without attempting to solve problems or avoid any unpleasant aspects of the immediate situation.

Such articulation and acknowledgement of suffering are, perhaps, the first tentative steps towards hope.

Can Something, Hope

Hopkins' wrestling with despair, in 'Carrion Comfort', demonstrates a steely determination, a rejection of the desire to succumb to easeful death.

> Not, I'll not, carrion comfort, Despair, not feast on thee;
> Not untwist—slack they may be—these last strands of man
> In me ór, most weary, cry I can no more. I can;
> Can something, hope, wish day come, not chose not to be. (Gardner, p. 60)

He considers, but firmly turns against, suicide. Hilary Pearson draws our attention to his recurring use of 'not' in these four lines. Especially striking is his final double negative in 'not chose not to be'. Here is 'a cry of desperate refusal to surrender to the darkness pressing in on him' (Pearson, p. 28).

Sartre's realisation of the contingency of existence leaves him floundering on the edge of anguish and nausea. But, paradoxically, the physical sensation of nausea becomes proof of his existence:

> I exist. It's sweet, so sweet, so slow. And light: you'd think it floated all by itself. It stirs. It brushes by me, melts and vanishes. Gently, gently. There is bubbling water in my throat, it caresses me - and now it comes up again into my mouth. For ever I shall have a little pool of whitish water in my mouth – lying low – grazing my tongue. And this pool is still me. And the tongue. And the throat is me. (Alexander, p. 134)

To paraphrase Descartes, we now have *vomito ergo sum*. Sartre's moment of deepest despair may also be the foundation of a new reality.

For both Burton and Sartre, change is possible. As an antidote to predestinarianism, the Calvinist view, prevalent in the 1620 s, of man's fatal necessity to sin, Burton allows his readers a degree of agency. He criticises the writers of religious tracts which are 'too tragicall, too much dejecting men, aggravating offences' and encourages us to believe that, whatever God's destiny for us may be, 'our will is free in respect of us, and things contingent'.[24]

Sartre sees no need for Burtonian caution. As Roquentin comes to realise, we are just here. He finds himself with a past, a body and a social situation that constrains him in what he can do. But—in a direct link with Burton—just being here is *contingent*, subject to chance. There is no prior justification or reason for his—or my—existence. What is distinctive about me as a human being is that I am capable of putting my own being in question by asking myself, for example, whether I want to be a person of a particular sort. I am free in the sense I have the ability to choose how I am going to interpret things. I constitute the world through my freedom, to the extent that my ways of doing things determine how reality will be sorted out and matter to me. At the same time, I constitute myself through my own choices.[25]

While modern general practitioners may not worry so much about religious determinism, we are certainly concerned about the extent to which bio-genetic or socio-economic background may limit our patients' freedom of action. We may wish to follow Burton's example in finding a via *media* between these competing world views; or take Sartre's more radical step and proclaim agency as paramount.[26]

Leave Comfort Root-Room

Self-care is central to Burton's perspectives. He puts this into practice in his own writing, which he sees as a form of personal therapy: 'I write on Melancholy by being busie to avoid Melancholy' (Faulkner et al., vol. 1, p. 6). The Second Partition of his *Anatomy* is an extensive programme of self-care, whose mainstays are self-control and a change of daily habits, undertaken alone or with non-medical assistance. They involve agency—'thou tenderest thine owne welfare' (Faulkner et al., vol. 3, p. 445)—and are preventative and holistic, being presented as a collection of complementary responses. Using a combination of Stoic philosophy and Christianity, Burton shows us how to live well in the face of sad and apprehensive states. He follows a tradition of *consolatio* writing which can be traced back to Seneca, Lucretius and Augustine, addressing the sickness of the soul which is the human condition.

He dismisses unlawful means 'from the devil, magicians, witches &c. by charms, spells, incantations, images, &c' (Faulkner et al., vol. 2, Synopsis to Partition 2). Lawful means begin with direct help from God, but he concentrates on three more worldly matters: the works of the physician 'in whom is required science, confidence honesty &c'; the attitude of the patient 'in woom is required obedience, constance, willingness, patience, confidence, bounty &c'; and the correct use of 'physick', which may be 'dietetical', 'pharmaceutical', or 'chirurgical' (Faulkner et al., vol. 2, Synopsis to Partition 2). Of all these, *dietetical physick* occupies most of Burton's attention, being discussed for almost two hundred pages. It consists not only in advice on food and drink but also information on how to address the other necessary causes of melancholia. He recommends exercise, both of the body 'as hawking, hunting, riding, shooting… walking in fair fields…' and of the mind 'as chess cards, tables &c to see plays, masks &c, serious studies, business, all honest recreations' (Faulkner et al., vol. 2, pp. 72, 79). The 'passions and perturbations of the mind' (Faulkner et al., vol. 2, p. 238) should be addressed 'by using all good means of help, confessing to a friend, &c, avoiding all occasions of his infirmity, not giving way to passions, but resisting to his utmost' (Faulkner et al., vol. 2, Synopsis to Partition 2). Friends are important. They provide 'counsel, comfort, good perswasion, witty devices', music of all sorts, 'mirth, and merry company' (Faulkner et al., vol. 2, Synopsis to Partition 2).

It is not just in the content, but also in the process of reading that Burton offers healing. As Mary Ann Lund notes, Burton's interest in the experience of reading 'takes his text beyond the normal scope of medical writing on disease, since it aims to perform a cure through its pages' (Lund, p. 2):

> like guilded pilles, which are so composed as well to tempt the appetite, and deceave the pallatt, as to help and medicinally worke upon the whole body, my lines shall not onely recreate, but rectifie the minde. (Faulkner et al., vol. 3, p. 5)

Reading can be enjoyed by many, and is more accessible than medicine. We can confirm, from our contemporary research, Burton's contention that the act of reading itself may have direct power in dispersing melancholy.[27]

And for care and kindness to the self in times of trouble, I am hard-pressed to find a more powerful example than Hopkins' sonnet 'My own heart let me have more pity on', composed in Dublin in 1885. It speaks for itself:

> My own heart let me more have pity on; let
> Me live to my sad self hereafter kind,
> Charitable; not live this tormented mind
> With this tormented mind tormenting yet.
> I cast for comfort I can no more get

By groping round my comfortless, than blind
Eyes in their dark can day or thirst can find
Thirst's all-in-all in all a world of wet.

Soul, self; come, poor Jackself, I do advise
You, jaded, let be; call off thoughts awhile
Elsewhere; leave comfort root-room; let joy size
At God knows when to God knows what; whose smile
's not wrung, see you; unforeseen times rather — as skies
Betweenpie mountains — lights a lovely mile. (Gardner, p. 63)

Be Not Solitary, Be Not Idle

So far we have articulated and acknowledged suffering, found the strength and determination to carry on despite it, and begun to take steps to address it through care of the self. But Burton, Hopkins and Sartre all show us how the practice and experience of hope may also take more positive forms.

Towards the end of the final volume of the Anatomy, Burton provides us with a brief admonitory summation of his life's work:

> Only take this for a corollary and conclusion, as thou tenderest thine own welfare in this and all other melancholy, thy good health of body and minde, observe this short precept, give not way to solitariness and idleness. Be not solitary, be not idle. (Faulkner et al., vol. 3, p. 445)

Both he and Hopkins take their pastoral work seriously and find solace and personal enrichment in it. Hopkins expresses this best in 'Felix Randal', written in 1881 while parish priest of St Francis Xavier, Liverpool. I find this poem resonates strongly with the real world relationships still enjoyed by the modern general practitioner; not only in his vivid descriptions of the crumbling from former power of farrier Felix Randall

his mould of man, big-boned and hardy-handsome
Pining, pining, till time when reason rambled in it, and some
Fatal four disorders, fleshed there, all contended? […]
How far from then forethought of, all thy more boisterous years,
When thou at the random grim forge, powerful amidst peers,
Didst fettle for the great grey drayhorse his bright and battering sandal!
(Gardner, pp. 47–48)

but also in the mutual benefits for both Hopkins and his parishioner that derive from his care of Felix as his death approached: 'This seeing the sick endears them to us, **us too it endears**' ([my emphasis] Gardner, p. 48). It is legitimate—and essential—to acknowledge that we ourselves receive comfort and an enhanced sense of wellbeing, as we offer comfort to others.

In stressing the two key elements of sociality and activity, Burton is more concise than the New Economics Foundation with its Five Ways to Wellbeing.[28] And he foreshadows Sartre's response to the bleak immensity of *Nausea*. In his subsequent philosophical writings, expressed in literary form through his *Road To Freedom* trilogy, Sartre argues for engagement and adventure. With the coming of the Second World War, and his capture and imprisonment by the Germans in June 1940, he changes from a thinker preoccupied with the personal into a very political animal. He challenges the intellectual and the artist to abandon their position as simple spectators and take part in real life. Engagement now means commitment and solidarity. Freedom is not a gratuitous activity that needs no particular aim or purpose to be of value. It is a tool for human struggle, involving social responsibility and political activity.

Mathieu Delarue, one of the principal characters in *Iron in the Soul*, has spent most of his life as an indecisive and ineffectual schoolteacher. Caught up in the war, he finds himself able to act decisively for the first time in his life. Deserted by their officers and trapped in a village clock tower, he and his company collectively make their last stand. Shooting a German infantryman is a freely chosen and deliberate act, for which Mathieu is solely responsible. It is deeply significant.

> For years he had tried, in vain, to act. One after another his intentions had been stolen from him: he had been no firmer than a pat of butter. But no one had stolen this! (Hopkins, p. 217)

Facing death, he realises his own freedom.

> Nothing more to ask of Fate now except one half-minute. Just enough time to fire at that smart officer, at all the Beauty of the Earth, at the street, at the flowers, at the gardens, at everything he had loved. Beauty dived downwards like some obscene bird. But Mathieu went on firing. He fired. He was cleansed. He was all-powerful, He was free. (Hopkins, p. 225)

This uncompromising, ecstatic act is the ultimate affirmation of Mathieu's freedom.[29] Finally, he achieves authenticity.

While this is an extreme example of freedom and authenticity, it makes sense to the life experience of Darren, whom I first meet as a bristling, frustrated 19-year old, piercings through lip, nose and eyebrows, scarring up both arms. He tells me about parental separation, fostering and sexual abuse, bullying in school; and how booze keeps him from feeling too much but leads to fights with friends, nightclub doorman and police. His only comfort is beating the hell out of his drum kit in the middle of the night. We have many conversations over the next few years, initially to ensure he stays alive and then to help him develop his relationships and his musical career. Beneath the anguish, I discover a person with a keen critical intelligence, great compassion for his family and friends and an utter disdain for what he sees as so much rhetorical '*political bullshit*'. Darren is determined to live his life genuinely, whatever the cost.

Dapple-Dawn-Drawn Falcon

Hope in its ecstatic form may also emerge from our appreciation of the unique beauty of the world around us. Here, Hopkins is our singular guide.

In his journals he coins the term *inscape* to refer to the charged essence, the absolute singularity that gives each created thing its being; the unified complex of characteristics that give each thing its uniqueness and that differentiate it from other things. His complementary term *instress* refers both to the energy that holds the inscape together and—importantly—the impulse from the inscape which carries it whole into the mind of the beholder.[30]

> There is one notable dead tree … the inscape markedly holding its most simple and beautiful oneness up from the ground through a graceful swerve below (I think) the spring of the branches up to the tops of the timber. I saw the inscape freshly, as if my mind were still growing, though with a companion the eye and the ear are for the most part shut and instress cannot come.[31]

For Hopkins, *inscape* and *instress* describe the overflowing presence of the divine within the temporal; the unique thingness of a thing equates to its sanctity, its purpose in the world. He presents this most perfectly in his own most favoured poem, 'The Windhover'.

> I caught this morning morning's minion, king-
>   dom of daylight's dauphin, dapple-dawn-drawn Falcon, in his riding
>   Of the rolling level underneath him steady air, and striding

High there, how he rung upon the rein of a wimpling wing
In his ecstasy! then off, off forth on swing,
    As a skate's heel sweeps smooth on a bow-bend: the hurl and gliding
    Rebuffed the big wind. My heart in hiding
Stirred for a bird, – the achieve of, the mastery of the thing!

Brute beauty and valour and act, oh, air, pride, plume, here
    Buckle! AND the fire that breaks from thee then, a billion
Times told lovelier, more dangerous, O my chevalier!

    No wonder of it: shéer plód makes plough down sillion
Shine, and blue-bleak embers, ah my dear,
    Fall, gall themselves, and gash gold-vermilion. (Gardner, p. 30)

We do not need to share Hopkins' religious convictions to gain profound hope from this sonnet. The beauty and joy of the falcon, ecstatically riding the wind, infuses with his energy not only Hopkins the poet but also our selves the readers. He reminds us to celebrate those—perhaps fleeting—moments in our own lives when we feel effortlessly magnificent and free. He inspires us to believe in a glittering luminous core to our own being, a core not suppressed by our daily strivings but rather brought by them to the surface, honed and sparkling in the sun. And all this is in full awareness that our existence is ephemeral and contingent, that danger and death await us; which knowledge serves only to heighten the intensity of our life in the present moment.

Notes

1. E. J. Cassel, 'The Nature of Suffering and the Goals of Medicine', *New England Journal of Medicine*, 306.11 (1982), 639–45.
2. I. McWhinney, 'Being a General Practitioner: What It Means', *European Journal of General Practice*, 6.4 (2000), 135–39.
3. R. M. Epstein and A. L. Back, 'Responding to Suffering', *Journal of the American Medical Association*, 314.24 (2015), 2623–24.
4. R. Bressan, E. Iacoponi, J. Candido de Assis, and S. Shergill, 'Hope Is a Therapeutic Tool', *British Medical Journal*, 359 (2017), j5469.
5. C. Dowrick, 'Suffering and Hope: Helen Lester Memorial Lecture 2016', *British Journal of General Practice Open* (15 February 2017). https://doi.org/10.3399/bjgpopen17X100605.

6. H. Riess, J. M. Kelley, R. W. Bailey et al., 'Empathy Training for Resident Hysicians: A Randomized Controlled Trial of a Neuroscience-Informed Curriculum', *Journal of General Internal Medicine*, 27.10 (2012), 1280–86.
7. M. S. Krasner, R. M. Epstein, H. Beckman et al., 'Association of an Educational Program in Mindful Communication with Burnout, Empathy, and Attitudes among Primary Care Physicians', *Journal of the American Medical Association*, 302.12 (2009), 1284–93.
8. H. B. Beckman, M. Wendland, C. Mooney et al., 'The Impact of a Program in Mindful Communication on Primary Care physicians', *Academic Medicine*, 87.6 (2012), 815–19.
9. H. Verweij, R. C. Waumans, D. Smeijers et al., 'Mindfulness-Based Stress Reduction for GPs: Results of a Controlled Mixed Methods Pilot Study in Dutch Primary Care', *British Journal of General Practice*, 66.643 (2016), e99–e105.
10. L. Rowe and M. Kidd, *First Do No Harm: Being a Resilient Doctor in the 21st Century* (New York: McGraw-Hill Medical, 2009).
11. C. Dowrick, *Beyond Depression*, 2nd edn (Oxford: Oxford University Press, 2009).
12. R. Burton, *The Anatomy of Melancholy*, ed. by T. Faulkner, N. Kiessling, and R. Blair, 3 vols. (Oxford: Clarendon Press, 1989–1994). Quotations range across vols. I–III.
13. G. M. Hopkins, *Poems and Prose of Gerard Manley Hopkins*, ed. by W. H. Gardner (London: Penguin Books, 1963).
14. J. P Sartre, *Nausea*, trans. by L. Alexander (New York: New Directions, 1964).
15. J. P. Sartre, *Iron in the Soul*, trans. by G. Hopkins (London: Penguin Books, 1963).
16. G. M. Hopkins, Letter to Robert Bridges, 17 May 1885, in Gardner, p. 202.
17. J. Radden, *Melancholic Habits: Burton's Anatomy and the Mind Sciences* (New York: Oxford University Press, 2017), p. 23.
18. H. Pearson, 'The Terrible Sonnets of Gerard Manley Hopkins and the Spirituality of Depression', *The Way*, 46.1 (2007), 23–37.
19. J. Saville, *A Queer Chivalry: The Homoerotic Asceticism of Gerard Manley Hopkins* (Charlottesville: University Press of Virginia, 2000).
20. J. P. Sartre, *Being and Nothingness: A Phenomenological Essay on Ontology*, trans. by H. Barnes (New York: Washington Square Press,1992).
21. J. P. Sartre, *Anti-Semite and Jew*, trans. by G. Becker (New York: Schocken Press, 1948), p. 90.
22. V. Schwarcz, 'The Pane of Sorrow: Public Uses of Personal Grief in Modern China', *Daedalus*, 125.1 (1996), 119–48.
23. J. P. Sartre, *Sketch for a History of the Emotions*, trans. by P. Mariet (London: Routledge, 1971), pp. 68–70.

24. M. A. Lund, *Melancholy, Medicine and Religion in Early Modern England* (Cambridge: Cambridge University Press, 2010), p. 184.
25. 'Authenticity in Stanford Encyclopaedia of Philosophy'. https://plato.stanford.edu/entries/authenticity/#SarDeBea. Accessed 16 November 2017.
26. C. Dowrick, ed., *Person-Centred Primary Care: Searching for the Self* (London: Routledge, 2018).
27. C. Dowrick, J. Billington, J. Robinson, A. Hamer, and C. Williams, 'Get into Reading as an Intervention for Common Mental Health Problems: Exploring Catalysts for Change', *Journal of Medical Humanities*, 38.1 (2012), 15–20.
28. 'Five Ways to Wellbeing', New Economics Foundation, 2008. https://issuu.com/neweconomicsfoundation/docs/five_ways_to_well-being?viewMode=presentation. Accessed 9 January 2018.
29. G. Cox, *Sartre and Fiction* (London: Bloomsbury Continuum Books, 2009).
30. A. Domestico, 'Inscape, Instress and Distress', *Commonweal*, 9 March 2009. https://www.commonwealmagazine.org/inscape-instress-distress?_ga=1.190997742.596395981.1472016212. Accessed 14 November 2017.
31. From Hopkins' Journal, 1871–72, in Gardner, p. 127.

3

The Sonnet 'Cure': Renaissance Poetics to Romantic Prosaics

Grace Farrington and Philip Davis

It was during the Elizabethan age, we contend in this chapter, that the foundation was laid for the future of English poetry both as a written craft and as an inner mental discipline productive of 'good health' in Burton's sense of that term. Verse was created in order to contain passionate feeling as well as struggling, conflicted thoughts, in ways that alleviated or consoled human sorrow through aesthetic achievement.

The Frame

The point of creative origin in Elizabethan poetics is when the poet makes order out of the forces and elements of human chaos within the form of the little world or multidimensional map offered by his or her poem. A place or site is founded:

> For the body of our imagination being as an unformed chaos without fashion, without day, if by the divine power of the spirit it be wrought into an orb

G. Farrington (✉)
The Reader, Liverpool, UK
e-mail: graceframe@thereader.org.uk

P. Davis
Centre for Research into Reading, Literature and Society, University of Liverpool, Liverpool, UK
e-mail: phildav@liverpool.ac.uk

J. Billington (ed.), *Reading and Mental Health*,
https://doi.org/10.1007/978-3-030-21762-4_3

> of order and form, is it not more pleasing to Nature, that desires a certainty and comports not with that which is infinite, to have these closes, rather than not to know where to end, or how far to go, especially seeing our passions are often without measure?[1]

Samuel Daniel does not want to be rid of imaginative or passionate power, but to show how it might be incorporated into a structure, where it can be put into channelled use. For without direction from some perspective above themselves human passions are likely to expand and run on, sustained by their own strength, until they become almost independent of the original motive or substance of feeling, or simply run out of energy. Daniel's model of poetry is a mental safeguard, a rhymed holdfast, against such chaos or entropy. On the one hand, the poet can get above and outside the lines as the maker of the little world in which they are contained by rhyme and form. On the other, the poet may simultaneously remain inside the poem at the level of the lines themselves, making up as they do the separate elements, compounds and conflicts experienced within their world.

Likewise, in Elizabethan structures, we are particularly conscious of reading both along the lines as distinct units and down them in the turns of the whole. So it is in Barnaby Googe's poem 'Out of Sight, Out of Mind', for example:

> The oftener seen, the more I lust,
> The more I lust, the more I smart,
> The more I smart, the more I trust,
> The more I trust, the heavier heart,
> The heavy heart breeds mine unrest;
> Thy absence therefore like I best.[2]

The poem, unhappily driven by the horizontal pressure of lust as it moves from line to line, generates in the end an ironic inversion of the longed-for return. It is 'absence' itself turned from being presence, which has now to be associated with 'like'. The aspiration lies in the words of Robert Southwell: 'What thought can thinke an other thought can mende'.[3] For what is offered is a model of something more finally complete than one might be able to see visually in the form of the line, with its move from left to right or from a to b. By the turns across the lines, in search of a resolution in sanity, the poet (though he must know he protests too much) here tries to prevent the poem going round and round in circles. As Ben Jonson writes of Shakespeare:

For though the poet's matter, nature be,
His art doth give the fashion. And, that he,
Who casts to write a living line, must sweat,
(Such as thine are) and strike the second heat
Upon the muses' anvil: turn the same,
(And himself with it) that he thinks to frame;
Or for the laurel, he may gain a scorn,
For a good poet's made, as well as born.
And such wert thou.[4]

The poem is a second world beaten out by a blacksmith with the powers of a lower Vulcan. In forming that second world, the poet offers some initial spark but needs a second heat, something made and not just innate, to beat out a form in which that first heat is reignited and made constructive. Then as the poet turns across a line, it is not just the line he crosses but something in his own mind ('And himself with it') that turns, changes, and may be reconstituted with it. Poetic creation in this period becomes just such a process of reappraisal and reassembly, down the vertical axis, involving turns and turning-points, from one line or one state to another that makes for vital transmutation and transformation.

This is a craft to be learned by the poet and reader. For the Elizabethan reader and analyst, George Puttenham, poetry is a craft that involves the same awareness of practical human constraints that one might see for instance in the work of a carpenter or a builder or Jonson's blacksmith:

> Now ye may perceive … that there is a band to be given every verse in a staff, so as none fall out alone or uncoupled, and this band maketh that the staff is said fast and not loose: even as ye see in buildings of stone or brick the mason giveth a band, that is a length to two breadths, and upon necessity divers other sorts of bands to hold in the work fast and maintain the perpendicularity of the wall. So, in any staff of seven or eight or more verses, the coupling of the more meters by rhyme or concord is the faster band; the fewer, the looser band.[5]

The structure which the poet has to work with in his composition of the poem is designed to ensure the poem holds together. In poetry the perpendicular 'band' has to follow *down* rather than just across the page, creating along with a set of internal links a kind of 'fast'-ness that will give that certain movement of which Daniel speaks. For both Puttenham and Daniel saw poetry as being at least three-dimensional in its body and constructed form.

Robert Frost was to talk of poetry as 'a momentary stay against confusion'.[6] The origins of that stay or hold lie partly in the defence of rhyme that Elizabethan poets such as Daniel mounted. It is rhyme 'whose known frame hath those due stays for the mind, those encounters of touch, as makes the motion certain, though the variety be infinite' (*English Critical Essays*, p. 66). Within the right frame there can be room for content which in its chaotic variety might otherwise feel 'without measure'. The mind requires those 'due stays', the linear pauses and holdfasts, which steady the writer and reader alike and provide a sense of something within the poem to rest upon. The formal achievement of rhyme contains this realisation of the infinitely unknown or indefinitely uncertain within manageable limits. So in Daniel's sonnet 'Let others sing of knight and palatines', he says of his own lines here, written to and for the beloved:

> These are the Arkes, the Trophies I erect,
> That fortifie thy name against old age:
> And these thy sacred vertues must protect,
> Against the darke and Tymes consuming rage.[7]

'Protect' there does not merely tame or stave off the threat: at the next line it includes 'the dark', letting it back in again with a line of its own, in counterpoint against the overall sentence.

By contrast, the language of prose goes forward without such holds, potentially shapeless. As Ben Jonson says of sentence-structure: 'Periods are beautiful when they are not too long, for so they have their strength too, as in a pike or javelin'.[8] Yet in Elizabethan verse, beauty is played out in the contrapuntal harmony across lines and between parts and wholes. Witness Jonson himself on the brevity of a young life which nonetheless had its own completed shape and self-contained quality:

> In small proportions, we just beauties see:
> And in short measures, life may perfect be.[9]

The form seeks to create perfection against the dark of time.

The lyric's solidity was to create that 'moment's monument'[10] which would enlarge, rather than reduce the meaning of an individual life. Puttenham applied this idea to the situation at court, where despite all the privilege of their position, princes

> have not one hour to bestow upon any other civil or delectable art of natural or moral doctrine, nor scarce any leisure to think one good thought in perfect and godly contemplation, whereby their troubled minds might be moderated and brought to tranquillity. (*The Art of English Poesy*, p. 111)

For the adult caught up in the business of the day, time institutes its own law of automatic follow-on from one thing to the next, without any institution of form or priority or 'closes'. Immediate considerations take over from higher ones, as if by necessity. But Puttenham feels that to be able to think 'one good thought' might in some way reset the balance, creating a fresh basis from which to carry on. Though the prince has not one hour for it, 'a sonnet is a minute' ('14 breaths and 70 heartbeats').[11] It is the perfect model, setting aside a single unit of time in which to develop and contain a complete thought.

The Healing 'Turn'

Puttenham introduces an analogy with the work of the physician in that same common-sense mode that had led him to think of the comparison with the mason. Again he is interested in proportion, and the pain caused by imbalances:

> Lamenting is altogether contrary to rejoicing: every man saith so, and yet is it a piece of joy to be able to lament with ease and freely to pour forth a man's inward sorrows and the griefs wherewith his mind is surcharged. This was a very necessary device of the poet and a fine: besides his poetry to play also the physician, and not only by applying a medicine to the ordinary sickness of mankind, but by making the very grief itself (in part) cure of the disease. (*The Art of English Poesy*, p. 135)

In early modern medical discourse the word 'cure' 'denoted a range of meanings, including 'a method of treatment … the relief of symptoms, and even sheer survival of an acute illness, as well as the modern sense of full recovery'.[12] For Puttenham the word seems to mean more than recovery back to a baseline. His description does imply a kind of acute experience of grief which is turned into something other than itself even by speaking of itself in song. Many situations in life are susceptible to ordinary cures, but poetry concerns those which have no answer or solution:

> Therefore, of death and burials, of the adversities by wars, and of true love lost or ill-bestowed, are the only sorrows that the noble poets sought by their art to remove or appease, not with any medicament of a contrary temper, as the Galenists use to cure *contraria contrariis* [opposites by opposites], but as the Paracelsians, who cure *similia similibus* [like by like], making one dolor to expel another, and in this case, one short sorrowing the remedy of a long and grievous sorrow. (*The Art of English Poesy*, pp. 136–37)

In the ancient world there would have been certain appointed times and places for lamentation, in the same way that collective rejoicing was provided for and expected at communal feasts and festivals. Temples and statues served as places that one could visit, where the kind of emotional expression that Puttenham describes would literally have found a place for ritual. The poem is here the less material version of such temples and monuments, the repository for inward sorrows more private and less immediately communal, and often humiliatingly belittling.

For his idea that poetry might be cathartic and therapeutic, Puttenham takes as his model not Galen, the second-century physician and surgeon, but Paracelsus, a Renaissance physician. Instead of aggressive intervention, surgical counters to disease, what Paracelsus offers is homoeopathy: 'similia similibus', a short intense form of the otherwise long linear suffering. So Puttenham cites Sir Walter Raleigh:

> With wisdom's eyes had but blind fortune seen,
> Then had my love, my love for ever been.

The secret lamentation 'my love, my love' internal to the second line in a way that turns against the mere linear movement left to right is an instance of epizeuxis or what Puttenham renames the cuckoo-spell (*The Art of English Poesy*, p. 285). It is like a little inner image of poetry, the repetition across the mid-point of the line almost lifting itself out of the ongoing account of what has been and is no longer. It is as if poetry finds a sudden place in which those little words which for so long had remained unspoken in loss are needed almost importunately by the voice of the poem.

'One short sorrowing the remedy of a long and grievous sorrow'. The act of 'sorrow-ing' offers to counter the silting up of sorrow as a noun, a process of calling out the dull inwardly constricted ache which is thus 'tunably running' in a form of music (*The Art of English Poesy*, p. 227). The transmutation is like that moment of relief when a person whom one knows to be suffering—and yet who will not speak of the cause—begins to cry.

The person may not be saying anything as yet, 'but at least there is some movement', one thinks. Only in the poetry the cry is made beautiful by a healing art: 'my love, my love'. Philip Sidney imagines the poet in a vineyard, holding out 'a cluster of grapes' to anyone who might venture in. He is confident that poetry's sweetness might work upon any reader, 'even those hard-hearted evil men' who 'know no other good but *indulgere genio* [to follow their own devices]', and who 'feel not the inward reason' upon which a philosopher's admonitions might be based.[13] 'My love, my love' is like that inward reason.

As Montaigne writes, 'we ought to grant free passage to diseases', rather than be forever fighting them, Galen-style.[14] In Chidiock Tichborne's 'Elegy' the young protagonist thus faces his own fate unflinchingly as it presents itself before him on the page. The poem, apparently written the night before his execution, seems to allow him a space in which to consider the foreshortening of his own life even at that point when nothing can be done to alter it:

> My tale was heard, and yet it was not told;
> My fruit is fall'n, and yet my leaves are green;
> My youth is spent, and yet I am not old;
> I saw the world, and yet I was not seen:
> My thread is cut, and yet it is not spun;
> And now I live, and now my life is done.[15]

Sorrow is contained here within the form: 'and yet, and yet, and now'. For whilst the poem is mapped out as if it were a riddle or a paradox, what it spells out very plainly is the truth of this poet's otherwise untold tale. 'The spring is past, and yet it hath not sprung', 'My youth is gone, and yet I am but young': these are terrible present tenses just about to become past, 'I saw the world, and yet I was not seen'. Only poetic time can hold onto individual time. Spring not sprung, youth gone but young: the very interplay of the words is the work of 'simila similibus'. Though the personal is thus contained within measure, it is still that fragile sense of the personal—its temporariness on earth, its vulnerability to loss—that remains the inner motive-force for the existence of poetry in the Renaissance. Antidotes against time, against the loss of tiny personal notes overwhelmed in anonymising obliviousness.

The purpose, says Sidney, is 'to move men', so as ultimately 'to make them know that goodness whereunto they are moved' (*An Apology for Poetry*, p. 87). Yet the taste of such goodness amidst bitter experience has to be sweet and the touch delicate in order to entice in the reader from other hungers and thirsts than those which a poem might be able to satisfy. In Shakespeare's sonnet 29

> When, in disgrace with fortune and men's eyes,
> I all alone beweep my outcast state

sweetness comes as a surprise to the 'sullen earth':

> Yet in these thoughts myself almost despising,
> Haply I think on thee, and then my state
> (Like to the lark at break of day arising)
> From sullen earth sings hymns at heaven's gate.
> For thy sweet love remembered such wealth brings
> That then I scorn to change my state with kings.[16]

Burrow notes how that sudden response out of the sullen contained in the word 'sings' has already been anticipated in 'despi*sing*' and 'ari*sing*' (Burrow, p. 438). The internal recall of those two earlier words signals the transformation of the despised self, that unhappy state previously spelt out as 'all alone' which in a matter of two lines has been almost forgotten. So much in Elizabethan verse thus depends on one thing contained in another—one word in a longer or harsher one, goodness within sadness, grace found in the midst of disgrace—so that a healing art might carry out its restorative work from within the grief itself. 'Usually these two stages have to be successive', George Santayana writes: 'first we suffer, afterwards we sing'.[17]

Sidney speaks more theologically of 'that second nature' which the work of a poet serves to activate:

> when with the force of a divine breath he bringeth things forth far surpassing [Nature's] doings, with no small argument to the incredulous of that first accursed fall of Adam: since our erected wit maketh us know what perfection is, and yet our infected will keepeth us from reaching unto it. (*An Apology for Poetry*, p. 86)

'These are the arks, the trophies I erect' wrote Daniel. It is that erecting that works against the infecting even by incorporating it. And in that it is nothing less than a small vital attempt to restore something pre-lapsarian to the post-lapsarian world, in the midst of the fallenness and not despite it. 'Against the dark'.

For Sidney the poem's 'embrace of nature'[18] is foundational to that higher purpose of developing 'another nature' (*An Apology for Poetry*, p. 85) which would purify the idea of pleasure from its fallen association with moral corruption. For the condition of a reflective human life is one of being caught between these higher and lower levels. This fallen 'soul' has to inhabit a universe with which it is not wholly in sync, and in which its very form feels like a debased memory of the original. What poetry seems to offer within this general human predicament is the capacity to hold the various levels together. And what is important is the transformation into song, harmoniously crying out loud and soft, within the music of poetry. The frame thus acts almost like a tuning fork, allowing the reader to hear where the sound is made truly perfect, and where the notes cannot be other than broken and distorted.

Giving Voice

Such poetry cannot attain its full effect simply through being seen from without. It also has to be performed, like an instrument that is sounded. As Richard Wistreich has argued, in the early modern period all written texts were understood as needing to be 'brought to voice' in order to complete the process of making them efficacious.[19] Poetry was regarded not only as an outlet for the mind, a way of mapping out its contents on the page. A poem was also a carrier of voice. Walter J. Ong has written thus on the sudden effect in the world of voiced words and live sound, even from its most brutal origins:

> In an oral culture, which knows words only in their natural habitat, that is, the world of sound, words necessarily carry with them a special sense of power. For sound always indicates the present use of power. A primitive hunter can see a buffalo, smell a buffalo, touch a buffalo, and taste a buffalo when the buffalo is dead and motionless. If he *hears* a buffalo, he had better watch out: something is going on. No other sensory field has this dynamism which marks the field of sound. So long as words are known only directly and without interference for what they ultimately are – sounds – and cannot possibly be imagined to be what they really are not – marks on a surface – they are sensed as physically powered events, happenings, of a piece with all present actuality.[20]

It is this presentness that Elizabethan verse transmutes when words are taken out of their natural habitat in the world and offered instead as notation on the page. Paradoxically, as in Shakespeare's sonnets, poetic notation represents 'my dumb thoughts, speaking in effect'. The condensed power of the Elizabethan lyric stems from its origins in 'unvoiced'[21] thought, as though the poem were produced out of the lack of any other means of expressing the inner voice. When those marks on the page are released back out again in performance, they trigger an echo in the auditor's or reader's own dumb thoughts. Perhaps the strangest thing about a lyric poem in the Elizabethan tradition is the way in which this echo from another person (living in another place and time) can seem to feel as if it came from inside its auditor, echoing his or her own thoughts, recalling the echo of his or her own forgotten or lost or hidden inner being (past and present). The Elizabethan lyric seems a generic individual, at once a single voice and yet resonant on behalf of the collective race. What is more, a poem *retains* this echo over time, so that it can be re-sounded again, inside and out, when the poem is read a second, and a third time; recollected in quietness, listened out for carefully. Douglas Oliver, twentieth-century poet and expert performer of poetry, explored the way in which feelings, recreated out of their natural habitat, get acted out in the process of poetry's live transmission where 'fictitious' emotions are 'mimed' in an intonation pattern 'almost perfectly suitable for their expression':

> The link between emotion and intonation pattern, even when mimed, is *extremely direct*, like that link between sight and cognitive awareness in perception, for it is sensuous once we begin the performance of a poem. What we do when we read a poem well is modulate our speed and emphasis of reading, so as to bring the conceptualised emotion into temporal consonance with the semantic field and to let emotion's necessary sensuous conjunction with sound create a unity between all three factors. It's almost as if the emotional and temporally accorded semantic concepts drag the sound directly and sensuously along with them: when we recite well we have almost to wait for the right instant to speak each syllable, delaying very minutely durations of vowels to make the tempo perfect.[22]

To read a good poem well is not simply to ride the wave of an already known emotion. It is to sense the minute shifts, delays and crescendos that the composer barely writes into the score, but which the musician senses to be of a piece with the music as it has been written. In practice it is as in the opening of the final farewell poem of Michael Drayton's life, which begins:

> Soe well I love thee, as without thee I
> Love nothing.[23]

The real gap seems to open up in between that repetition of 'thee', and the 'I' that follows afterwards, even in advance of the line break. It is a kind of hidden partition—the telegraphese of 'without thee' again musically disrupting with delicacy the otherwise straightforward left to right movement—that is only made present in the careful reading out-loud, even be it sub-vocally within one's own head.

What is at stake here is the almost physical way in which a hidden inner emotional mentality is quietly released in response to the outer sonic motion: similia similibus. The word rebounds upon its writer or hearer as if disclosing inside-out the hidden and veiled inner meaning which they could not otherwise find. It is this double speech, the outer sound and the resounding inner message, that is the resonance of such poetry. It is that which, in a later time, William Wordsworth heard from the solitary reaper:

> The music in my heart I bore,
> Long after it was heard no more[24]

or from an ordinary anonymous woman casually saying to him, 'What you are stepping westward?'

> The echo of the voice enwrought
> A human sweetness with the thought
> Of travelling through the world that lay
> Before me in my endless way.[25]

This is, in its last two lines also echoing Milton, a version of poetry's paradise regained through erected wit. 'My own voice cheared me, and, far more, the mind's/Internal echo of the imperfect sound'.[26]

Indeed, Wordsworth, we suggest, at the close of this chapter, was the Romantic transmitter and re-beginner of the Elizabethan lyric tradition that (as he puts it in *The Prelude*) 'through the turnings intricate of verse' effected 'a sorrow that is not sorrow to hear of' (1805, vol. 627; XII, pp. 245–47). It is possible even to pinpoint an explicit place of influence. It occurs, in the midst of social turmoil, in Book 4 of *The Excursion* (1814) where (unusually) Wordsworth quotes a poet at length, the poet being Samuel Daniel, in order to recentre himself:

> "Knowing the heart of Man is set to be
> The centre of this World, about the which
> Those revolutions of disturbances

Still roll; where all the aspècts of misery
Predominate; whose strong effects are such
As he must bear, being powerless to redress;
And that unless above himself he can
Erect himself, how poor a thing is Man!"[27]

It was Wordsworth's ambition, without ever forsaking what is down to earth, prosaic and common, to find the extraordinary in the ordinary, the poetry within the prose, the ability of the creative mind not wholly to become what circumstances were conspiring to make it. The great cause set out in the *Lyrical Ballads* and its famous Preface—the poet as man speaking to men, the need to wipe poetry clean again of its accumulated verbal artifice, the belief in humble life as subject matter—is a descendant of the Renaissance effort to establish the very basis of what was poetry.

This is what Coleridge, who had introduced Wordsworth to Daniel, recognised when in *Biographia Literaria* (1817) he described Daniel's work, alongside Wordsworth's, as occupying 'the neutral ground of prose and verse, common to both'.

> Mr Wordsworth strikingly resembles Samuel Daniel, one of the golden writers of our golden Elizabethan age, now most causelessly neglected: Samuel Daniel, whose diction bears no mark of time, no distinction of age, which has been and, as long as our language shall last, will be so far the language of the to-day and forever, as that it is more intelligible to us than the transitory fashions of our own particular age. A similar praise is due to his sentiments. No frequency of perusal can deprive them of their freshness. For though they are brought into the full daylight of every reader's comprehension, yet are they drawn up from depths which few in any age are privileged to visit, into which few in any age have courage or inclination to descend.[28]

The same purity, principle and commitment impelled Wordsworth to make a new beginning again. That is why he would look at over-elaborate poems and try to paraphrase them, try to see whether beneath their fattened flesh there remained the skeleton of real feeling. Too often he found the basis of a genuine original lost beyond recognition: 'there is no under current, no skeleton or stamina, of thought and feeling'.[29]

O reader! had you in your mind
Such stores as silent thought can bring,
O gentle reader! you would find
A tale in every thing.[30]

That remained Wordsworth's centre: honour to the fundamentally human and honour to the ostensibly prosaic were alike the task of poetry in its fresh revolution. As Iain McGilchrist dares to put it, in referring to what he takes to be the great turning-points or re-beginnings in his model of the modern Western mind: 'It is notable that it is at times when, according to my view, there has been a period of "release" in the right hemisphere – the Renaissance and Romanticism – that there has been an interest in the long view, and the high view, of life'. It is an extended view that becomes necessary, he argues, 'if one is aware of the uniqueness of individual people and things', for then one is also 'inevitably forced to confront separation and loss'.[31] Against such loss, poetry locates 'something ever more about to be' (*The Prelude*, 1805, VI, 542)—'something', even thus unnameable, from within the ordinary world that can transcend it.

Notes

1. S. Daniel, 'A Defence of Rhyme' (1603), in *English Critical Essays (Sixteenth, Seventeenth and Eighteenth Centuries)*, ed. by E. D. Jones (London: Oxford University Press, 1947), pp. 61–87 (p. 69).
2. B. Googe, 'Deuli augent dolorem', in *Eclogues, Epitaphs, and Sonnets* (1563), ed. by J. M. Kennedy (Toronto: University of Toronto Press, 1989), p. 97.
3. R. Southwell, 'Looke Home' (from *St Peter's Complaint*, 1595), in *Collected Poems*, ed. by P. Davidson and A. Sweeney (Manchester: Carcanet, 2007), p. 49.
4. B. Jonson, 'To the Memory of My Beloved, the Author Mr. William Shakespeare: And What He Hath Left Us' (1623), in *The Complete Poems*, ed. by G. Parfitt (New Haven: Yale University Press, 1982), p. 265.
5. G. Puttenham, *The Art of English Poesy: A Critical Edition* (1589), ed. by F. Whigham and W. A. Rebhorn (Ithaca: Cornell University Press, 2007), p. 178.
6. 'The Figure a Poem Makes' (1939), in *Selected Prose of Robert Frost*, ed. by H. Cox and E. C. Latham (New York: Collier Books, 1968), pp. 17–20 (p. 18).
7. S. Daniel, 'Sonnet 52' (from *Delia*, 1592), in *The Penguin Book of Renaissance Verse 1509–1659*, ed. by H. R. Woudhuysen (London: Penguin, 1993), pp. 250–51.
8. B. Jonson, 'Notes on Literature', in *English Renaissance Literary Criticism*, ed. by B. Vickers (Oxford: Clarendon Press, 2003), pp. 558–89 (p. 577).
9. B. Jonson, 'To the Immortal Memory and Friendship of That Noble Pair, Sir Lucius Cary and Sir H. Morison' (1629), in *The Complete Poems*, p. 214.

10. D. G. Rossetti, 'Sonnet on the Sonnet' (from *The House of Life*, 1881), in *Collected Poetry and Prose*, ed. by J. McGann (New Haven: Yale University Press, 2003), p. 127.
11. S. Haldane, 'Note on Pulsation and Poetry', *The Reader*, 48 (2012), 41–43 (p. 43).
12. M. A. Lund, *Melancholy, Medicine and Religion in Early Modern England: Reading the Anatomy of Melancholy* (Cambridge: Cambridge University Press, 2010), p. 99. Lund refers here to a 1974 essay, 'Clinical Medicine', printed in *Medicine in Seventeenth-Century England: A Symposium Held at UCLA in Honor of C. D. O'Malley*.
13. P. Sidney, *An Apology for Poetry, or the Defence of Poesy* (1595), ed. by G. Shepherd (Manchester: Manchester University Press, 2002), p. 95.
14. 'Of experience' (1575), in *The Essays of Michael, Seigneur de Montaigne*, trans. by C. Cotton (London: Ward Lock & Co., undated), pp. 849–92 (p. 869).
15. C. Tichborne, 'Elegy' (1586), in *Elizabethan Lyrics*, ed. by N. Ault (London: Faber and Faber, 1986), p. 120.
16. 'Sonnet 29', in *The Oxford Shakespeare: The Complete Sonnets and Poems*, ed. by C. Burrow (Oxford: Oxford University Press, 2002), p. 439.
17. G. Santayana, *The Sense of Beauty: Being the Outline of Aesthetic Theory* (1896) (New York: Dover, 1955), p. 139.
18. C. Coch, 'The Woman in the Garden: (En)gendering Pleasure in Late Elizabethan Poetry', *English Literary Renaissance*, 39 (2009), 97–127 (p. 101).
19. R. Wistreich, 'Reading the Voice: The Anatomy and Physiognomy of Speaking and Singing', Paper given at *Symposium on Reading and Health in Early Modern Europe, 1500–1800* (Newcastle University, July 2013).
20. W. J. Ong, 'Foreword' to Pedro Laín Entralgo's *The Therapy of the Word in Classical Antiquity*, ed. and trans. by L. J. Rather and J. M. Sharp (New Haven: Yale University Press, 1970), pp. xiii–xiv.
21. G. T. Wright, 'The Silent Speech of Shakespeare's Sonnets', in *Shakespeare and the Twentieth Century: The Selected Proceedings of the International Shakespeare Association World Congress, Los Angeles, 1996*, ed. by J. Bate, J. L. Levenson, and D. Mehl (London: Associated University Presses, 1998), pp. 314–35 (p. 316).
22. D. Oliver, *Poetry and Narrative in Performance* (Basingstoke: Macmillan, 1989), p. 107.
23. 'Verses Made the Night Before He Dyed', in *Poems of Michael Drayton*, ed. by J. Buxton (London: Routledge & Kegan Paul, 1953), p. 286.
24. W. Wordsworth, 'The Solitary Reaper' (*Poems*, 1807), in *The Major Works*, ed. by S. Gill (Oxford: Oxford University Press, 2000), pp. 319–20.

25. W. Wordsworth, 'Stepping Westward' (*Poems*, 1807), in *The Major Works*, pp. 313–14.
26. W. Wordsworth, *The Prelude: 1799, 1805, 1850*, ed. by J. Wordsworth, M. H. Abrams and S. Gill (New York: W. W. Norton, 1979), 1805, I, pp. 64–65.
27. 'The Excursion' (1814), in *The Poems of William Wordsworth*, ed. by Jared Curtis, 3 vols. (Ithaca: Cornell University Press, 2009), II, pp. 298–570 (pp. 400–401).
28. S. T. Coleridge, *Biographia Literaria*, ed. by George Watson (London: J. M. Dent & Sons, 1960), p. 267.
29. 'Essays Upon Epitaphs', in *The Prose Works of William Wordsworth*, ed. by W. J. B. Owen and J. W. Smyser, 3 vols. (Oxford: Clarendon Press, 1974), II, pp. 63–79 (p. 75).
30. 'Simon Lee, the Old Huntsman' (from *Lyrical Ballads*, 1798), in *The Major Works*, p. 87.
31. I. McGilchrist, *The Master and His Emissary: The Divided Brain and the Making of the Western World* (New Haven: Yale University Press, 2009), p. 365.

4

The Victorian Novel: Laying the Foundations for 'Bibliotherapy'

Grace Farrington, Philip Davis and Josie Billington

The Victorian Novel as the Original 'Reader Outreach Project'

The Victorian age had a more anxious interest than did the Renaissance period in the place that literature might occupy within the wider world as a regenerative force for good. It is a concern that manifests itself in the rise of the realist novel during the formation of what was to become a modern mass-industrial democratic society. The twinned ideals of the nineteenth-century novel were continuing the Renaissance and Romantic dedication to a high form of serious literature yet modified by the need to be able to increase its reach within the everyday world. The realist novel, the great innovation of the Victorian era, had to rebegin in its own form the argument of Wordsworth's Preface to *Lyrical Ballads* in the commitment of literature to ordinary experience or to the extraordinariness—and often deep

G. Farrington (✉)
The Reader, Liverpool, UK
e-mail: graceframe@thereader.org.uk

P. Davis · J. Billington
Centre for Research into Reading, Literature and Society,
University of Liverpool, Liverpool, UK
e-mail: phildav@liverpool.ac.uk

J. Billington
e-mail: jbilling@liverpool.ac.uk

J. Billington (ed.), *Reading and Mental Health*,
https://doi.org/10.1007/978-3-030-21762-4_4

and troubled seriousness—lodged within it. This chapter offers an account, albeit a broadly suggestive one, of the challenging social circumstances for the maintenance of a place for reading serious literature which are inherited even at the present time from the Victorian crisis.

Reading, Literature and 'Culture' in the Victorian Period

Whilst the climax of the Renaissance movement in England during the Elizabethan period had been prepared for by a revival of classical or ancient philosophy and culture, entirely new pressures affected the Victorian ability to revive and maintain origins and traditions. The theory of advance and progress, fuelled by the Industrial Revolution, seemed to require a change in direction, a looking forward rather than back. In the face of such movement, there was a major task to be undertaken in determining those ideals which might be preserved as constant supports in a hastening future. What was required, said John Ruskin—who more than any thinker kept the spirit of Romanticism alive in the Victorian period[1]—was 'to go to [books] for help', 'to consult with the wisest and the greatest men on all points of earnest difficulty', and to be 'led by them into wider sight'.[2]

For Ruskin, art itself begins with vision. The person who has the vision might not always understand its content; it is enough that the artist seeks to convey it. As Mary Jacobus writes of John Clare, he 'not only observed nature minutely', but 'saw more than he knew, and perhaps knew more than he could see'.[3] The vision takes on the quality of a felt truth, a kind of embodied revelation: 'to see clearly', said Ruskin, 'is poetry, prophecy, and religion,—all in one' (*Modern Painters* iii, in *Works*, V, p. 333). In that endeavour, where a moment of insight may now have to stand in place of a whole lost framework of understanding, the impatient imagination of Ruskin will even risk the 'sacrifice' of the perfection of form in order that there may be a present realisation of expansive content.[4]

For risks are now necessary when vision is giving way to blunter sight, when the quickening sense of the imagination is in danger of being overwhelmed by the governing trend of materialism:

> The imagination would on the whole rather have it *not* there; - the reality and substance are rather in the imagination's way; it would think a good deal more of the thing if it could not see it. Hence, that strange and sometimes fatal charm, which there is in all things as long as we wait for them, and the moment we have lost them; but which fades while we possess them;

> - that sweet bloom of all that is far away, which perishes under our touch. Yet the feeling of this is not a weakness; it is one of the most glorious gifts of the human mind, making the whole infinite future, and imperishable past, a richer inheritance, if faithfully inherited, than the changeful, frail, fleeting present: it is also one of the many witnesses in us to the truth that these present and tangible things are not meant to satisfy us. (*Modern Painters* iii, in *Works*, V, pp. 181–82)

It is not enough for sight to be limited to 'substance'—to what one might touch—nor for a person or an age sufficient to itself. What is needed is a larger range, a wider expanse, 'a richer inheritance' than can be gleaned from the present. There is risk here of mere nostalgic loving of loss, a retreat into what is past and absent. But for Ruskin our needs are more finely tuned than we often realise: we are not satisfied by the tangibly useful, but carry other desires for the 'sweet bloom' of what cannot be possessed for any length of time.

Art might be a way of bringing back into the world what is not wholly of it. But taking place within the world, art has to be a form of work, contributing to that world, and being affected by its conditions. Not even the artist can work in a rarefied atmosphere, closed off from the world, for the artist shares the same character as any other kind of worker: 'whatever bit of a wise man's work is honestly and benevolently done, that bit is his book or his piece of art' ('Sesame and Lilies', *Works*, XVIII, p. 61). And if art is a form of work, this in turn raises the value of work, making labour itself akin to art.

But in Ruskin's modern civilised world the worker was becoming no longer a craftsman, but an invisible 'cog' in an inhuman machine, in peril of forgetting what he himself was made for.

> You must either make a tool of the creature, or a man of him. You cannot make both. Men were not intended to work with the accuracy of tools, to be precise and perfect in all their actions. If you will have that precision out of them, and make their fingers measure degrees like cog-wheels, and their arms strike curves like compasses, you must unhumanize them. All the energy of their spirits must be given to make cogs and compasses of themselves … and so soul and sight be worn away, and the whole human being be lost at last – a heap of sawdust, so far as its intellectual work in this world is concerned. (*The Stones of Venice* ii, *Works*, X, p. 192)

If workers are made to channel 'soul' into the machine-like structure of a system, the soul can only eventually die out, leaving behind the husk-like form of a dispirited and depressed creature. The accumulated human potential, that inheritance from generation to generation of a characteristically human spirit, is worn down in the one individual, to the part or segment that he represents within a whole that he cannot see and has no belief in. Or else the better-off young person is trained and made fit for a humanly devised '*station in life*' ('Sesame and Lilies', *Works*, XVIII, p. 54) as if there were nothing more to living than the effort of finding a class-position to fill. In contrast, said Ruskin, walk into any great building from the Gothic age. In the visible marks of the original mason one can see a person coming alive in his work, making the work itself a route towards something greater, rather than a diminishing act of slavery.

Ruskin showed how reading might achieve a similar effect, so long as the reader *worked* at discovering the author's 'hidden' meaning:

> When you come to a good book, you must ask yourself, 'Am I inclined to work as an Australian miner would? Are my pickaxes and shovels in good order, and am I in good trim myself, my sleeves well up to the elbow, and my breath good, and my temper?' The metal you are in search of being the author's mind or meaning, his words are as the rock which you have to crush and smelt in order to get at it. And your pickaxes are your own care … Often you will need sharpest, finest chiseling … before you can gather one grain of the metal. ('Sesame and Lilies', *Works*, XVIII, pp. 63–64)

The fact that even the life-giving work might still feel like painstaking activity is for Ruskin a necessary reminder of the worth and purpose of it: that there is something that the miner is trying to 'get at', however long it takes.

For Ruskin that 'something' was to be found within the consolidated tradition of great representative classic literature (the Bible, Milton and Shakespeare, Dante and Homer, Chaucer and Spenser) for which he coined the phrase 'the books of all time' ('Sesame and Lilies' in *Works*, XVIII, p. 60). It was to be found also in those authors to whom he was personally indebted as a writer, including, principally, Wordsworth. These 'books of high caste',[5] are not 'high' by virtue of their status within the contemporary social world. 'High' does not mean 'inaccessible'. Rather, these works from another age bear 'words of true descent and ancient blood'. They are members of the '*peerage* of words' ('Sesame and Lilies', in *Works*, XVIII, p. 65) which, whilst retaining their sense, are thus capable of regenerating the newer contexts into which they are brought as 'living powers'.[6] The words are like relics from another age, bearing a profusion of meaning, like the effect of Gothic handiwork in a cathedral. Ruskin used them to bring into being the kind of world that he believed in.

So too, Matthew Arnold, whose *Culture and Anarchy* is the most famous Victorian statement of the noble heritage passed on via books and transmitted with the force of a living idea.

> The great men of culture are those who have had a passion for diffusing, for making prevail, for carrying from one end of society to the other, the best knowledge, the best ideas of their time; who have laboured to divest knowledge of all that was harsh, uncouth, difficult, abstract, professional, exclusive; to humanise it, to make it efficient outside the clique of the cultivated and learned, yet still remaining the *best* knowledge and thought of the time, and a true source, therefore, of sweetness and light.[7]

For Arnold, however, by contrast with Ruskin, the central tension between historically founded cultural tradition and the new pattern of Victorian social formation was not caused by dehumanising industrial capitalism but by its political equivalent, democracy.

> The difficulty for democracy is, how to find and keep high ideals. The individuals who compose it are, the bulk of them, persons who need to follow an ideal, not to set one; and one ideal of greatness, high feeling, and fine culture, which an aristocracy once supplied to them, they lose by the very fact of ceasing to be a lower order and becoming a democracy. Nations are not truly great solely because the individuals composing them are numerous, free, and active; but they are great when these numbers, this freedom, and this activity are employed in the service of an ideal somewhat higher than that of an ordinary man, taken by himself. ('The Popular Education of France', 1861, *Prose Works*, II, pp. 17–18)

'I am, above all, a believer in culture' (*Culture and Anarchy, Prose Works*, V, p.88). For Arnold the only way to establish the 'best',[8] a keyword throughout his writings in the discrimination of quality, was to work from the top down, beginning with the achieved ideals of human thought. As a critic and a thinker Arnold wanted 'an adequate world over-view',[9] in which the current social issue of class could be redeemed from its degeneration by older literary versions of itself. Homer's 'grand style' is 'the chief virtue of a healthy and uncorrupted aristocracy' in which 'elevation of character' and a 'noble way of thinking and behaving' is 'generated in whole classes of men' by 'the importance and responsibility of high station and habitual dealing with great things' ('The Popular Education of France', *Prose Works*, II, pp. 5–6).

It was culture that was the reminder of the larger, greater, grander human concerns—crucially, culture itself far more than the cultured prophetic

Ruskinian individual. But it requires a human act of translation—a democratic educating mediator—to find a way for the meanings to be transmitted. It was 'the great teachers' that were needed, in the role of the writer and the reader both (Ruskin, 'Sesame and Lilies', *Works*, xviii, p. 78). Only they, as carriers of pre-digested wisdom, could raise the level of thinking above that of the 'ordinary self', the thinking common to one's own class (Arnold, *Prose Works*, v, p. 145).

And it was the new arising middle class, and the extension of education, which seemed to Arnold the most ready vehicle for its spread, for all that the spread brought its own risks. In the role of inspector of schools, Arnold was adamant that mass education's requirement for minimum standards of reading should not empty the books of that larger transmitted life. In his annual reports on his work in elementary schools, he observed how the criteria for examination were affecting the teaching of reading. Learning to read means more than being able to read a single examination text; it is about developing 'a real love for reading and literature', 'in itself the greatest power available in education'.[10] 'The only way in which such a love is ever really inspired' is 'by animating and moving' the student-reader (*Reports*, p. 83). Books need to be chosen which appeal to the reader at a primary human level, not just as a matter of factual interest in a particular subject: 'the atmosphere, the steam-engine, or the pump'. It is the same with poetry:

> If a child is brought, as he easily can be brought, to *throw himself into* a piece of poetry, an exercise of creative activity has been set up in him quite different from the effort of learning a list of words to spell, or a list of reigns and battles, capable of greatly relieving the strain from learning these and of affording a lively pleasure. (*Reports*, pp. 228–29)

The focus on the 'little things', the dogged rote learning of lists and spellings, is always draining, because of the way in which the larger meanings have already been drained out. The very energy of the child requires something that he or she may be able to 'throw' themselves 'into', not with increased effort, but with a childlike joy. As Ruskin had emphasised in relation to art, mechanical perfection cannot take care of everything; at worst it risks missing the very thing that matters.

This is why the term 'culture' becomes so important to Arnold. It gives a name, 'a single watchword',[11] which works beyond the literal definitions, measurable skills and strict classifications by which formal education and the social world was often ordered.

> What we are concerned for is the thing, not the name; and the thing, call it by what name we will, is simply the enabling ourselves, by getting to know, whether through reading, observing, or thinking, the best that can at present be known in the world, … and thus to get a basis for a less confused action and a more complete perfection. (*Culture and Anarchy Prose Works*, v, p. 191)

In itself the name is simply a 'convenient' prompt, a nuanced tactic broadly indicating 'a complex of features plainly listed'[12]:

> culture … places human perfection in an *internal* condition, in the growth and predominance of our humanity proper, as distinguished from our animality. It places it in the ever-increasing efficacy and in the general harmonious expansion of those gifts of thought and feeling, which make the peculiar dignity, wealth, and happiness of human nature … Not a having and a resting, but a growing and a becoming, is the character of perfection as culture conceives it. (*Culture and Anarchy, Prose Works*, v, p. 94)

The 'thing', the 'becoming'—the phenomenon and process of culture—as it is located in reading practices today (informal, educational; group-led and private) partly derives from an amalgam of the ideas of Ruskin and Arnold.

The Victorian Realist Novel

In the first part of this chapter, we have indicated the difficulties for culture and reading which arose in the Victorian age. We turn now to the key literary response to those same difficulties in the creation of a new form and a new power—the novel. In generating an unprecedented excitement and interest around books amongst large swathes of the population, the rise of the novel revolutionised reading. The realist novel in particular, we shall argue, in its sub-vocal language in partial contrast to the musical voicings of poetry, laid a new foundation for literature to reach what Arnold called the 'internal condition' and needs of its reader. But the special influence of the novel cannot be separated from the popular appeal which made it seem, to the high priests of culture, only another part of the demotic ephemera of the times.

It was the marketplace which was bringing about the greatest change. New high-speed printing presses were increasing the efficiency of the book market. Not only was the number of readers growing but so too the number of books and periodicals of all kinds, of all orders, indiscriminately available to readers. John Stuart Mill noted with concern:

> The world reads too much and too quickly to read well. When books were few, to get through one was a work of time and labour: what was written with thought was read with thought, and with a desire to extract from it as much of the materials of knowledge as possible. … Nothing is now read slowly, or twice over. Books are run through with no less rapidity, and scarcely leave a more durable impression, than a newspaper article. It is for this, among other causes, that so few books are produced of any value.[13]

The notion of the book itself was being cheapened, as the actual cost was brought down. Readers began to consume rather than to read books. Reading itself was beginning to function as a sign of absorption within the mass, not a function of independent thinking. As the new railways aligned progress with getting somewhere faster, so readers seemed carried along by the excitement of this newly invented technology rather than stopping to work out where it might be taking them. Though he enjoyed reading them, Arnold 'felt mildly, very mildly, ashamed' of his 'weakness for novels'.[14] He felt he could not even give sufficient credit to the novels he did admire, amidst the formless rush of a phenomenon to which the plentiful supply of books was now giving rise:

> to contemporary work so good as *David Copperfield*, we are in danger of perhaps not paying respect enough, of reading it (for who could help reading it?) too hastily, and then putting it aside for something else and forgetting it. ('The Incompatibles', 1881, *Prose Works*, IX, pp. 238–85, 273)

In fact, neither Arnold nor Ruskin was fundamentally interested in the novel. Though there were certain exemplary instances of the form that both would praise, the form itself was not felt to match the 'best' and the 'highest', the work of the poets, upon which the category of literature and the idea of culture had been formulated. For Arnold such criteria had an ancient standing: the ideal model was still that of Athens high culture. 'What Arnold wants to present as a universal experience was in practice socially exclusive'.[15] Yet the root of that sense of mission and purpose shared in their differing emphases by both Ruskin and Arnold was the idea of art and culture as a mode that might persist beyond the divisions and differences within society in order further to benefit the whole. It is a mode that was related to the democratising drive behind the realist novel. Arguably, then, the real descendants of Arnold and Ruskin as champions of literary reading that is wide in its reach and deep in its effects are the realist novelists themselves—the writers who were not just speaking *about* literature, but advocating for its unique purpose from within its apparent new ordinariness.

Dickens: Breaking Through from Below

In the midst of the nineteenth century, Dickens *was* the novel, was the force it constituted in opening up a nation both within his pages and in the readership of them. In 1849 Hugh Miller could already see the extent of the change that had been brought about during his own lifetime:

> The great-grandfathers and great-grandmothers of the present reading public could sympathize in the joys and sorrows of only kings and queens; and the critics of the day gave reasons why it should be so. Humble life was introduced upon the stage, or into works of fiction, only to be laughed at; or so bedizzened with the unnatural frippery of Pastoral, that the picture represented, not the realities of actual life, but merely one of the idlest conventualities of literature. But we have lived to see a great revolution in these matters reach almost its culminating point.[16]

That great revolution had begun with Dickens and 'the seriousness with which he took his own popular art'.[17] It was Dickens who desired to make the work of the novel a familiar presence to his readers, an influence that might reach right into 'all homes, and all nooks and corners', and be found positioned 'at the window, by the fire, in the street, in the house' (John, p. 31). He was not in the least concerned by the fact that reading goes on within life, in amongst the prosaic concerns and unpoetic business of the day. Rather than subtracting from the attention that one might be able to give to books, Dickens took the potential of ordinary relevance as an invitation to involve himself in his readers' lives. He would play the role of a 'fellow traveller'[18] on life's journey, making his presence known as a regular feature of life, via the instalments of each new novel. The drive was to become 'from infancy to old age, everyone's inseparable companion' (John, p. 32). The public readings of his novels allowed Dickens to recreate live what he had been attempting to enact across the nation via the serialisation of his novels: a 'public event' (Andrews, p. 13) during which the resonance of each passage might be felt at the same time by each person as part of a collective family. Dickens, wanting to know that his audience was with him, would therefore say, in his introduction to the readings:

> If you feel disposed as we go along to give expression to any emotion, whether grave or gay, you will do so with perfect freedom from restraint, and without the least apprehension of disturbing me. (Andrews, p. 70)

The emotional response was vital to Dickens's sense of his success with his readers, of his having served them well, and of having made them feel along with him and in 'communion' with each other (John, p. 150). It was the root meaning of 'community' that he wanted to sustain: 'to commune with you, in any form, is to me a labour of love' (Andrews, p. 9). Charles Lamb observed that Dickens was able to make 'the pulse of a crowded house beat like the pulse of one man' (John, p. 150). In his study of the reading lives of the working class, Jonathan Rose shows how Dickens likewise achieved for families in a whole variety of circumstances a sense of being knit together (almost in defiance of those circumstances).

> George Acorn ... scraped together 3 ½ d. to buy a used copy of *David Copperfield*. His parents punished him when they learned he had wasted so much money on a book, but later he read it to them: 'And how we all loved it, and eventually, when we got to "Little Em'ly," how we all cried together at poor old Peggotty's distress! The tears united us, deep in misery as we were ourselves. Dickens was a fairy musician to us, filling our minds with a sweeter strain than the constant cry of hunger, or the howling wind which often, taking advantage of the empty grate, penetrated into the room'.[19]

The reading offers more than a distraction from the penetrating, 'howling wind'. It produces a new kind of emotional atmosphere, even in the midst of the empty want and lack. In the boy's offer to share it out loud, the book remakes the family, transforming it into a united 'we', even after the initial punishment by the parents. It is as though the book's true value is now revealed in place of its monetary cost.

Dickens is repeatedly drawn to the survival of human feeling even in the lowest, least ideal and most unlikely of places, where the circumstances seem to militate against it, and where it tends to go unthought of. In *Bleak House*, Esther, accompanying Mrs Pardiggle on her charitable visit to the brickmaker's house, recognises how wide the gap is that separates them both from the ostensible objects of their charity. Whilst she is there, she observes the response to the sudden yet not surprising death of the child whom one of the group is holding:

> An ugly woman, very poorly clothed, hurried in while I was glancing at them, and coming straight up to the mother, said, 'Jenny! Jenny!' The mother rose on being so addressed, and fell upon the woman's neck.
>
> She also had upon her face and arms the marks of ill-usage. She had no kind of grace about her, but the grace of sympathy; but when she condoled with the woman, and her own tears fell, she wanted no beauty. I say condoled, but her only words were 'Jenny! Jenny!' All the rest was in the tone in which she said them. I thought it very touching to see these two women, coarse and

> shabby and beaten, so united; to see what they could be to one another; to see how they felt for one another; how the heart of each to each was softened by the hard trials of their lives. I think the best side of such people is almost hidden from us. What the poor are to the poor is little known, excepting to themselves and GOD.[20]

Esther is a sincere and feeling witness, and yet even her attempt to relay the import of the glimpse that she has had of these lives ('I thought it very touching …') risks saying too much. The 'almost hidden' and the 'little known' means more for remaining so, a realism loyal to the limited reality it half augments, half reproduces. The 'little' signs that hold the capacity to 'mean more' create an excitedly asymmetrical or disproportional indicator of literary value disruptive of conventional forms. And so more important than Esther's reflection on the softening of hearts, or even the social issue of 'the poor' as a 'little known' class, is the almost musical tone in which the one woman still calls out the name of the other. Dickens makes the reader stay with it, quoting it twice, as if feeling that this is the only thing that can be said, and the very thing that must be preserved by a sub-vocal language of the novelist's art that existed to protect the vulnerable ordinary things of this world. Dickens treated his characters as if one could not make a true estimation of them until one had got inside, and felt what it was like to carry the weight of that particular human story. The external definitions (of 'types' and 'classes' in Dickens's case) can only give an approximation to the truth. It is as if the democratic project of the novel has to go deeper than this, to get even to the 'inmost heart'[21] of things, and to rescue it before the reader passes on by. It is literature on behalf of those who have no voice, who do not seem worthy subjects of traditional writings. For what stands out to Dickens, as if this were almost a paradox, is the extent of the suffering that goes on within such places of apparent insignificance: suffering which cannot finally be expurgated as it might have been in tragic drama, but which is to be witnessed as holding off of this speechpart of an ongoing daily reality. His aim was to draw on the pre-articulate sense of the inner life and breath of a person, the beating heart, so as to recreate via his readers 'an external community in which such innerness has a human home'.[22]

The small was innerly bigger than it seemed uncaringly from without. The moral shape of the world was utterly different from the form society distortingly imposed upon it. In thus challenging form by inner content, the danger was that the crowded novels might appear 'formless' and therefore 'void' as literature: not much more than 'large loose baggy monsters'.[23] But for Dickens there was a reason why the novel had had to grow and to adjust the proportions according to the content, suddenly finding form and connection in the midst of itself. For the effort to discover form from within crowdedness and to determine where characters fit in relation to one another is often a major part of the deeply emergent and shifting structure of a Dickens novel. It is as though the guide for the story itself is not so much a predetermined plan but the presence of a novelistic instinct for significance.

Even in an Elizabethan lyric, where the smallest number of words can be made to effect the greatest transformation, form had represented more than a 'container' of content. It is the very manner in which these forces of form and content interact, in formation itself, that makes for a strong but supple poetry. In Dickens's novels these creative forces are translated back out again at the larger level of character, where individual people are repeatedly found and refound from within the crowded world of human activity to make and remake the form of the novel's world as it shifts from one catalytic human centre to another.

In *Bleak House* the interconnections are so many and so thickly interwoven that the risk is that some of these will be picked up at the wrong time or by the wrong person, as if by chance they should suddenly fall into line in a person's mind. Thus when Guppy presents the results of his investigations into Esther's history and parentage to Lady Dedlock, it seems almost importunate of a man who ought only to have a minor role in this novel as a failed suitor to Esther, to be tying up the threads of a story which concerns some of the major characters so profoundly. As a reader himself of the situation, Guppy might represent the response of a reader who is still trying to piece together what he cannot yet understand. He thus relates the tale of his first discovery to Lady Dedlock: 'I found … such a resemblance between Miss Esther Summerson and your ladyship's own portrait, that it completely knocked me over; so much so, that I didn't at the moment even know what it *was* that knocked me over. And now I have the honour of beholding your ladyship near … it's really more surprising than I thought it' (*Bleak House*, p. 462). Dickens will deliberately arrange these moments when a reader might almost be 'knocked over' by the information that he or she suddenly seems to see presented before them. And yet Dickens wants a reader who will not just exclaim upon the plot connection, but who will feel with him the emotional implication of that moment. For Guppy is too cleverly self-absorbed to care very much about the effect of his words upon Lady Dedlock, who will be left at the end of this chapter as 'a wild figure on its knees', uttering an unheard cry. It is only the space accorded here to that voice by the novel which rescues it from secret hiding. The repetition is unwitnessed this time by anyone save the reader: 'O my child, my child! … O my child, O my child!' (*Bleak House*, p. 466)

When those words are again uttered near the end of the novel, it is by a different mother, to a son whom she had little hoped to be able ever to see again. This time the observer in the scene, Mrs Bagnet, is herself a mother, and it is she who for some time has acted as the mother figure to whom George, the son, has most often turned for help. Mrs Bagnet thus looks on as Mrs Rouncewell is initially silent upon entering the room, and George remains unaware that anyone is there:

> Not a rustle of the housekeeper's dress, not a gesture, not a word betrays her. She stands looking at him as he writes on, all unconscious, and only her fluttering hands give utterance to her emotions. But they are very eloquent; very, very eloquent. Mrs Bagnet understands them. They speak of gratitude, of joy, of grief, of hope; of inextinguishable affection, cherished with no return since this stalwart man was a stripling; of a better son loved less, and this son loved so fondly and so proudly; and they speak in such touching language, that Mrs Bagnet's eyes brim up with tears, and they run glistening down her sun-brown face. 'George Rouncewell! O my dear child, turn and look at me!' (*Bleak House*, p. 805)

As Mrs Bagnet's eyes brim up it is almost a sign of the overflow of this scene, which carries within it those long years of separation between the mother and son, and all the emotion of that time which only Mrs Rouncewell's fluttering hands have been able regularly to give expression to. Thus the gesture of the hands and the tears have to come before anyone speaks here. And yet the holding off of this speech throughout the quoted paragraph, as a reminder of that much longer wait which Mrs Rouncewell has already endured, only gives a greater force to that eventual calling out of the mother to her son. The reader moves from Mrs Bagnet's glistening face to the as yet undisclosed face of George, which Mrs Rouncewell must now see. It is like a turning point not between or within the lines, as in a poem, but between and amongst each one of these characters and across the multiple resonances of mothering in this book. For it is Mrs Rouncewell who must ask George to turn *back* to the mother from whom he had turned away so long ago.

The power of such moments emerges out of the saturated solutions which Dickens creates in his novels, where the chemical structure of the novel reaches a stage when it becomes ripe for explosion. Apparently bound to the limiting framework of common language and ordinary event, the novel creates a field *inside* its mundane human material, whereby the novel's half-events, picked up across the implicit vital memory of the whole work, suddenly come together, through a connection emotionally found as much as formally required. The whole experiment of realism might be regarded less as an attempt to transcribe reality than an effort to find space for a bigger quality that lies behind it all: the poetry buried secretly beneath its ostensibly undiscriminating continuities, with power to reveal that concealment at moments of transcendent reality, even through loyalty to the temporal-prosaic medium. It is a literary mission which lays a foundation and provides a template for the diverse modes of Shared Reading out in the world which is the subject of Part Two of this book.

George Eliot: Hearing Characters Think: The Realist Novel as a Prototype for Psychoanalysis

In Dickens's novels, the unspoken is often identified with those secrets which particular characters have to guard, as the ghostly residue of their own or others' pasts. It is also wincingly associated with social neglect and private vulnerability. In George Eliot's work, most of what goes unspoken happens live in front of the reader. The substance of those thoughts which the characters cannot share openly with one another is transmitted by the writer into a form that can be rendered in the present, on the page. In the novel's extension of the subject matter of art, the capacity to listen in to one's fellow beings would test the very limits of what a human person might be able to tolerate:

> If we had a keen vision and feeling of all ordinary human life, it would be like hearing the grass grow and the squirrel's heart beat, and we should die of that roar which lies on the other side of silence.[24]

As a writer, what George Eliot represents is the function of being a great reader of human beings, the ideal reader of her own novels, perhaps the ideal reader of any human work. This was a matter of developing not only a psychologically analytic language but a new method of translating the inner world—finding out, as Roy Pascal put it

> how to render inner movements, perceptions, reactions at the levels that precede thought and words, before they have found the way to consciousness and articulate utterance.[25]

The principal tool used to carry out this work within the classic realist novel is an extension of the narrating voice which, from Jane Austen to Dickens, reaches culmination in George Eliot as free indirect discourse. It is the great instrument of the reader of innerness serving the middle ground between the interpretative report or comment of the narrator (the mode in which George Eliot will speak out) and the direct speech and overt thoughts of a character (the chief mode of the epistolary novel). The effect of free indirect discourse is usually momentary, just as the glimpse of the 'almost hidden' lives of the two women at the brickmaker's house in the Dickens' scene had been. The linguistic marker of this discourse is the sudden syntax of indirect speech, whilst the statement is referred back to the character as if coming from inside him or her, as an inner voice (Pascal, pp. 8–9). It is a 'fusing' (pp. 26, 55) or 'melding'[26] of modes, creating 'the very special two-in-one effect' that for Dorrit Cohn ought not to be seen either as exclusively 'dual' or 'single' (Cohn, p. 112). It is at once inside the character and yet also outside him or her. This may be illustrated by an example from *Middlemarch*, a novel in which even the title suggests how important the middling, in-between stages will be to the kinds of mundanely hidden stories that will be told within it.

Chapter 50 opens with two sisters sitting together watching a baby play. It is the first time that we have seen Dorothea since the death of her husband Casaubon, and there is a painful sense in the opening pages of that lapsed quiet when there is nothing ahead as yet to move on to, and the past is all raw and unresolved. It is accentuated by the contrast with Celia, who is comfortably married, and mother to the baby. As they are talking, Celia, in a moment of determination, decides to tell Dorothea about the details of Casaubon's will, shockingly conditional upon the widow not marrying Ladislaw. In the aftermath of the conversation Dorothea is left alone for a moment:

> Dorothea by this time had turned cold again, and now threw herself back helplessly in her chair. She might have compared her experience at that moment to the vague, alarmed consciousness that her life was taking on a new form, that she was undergoing a metamorphosis in which memory would not adjust itself to the stirring of new organs. Everything was changing its aspect: her husband's conduct, her own duteous feeling towards him, every struggle between them – and yet more, her whole relation to Will Ladislaw. Her world was in a state of convulsive change; the only thing she could say distinctly to herself was, that she must wait and think anew. (*Middlemarch*, pp. 531–32)

This is form emergent from within the character herself. Yet it takes several sentences before Dorothea can 'say' anything to herself 'distinctly', in a world in which the problem will have to be presented to herself and worked out inwardly over time, before anything can be said to others out loud. It is as if the 'stirring of new organs' in response to a changing form of life creates an accompanying need for the invention of a new literary form or technique, a need for '*close writing*' as much as close reading.[27] For there are new meanings to be deciphered here, which free indirect discourse registers by keeping company with the character even where she is most alone.

This is an instance of what the psychoanalyst Wilfred Bion called the 'really real', and which he designated '0'[28] in recognition that no ordinary definition or discourse would serve for what exists prior to language and cannot be 'contained' by it. 0 cannot be truly known except by experience or discovery. It 'does not fall in the domain of knowledge or learning save incidentally'; it can be 'become' (its presence can be recognised or felt), but it cannot be abstractly comprehended except in the moment of happening (Bion, 1970, p. 26). The really real is immersively lived, experienced in absorption, or in the convulsive 'undergoing' of a Dorothea. Yet it is precisely at such moments, says Bion, that thinking, or rather proto-thoughts, begin. These inchoate, half-commenced thoughts originate in 'vague' unnameable crises when the normative framework is lost and there is nothing yet to replace it. Instead there is only the existence of something incontrovertibly wrong yet not identifiably there. If there is 'no thing', then 'no thing' is 'a thought'.[29] Such thoughts 'wait', like Dorothea, for a thinker.

Bion called these embryonic thoughts 'beta' elements and the capacity to think them, 'alpha function'.[30] Unmetabolised experiences need to be operated on, converted, digested, given a substance by thinking and thus be made available for use and translation into action as 'alpha elements' (Bion, 1967, p. 117). It is an axiom of Bion's theory that the inability 'to "think" with one's thoughts' is a catastrophic 'deprivation of truth' where truth is 'essential for psychic health' (Bion, 1962, pp. 56, 84). 'Failure to eat, drink or breathe properly has disastrous consequences for life itself. Failure to use the emotional experience produces a comparable disaster in the development of the personality' (Bion, 1962, p. 42). But Bion also knew that thinking one's thoughts—thinking 0—could be almost impossibly hard to achieve. Indeed, for Bion, the discovery of psychoanalysis was itself a symptom of the fact that thinking and the tasks of self-knowledge had been forced upon a mentality ill-suited and undeveloped for the purpose. Real thinking 'is embryonic even in the adult and has yet to be developed fully by the race' (Bion, 1962, p. 57). So it was that the 'practical task' of psychoanalysis, according to Freud, was 'to return to the ego the lost zones of the psyche'. In return for the ego's full honesty, the analyst 'puts at its service our experience in interpreting the material influenced by the unconscious. Our knowledge is supposed to compensate for its *lack* of knowledge'.[31] The analyst's knowledge or interpretation, thus deployed *on behalf of* the patient to 'compensate' for a 'lack' *within* the patient, precisely expresses, analogously, the position of the writer in relation to the character in George Eliot's work. Indeed, the author shared with Freud a common touchstone in the philosophy of Spinoza.[32] George Eliot translated *Ethics*, in which the necessity of 'thinking' one's emotion and experience in order to free them for use is as sternly urged as in Bion's psychoanalytic theory.

> Our mind is necessarily active so far as it has adequate ideas … necessarily passive so far as it has inadequate ideas…. The better we know or understand an emotion … the more it is in our power, and the less the mind suffers from it … That mind suffers most … which chiefly consists of inadequate ideas, so that it is characterised more by what it suffers than by what it does.[33]

Dorothea's 'vague, alarmed consciousness' demonstrates why we need George Eliot's language to release the meaning of Dorothea's predicament. In expressing what was inexpressible by the subject herself, articulating thoughts which Dorothea cannot yet formally think, George Eliot was not only anticipating, but *performing* the function of psychoanalysis. And free indirect mode was this novelist's analytical precision tool from the first.

Indeed, George Eliot's earliest work of fiction, *Scenes of Clerical Life*, demonstrates how free indirect discourse was not so much a new invention as a continuation or translation of older expressive practices. In *Janet's Repentance* especially, we seem to see this literary tool taking over from the confessional mode whence it derived (Cohn, p. 113). The protagonist, Janet Dempster, is driven to alcohol addiction by the brutality she has suffered at the hands of her abusive husband. Twice at moments of deep and dangerous despair, Janet's trouble finds expressive relief in the form of confession to the minister, Mr Tryan:

> She was unable to utter any words of mere politeness, or even of gratitude; her heart was too full of other words that had welled up the moment she met his pitying glance, and felt her doubts fall away. …
>
> In this artificial life of ours, it is not often we see a human face with all a heart's agony in it, uncontrolled by self-consciousness; when we do see it, it startles us as if we had suddenly waked into the real world of which this everyday one is but a puppet-show copy. For some moments Mr. Tryan was too deeply moved to speak.[34]

Religious confession, substituting both for lonely silence on the one hand and the 'mere politeness' of conversation on the other, is offered in this work as the only available serious language in which Janet can discharge the hidden burden of her hitherto unused 'other words'. Yet, as George Eliot's narrating voice explicitly recognises at this moment, this deep heart-language, the essential register of reality amid artificiality, is simply not available under ordinary life conditions: 'In our moments of spiritual need, the man to whom we have no tie but our common nature, seems nearer to us than mother, brother or friend' (Billington, 2015, p. 279). Significantly, free indirect discourse occurs in the novel at precisely those crises when Janet's literal confessor, Tryan, is absent. So when, with Dempster now dead, and whilst Janet is still fighting her addiction, she inadvertently discovers a decanter of Dempster's brandy. Desire overwhelms her, and she dashes it to the ground and flees.

> Where should she go? In what place would this demon that had re-entered her be scared back again? … The temptation would come again – that rush of desire might master her the next time– she would slip back again into that deep slimy pit from which she had once been rescued, and there might be no deliverance for her more. (Noble and Billington, 2015, pp. 318–19)

In this interval between crisis and explicit confession, free indirect discourse—'Where should she go?' 'The temptation would come again'—takes the place of the ancient religious practice of confession as an emotionally attuned verbal witness. At once a descendant and a secular, prosaic replacement for religious discourse, free indirect mode was especially equipped to 'listen in' to the kind of spiritual crisis which is now called 'depression',[35] in anticipation of the secular listener we find in Freud's analyst.

In 'An Outline of Psychoanalysis', Freud himself acknowledged the similarity of the role of the confessor to that of the analyst, enabling 'total honesty in return for complete discretion'. But there is this 'great difference', said Freud: 'we don't simply want to hear from the patient the things he knows and hides from others: he also has to tell us what he *doesn't* know' (Freud, 2003, p. 202). Analogously, free indirect discourse tells the experience of a person's life as he or she never quite lives it (Miller, 2003). For Janet, at this moment, the only reality is her weakness, the overwhelming sense of all that she cannot be or do. Indeed, from any point of view other than that of the novelist, Janet's life is more or less a failure. Only the novel, by subvocally capturing the deeper reality of hidden struggle, with its agonies *and* its brave resistances, can find in Janet's story a narrative of heroic achievement. This is what the patient seeks from the analyst. Tell me the true story about myself:

the one I cannot see and most need to have. As Ricoeur puts it in 'Life: A Story in Search of a Narrator': 'The goal and outcome of analytic sessions' is that the person analysed 'presents the psychoanalyst with bits and pieces of lived histories' and 'draws from these bits and pieces a narrative that is both more bearable and more intelligible'.[36] The burden of high Victorian realism was always thus analogous to that of psychoanalysis: finding means to release into expression the intimate human matter which is otherwise lost to the subterranean inwardness of a private and more or less neurotic psychology. It is the emotionally attuned verbal witness, needed but missing in ordinary life, which brings the hidden roar partially to voice.

Yet neither free indirect discourse, nor the so-called omniscience of author-narrator, are of course truly 'there' for Janet herself in any sense. Free indirect discourse is not offered as a consolatory technique. It is not an extra presence that the characters in the novel can benefit from, for they cannot know that it exists or that the suffering which they experience in private can be perceived by anyone outside of themselves. Indeed, in *Middlemarch*, in the culminating crisis of the relationship between Dorothea and Casaubon, shortly before the latter's death, it is the special work of free indirect speech not simply to articulate thoughts which characters might need but to offer thoughts which perhaps no human could ever want.

At the crucial centre of the novel, Dorothea, following a further cruel rejection, has to begin to admit her unhappiness as Casaubon's wife, even whilst he is still alive:

> She was in the reaction of a rebellious anger stronger than any she had felt since her marriage. Instead of tears there came words: -
>
> 'What have I done – what am I – that he should treat me so? He never knows what is in my mind – he never cares. What is the use of anything I do? He wishes he had never married me'.
>
> She began to hear herself, and was checked into stillness. Like one who has lost his way and is weary, she sat and saw as in one glance all the paths of her young hope which she should never find again. And just as clearly in the miserable light she saw her own and her husband's solitude—how they walked apart so that she was obliged to survey him. If he had drawn her towards him, she would never have surveyed him—never have said, 'Is he worth living for?' but would have felt him simply a part of her own life. (Carroll, 1997, p. 421)

Dorothea's own words chasten her into silence not only because they begin to say too much too bitterly and distortingly, but because they summon a partner thought too devastating to be borne. It is one which George Eliot will later articulate on Lydgate's behalf in relation to his own wife,

Rosamond. 'In marriage, the certainty, 'She will never love me much', is easier to bear than the fear, 'I shall love her no more' (Carroll, 1997, p. 702). The point at which the character cannot bear to 'hear herself' is the point where George Eliot has to listen in more closely, to hear *for* Dorothea that terrible question which exists inchoately or resistingly *inside* her—'Is he worth living for?' Where in the previous examples offered, the author and reader might wish that the characters *could* 'hear' the thoughts uttered on their behalf, and have access to their own true story, here it almost has to be the writer and not the character in whom intuition crystallises into new recognition. For how could one ever be one's own witness to this and simply carry on? How is this deeply inconsolable recognition even possible as a thought, as a 'solid' idea, for the person to whom it belongs? It is something barely thinkable except inside the book and an instance of realism's power to hold thoughts which humans feel it would almost kill them to contain in themselves.

This is what George Eliot's literary language might do on behalf of the species. 'The only effect I ardently long to produce by my writings', she wrote, 'is that those who read them should be able to *feel* the pain of those who differ from themselves in everything but the *broad* fact of being struggling, erring creatures'.[37] *Middlemarch* is an important image of how literature, as a way of thinking, helps create a reality deeper than the normal social world but contained within it and thus in need of art's supportive articulation.[38] The realist novel is less 'real life' than art's rescuing corrective to life. In place of the old religious language of confession, and in advance of psychoanalysis, such silent language, heard beneath the apparent loudness of the ordinary world, is the realist novelist's way of producing the most serious language that can be found for the communication *and* lack of communication between one human being and another. It is the great language of *reading*—of interpretation between the lines, beneath the surfaces, across the gaps.

These characteristics of Victorian realism will be seen in practice in Part Two of this volume—not only in examples of group reading of prose fiction but in the very processes of the reading groups themselves, ordinary people struggling to interpret equivalent lives in a literary model.

Notes

1. G. P. Landow, *Aesthetic and Critical Theory of John Ruskin* (Princeton: Princeton University Press, 1971).

2. J. Ruskin, 'Sesame and Lilies' (1865), in *The Works of John Ruskin*, ed. by E. T. Cook and Alexander Wedderburn, 39 vols (London: George Allen, 1903–1912), XVIII, pp. 53–187 (p. 112).
3. M. Jacobus, 'Cloud Studies: The Visible Invisible', in *Romantic Things: A Tree, a Rock, a Cloud* (Chicago: University of Chicago Press, 2012), pp. 219–47 (p. 224).
4. J. Billington, *Faithful Realism: Elizabeth Gaskell and Leo Tolstoy, A Comparative Study* (London: Associated University Presses, 2002), p. 102.
5. W. E. Gladstone et al., *Books Which Have Influenced Me* (London: Hodder and Stoughton, 1897), p. 45.
6. See R. C. Trench, *On the Study of Words* (London: Macmillan, 1882), p. 2.
7. M. Arnold, 'Culture and Anarchy' (1869), in *The Complete Prose Works of Matthew Arnold*, ed. by R. H. Super, 11 vols (Ann Arbor: University of Michigan Press, 1960–1977), V, p. 113.
8. M. Arnold, 'The Study of Poetry' (1880), in *Prose Works*, IX, pp. 161–88 (p. 163).
9. P. Davis, 'Arnold or Ruskin?', *Journal of Literature & Theology*, 6 (1992), 320–44 (p. 323).
10. M. Arnold, *Reports on Elementary Schools 1852–1882*, first published 1889, ed. by F. S. Marvin (London: Wyman and Sons, 1908), p. 142.
11. R. Williams, *Culture and Society, 1780–1950* (London: Chatto & Windus, 1958), p. 114.
12. J. Holloway, *The Victorian Sage: Studies in Argument* (London: Macmillan, 1953), p. 224.
13. J. S. Mill, 'Civilization', *The London and Westminster Review*, 3 (1836), 13–40 (p. 37).
14. C. Ricks, 'Matthew Arnold and the Novel', *Salmagundi*, 132 (2001), 76–95 (p. 83).
15. D. Birch, *Our Victorian Education* (Oxford: Blackwell, 2008), p. 30.
16. H. Miller, 'Literature of the People', in *Essays, Historical and Biographical, Political and Social, Literary and Scientific* (Edinburgh: Adam & Charles Black, 1862), pp. 291–99 (p. 291).
17. J. John, *Dickens and Mass Culture* (Oxford: Oxford University Press, 2010), p. 14.
18. M. Andrews, *Charles Dickens and His Performing Selves: Dickens and the Public Readings* (Oxford: Oxford University Press, 2006), pp. 23–24.
19. J. Rose, *The Intellectual Life of the British Working Classes* (New Haven: Yale University Press, 2001), p. 111.
20. C. Dickens, *Bleak House* (1853), ed. by Norman Page (London: Penguin, 1971), pp. 160–61.
21. C. Dickens, *Little Dorrit* (1855–1857), ed. by Harvey Peter Sucksmith (Oxford: Oxford University Press, 1999), p. 68.
22. P. Davis, *Why Victorian Literature Still Matters* (Chichester: Wiley-Blackwell, 2008), p. 135.

23. H. James, Preface to 'The Tragic Muse' (1890), in *The Art of the Novel: Critical Prefaces* (New York: Charles Scribner's Sons, 1934), pp. 70–97 (p. 84).
24. G. Eliot, *Middlemarch*, ed. by D. Carroll (Oxford: Oxford University Press, 1997), p. 483.
25. R. Pascal, *The Dual Voice: Free Indirect Speech and Its Functioning in the Nineteenth-Century European Novel* (Manchester: Manchester University Press, 1977), p. 59.
26. D. Cohn, *Transparent Minds: Narrative Modes for Presenting Consciousness in Fiction* (Princeton: Princeton University Press, 1978), p. 125.
27. D. A. Miller, *Jane Austen, or The Secret of Style* (Princeton: Princeton University Press, 2003), p. 58.
28. W. R. Bion, *Attention and Interpretation* (London: Maresfield Library, 1970), p. 26.
29. W. R. Bion, *Learning from Experience* (London: Maresfield Library, 1962), p. 35.
30. W. R. Bion, *Second Thoughts* (London: Maresfield Library, 1967), p. 117.
31. S. Freud, *An Outline of Psychoanalysis* (London: Penguin Books, 2003), p. 201.
32. J. Neu, *Emotion, Thought and Therapy* (London: Routledge and Kegan Paul, 1977), p. 151.
33. B. de Spinoza, *Ethics* (1677), trans. by George Eliot, ed. by T. Deegan (Salzburg: University of Salzburg, 1981), pp. 93, 219–20, 229.
34. G. Eliot, 'Janet's Repentance', in *Scenes of Clerical Life* (1857), ed. by T. Noble and J. Billington (Oxford: Oxford University Press, 2015), pp. 185–334 (pp. 283–84).
35. C. Dowrick, *Beyond Depression*, 2nd edn (Oxford: Oxford University Press, 2009). See Chapter 2.
36. P. Ricoeur, *On Psychoanalysis* (Cambridge: Polity Press, 2012), p. 197.
37. G. Haight, ed., *The George Eliot Letters*, 9 vols (New Haven: Yale University Press, 1954–1978), vol. iii, p. 111.
38. See J. Billington and P. Davis, 'Realism's Concealed Realities', *Synthesis, Special Issue: Experiments in Realism* (2011).

Part II

Practices

5

Reading for Depression/Mental Health

Clare Ellis, Eleanor McCann and Anne Line Dalsgård

Clare Ellis, 'Reading the Renaissance Lyric in Mental Health Contexts'

Over a 12-month period, Clare Ellis ran two Shared Reading groups for people with a confirmed diagnosis of depression – one in a GP surgery, the other in a mental health drop-in centre, both in an urban setting. The reading groups were part of a research study funded by the Liverpool Institute of Health Inequalities Research.[1] *Transcribed audio-recordings, as well as her own weekly diary of the group sessions, formed part of the primary data for the research study. Here, Clare returns to these records as an aide memoire.*

A question I am often asked by practitioners who are new to Shared Reading is how the literature I read with groups has been chosen. Typically, in The Reader model (see Chapter 1, p. 4), the material is very varied. Choice is based on the seriousness and quality of the literature, past experience of 'what works' in read aloud groups, and the agreed taste and interests

C. Ellis (✉) · E. McCann
The Reader, Liverpool, UK
e-mail: clareellis@thereader.org.uk

E. McCann
e-mail: eleanormccann@thereader.org.uk

A. L. Dalsgård
Aarhus University, Aarhus, Denmark
e-mail: ald@cas.au.dk

J. Billington (ed.), *Reading and Mental Health*,
https://doi.org/10.1007/978-3-030-21762-4_5

of the group members themselves. A new group will be exposed to a wide range of material, crossing century and genre, through 'tasters'—of poetry, short stories or extracts from longer novels—before settling by mutual decision on one work to stay with for an extended period. Opportunity for (informed) choice takes priority over prescriptiveness in respect of reading matter in order to give the group a sense of ownership of, and responsibility for, their reading experience.

In the case of the groups I ran for depression sufferers, the diversity proved particularly vital in encouraging participants to engage in discussion and thinking which called on the 'whole' person rather than just the 'depressed' part. Indeed, the importance of the range of material was illustrated very early in the life of the GP surgery group. Several members clearly viewed themselves, in this context, as depression sufferers who had come to the reading group seeking an alternative or complementary 'treatment'. Thus, they expected and asked for literature which, in their view, would be of direct benefit to their condition—works which either directly addressed their feelings of depression or which, conversely, were uplifting. But very soon, after only a few weeks, group members were expressing appreciation of the literature for its own sake rather than as a 'remedy' and, from that point, contributed and interacted as interested members of a reading group rather than as 'patients'. Increasingly, they were able to enjoy and indicate preferences that were stimulated by the intrinsic interest of the book, regardless of topic or difficulty or relative remoteness in time (choosing Charles Dickens's classic *Great Expectations*, for example, over the option of a more contemporary novel). The Reader model's custom of offering a rich rather than a narrow diet was found by the research study to be one of the most important components of the intervention's value for these readers. It allowed participants both 'to discover new, and rediscover old or forgotten, modes of thought, feeling and experience' that may have been suppressed or made difficult to access when suffering from depression.[2,3]

Prose and poetry were also observed to have distinctive, yet mutually complementary, functions and benefits, which were emphasised by their combination in each session. Broadly speaking, fiction-reading produced relaxation and calm in participants, as the extended continuity of the narrative mode enabled readers to inhabit a life other than their own for a space, away from distracting anxieties. Poetry, on the other hand, produced alert concentration, renewed mental effort and intensity (Billington, pp. 6, 29–33; Dowrick, p. 17). This finding certainly tallied with my own experience. I was particularly conscious in these specific groups of the concluding poem both signalling and producing satisfying completion: the poem gave a sense of the reading session as a defined happening and unit of meaning in the life of the group members. The weekly poem ritualised a 'transitional space' between life inside and outside the reading group. After a reading of Philip Larkin's 'I Go Among Trees and Sit Still', one group member said: 'I'm going to go home now and think about this. I'd just be sitting at home if I wasn't here in the reading group. It gets me out and it gets me thinking and afterwards I go out of the room still thinking about the poems we've read' (Billington, p. 17).

One striking phenomenon, here and generally, was that the difficulty of the material—and the poems always were, to some degree, 'difficult'—was never in itself an obstacle but more often appeared a cooperative challenge. The following extracts show each group reading Shakespeare's Sonnet 29, a favourite sonnet in Shared Reading. Reading the text aloud, slowly and quietly, is always the first step. When I read aloud, I am conscious of wanting to give this poem my best shot. This may well be the first and only time the people in the group will read this great poem. It is important, even on a first reading, that there is potential for people to begin to feel a connection to the words. Even if they do not have the language to describe that connection, something deep down might resonate. What I am trying for most of all is to allow the 'third voice' of the poem (neither my own, nor that of the group members) to come through. When I myself have a close connection to the poem, it feels as though a different human voice is coming through me as I read. It is the poem that is speaking. [It is worth noting that the group leader's expressive reading and interpretation of the literature, creating an atmosphere of serious attention through reading the poetry 'live', was found to be a crucial component of Shared Reading's value for depression sufferers (Billington pp. 6, 10, 34–42; Dowrick, p. 18)].

The group's first experience of Shakespeare's sonnet, then, is hearing that 'third voice' as they read from their own printed copy:

When, in disgrace with Fortune and men's eyes,
I all alone beweep my outcast state,
And trouble deaf heaven with my bootless cries,
And look upon myself and curse my fate –
Wishing me like to one more rich in hope,
Featur'd like him, like him with friends possess'd,
Desiring this man's art and that man's scope,
With what I most enjoy contented least;
Yet in these thoughts myself almost despising
Haply I think on thee, and then my state,
Like to the lark at break of day arising

12 From sullen earth, sings hymns at heaven's gate:
For thy sweet love remember'd such wealth brings
That then I scorn to change my state with kings.[4]

In the GP surgery group, May, one of the older and (often anxiously) chatty members of the group is the first to speak:

May: That is very conflicting. You know, at the beginning, it's really down and out, and yet at the end it's on top of the world. Just in the matter of those –
Clare: Yes, there are two movements to the poem, aren't there?
May: Yes, you don't know why you bother at the beginning but at the end, he's got everything to live for. A complete turnaround.
Clare: And it turns around by his having a thought of something else, someone else.
John: Think on thee.
Clare: Yes, line 10.

May and Barbara have quickly found a way into the poem: they intuit the poem's key emotional movement and shape of thought. May's quick intelligence perhaps comes close to summarising *too* quickly what the poem is 'about'; Barbara quotes the words of the poem almost at its turning point. It is this more specific thinking, more attuned to the poem's small internal workings, that I want to encourage. In order thus to slow it all down, to allow us to inhabit the space for thinking that the poem creates, I re-read the first quatrain.

When, in disgrace with Fortune and men's eyes,
I all alone beweep my outcast state,
And trouble deaf heaven with my bootless cries,
And look upon myself and curse my fate – 4

There is thoughtful silence for a few seconds before one of the group-members now instinctively rereads

Ann: Trouble deaf heaven with my bootless cries—trouble *deaf* heaven. He knows himself it's pointless. He knows he's done wrong or whatever.
Clare: I hadn't thought about that word trouble. Now you mention it, it's not like 'I talk to heaven or I reach out to heaven' but *trouble* –
John: Trouble deaf heaven with my bootless cries—He's not being listened to, he's not being heard is he?
Ann: It's almost like he feels like he's not worth troubling heaven.

One person's 'chewing' on a word ('trouble') has now become a shared group questioning. It is often the case that puzzlement or difficulty itself initiates group meaning-making. The transcripts help make visible how my function as group leader is not so much to direct, as to hold, or hold open, thoughts and ideas. Sometimes I capture aspects of participant contributions which help whole group understanding or which return us to a tiny detail—a word, phrase or line ('I hadn't thought about that word "trouble"'). Just as critical, however, is that the mode and quality of human attention to the participants is analogous to the attention given to the book or poem. The group leader must be an alert witnessing presence in relation both to the literature and the individuals.

In the GP surgery group, there was a particularly vulnerable woman, Dawn, who, now in her fifties, and educated to degree level, had suffered with depression most of her adult life. Once an avid reader, she had ceased reading altogether before joining the group, because she could not concentrate for long periods. The only reading experience available to her, therefore, was provided by the weekly group. In the first few weeks, Dawn had difficulty even staying in the room for the duration of the session. She always sat apart from the group, close to the door, and was rarely still—usually fidgeting or wiping her eyes. She became upset quickly, sometimes out of frustration at her inability to concentrate and from feeling that everyone else was able to participate in the discussion and 'get things out' of the story/poem while she was not. At times, she was so moved by the content of the literature that she would leave the room abruptly, crying, and I would have to alert the GP. The fact that this new 'treatment' wasn't 'working' for her added to Dawn's anxiety in the first few weeks.

But Dawn now joined in the discussion of that line—'and trouble deaf heaven with my bootless cries':

Dawn: Does bootless mean that he doesn't stop crying? Like when it won't stop?
Clare: The crying won't stop? Boot*less* - it's not contained in any way –
Dawn: There's no end to it.

This is a good example of how the very difficulty of an older language offers an obstacle to Dawn's default response. Dawn emotionally tunes in instinctively to the syllable—'less'—which speaks to her own sense of a limitless pain which has neither an end in time nor a purposeful point. Yet, pondering the unfamiliar word means that, for an instant—for the very first time in her attendance at the reading group—Dawn is 'thinking' her pain and not merely suffering it (see Chapter 4). The poem's *language* of crying momentarily takes the place of crying itself in Dawn. These tentatively verbalised efforts—so small as to be easy to miss—always need delicate encouragement, precisely because they are rarely recognised as achievements, least of all by the persons themselves.

At times, the breakthrough moment is virtually subvocal, as in this instance from the group in the mental health drop-in centre. Lorraine is in her early 50s. She has learning disabilities in addition to the depression and anxiety she suffers. She lives alone (her daughter is currently in care) and she feels isolated in her community and local neighbourhood. Due to past experiences, Lorraine is nervous about going out by herself, outside of her local area. She says she finds it difficult to trust people. The drop-in centre is one of the few places she feels safe.

Up to this point in the reading group, Lorraine had been very shy and reluctant to talk.

In this session, after the first reading of Sonnet 29, she had remained silent, looking intently at the poem, as group members first pondered the speaker's plight: 'about a man with nothing isn't it? Or could be somebody who has lost everything'; 'he feels as though he is like an outcast on an island, crying for help and there is nobody'. On a second reading, the group begin to see that it is a before a before-and-after poem, signalled by the change of the language of line 2 ('my outcast state') to the language of lines 9–11 ('and then my state,/Like to the lark'). 'The poem changes', says someone. 'Where?' I ask. 'When I think of thee: someone, could even be something I love'. Then Lorraine speaks for the first time, barely audible:

> Lorraine: That bit there. It says 'From sullen earth sings hymns at heaven's gate; For thy sweet love remembered …' It's there. Can't explain.

What Lorraine says at that moment is also, bravely, what she does: her words seemed to surface in involuntary witness to her instinct—prior to articulation ('Can't explain')—for pinpointing the very instant where the poem launches itself out of its outcast state into uplift: 'From sullen earth'. It seems crucial that Lorraine, was not, here, alone, outcast. Her finding of the poem's almost invisible point of transition (not the conventional sonnet 'turn' at line 9 which more articulate cleverness might have insisted upon), was made possible only by the protective presence of the group. Lorraine, reading alone, if she had read at all, might so easily have become discouraged. Here was safety not in numbers merely but in a shared effort after enabling human meaning. I had recognised before that live group reading was always still *personal* reading but had not appreciated the degree to which one enabled the other or how the secure freedom to pursue personal meanings in relation to the literature ('Can we keep this one?' was Lorraine's final moving contribution at this session) are the gift of a reciprocal act of trust bringing persons and poem uniquely together. 'The reading group gets it out in the open', Lorraine said to me after the first months: 'Whatever is hidden up and out - if you've got feelings put down they've got to come up and out otherwise your head would explode'.

In the GP surgery, the change is felt across the group.

> Ann: 'Haply I think on thee, and then my state,/Like to the lark at break of day arising'—isn't that a beautiful verse. Isn't that lovely?
> Clare: Shall we stay with that? What's the feeling there?
> May: It's the birds singing—first thing in the morning. It's a new beginning.
> John: Sings hymns at heaven's gate.
> Dawn: That's what the lark does—goes right up to heaven. Larks sing right up there you can't even see them, but you can hear them.

When Dawn follows the lark in its imagined flight, a new release of energy, out of pained self-absorption a sense of awakened life and vitality—in Dawn and in the room—is palpable. The linguist on the research team, Andrew Hamer, was interested in how participants would often 'mirror' one another, repeating one another's words or syntax (Billington, pp. 49–50; Dowrick, p. 18). Here, in a subtle variation of this phenomenon, the group members have multiple related thoughts ('break of day arising', 'first thing … new beginning', 'heaven's gate', 'goes right up') all pointing in the same (transcendent) direction. This group uplift signalled a move away from mutual consciousness of the participants' common medical condition (very strong, as I have said, when the group began) to a close in-tune-ness with one another's fuller selves through responsiveness to the book or poem. The GP was the only one of the research team who knew the group members' personal mental health history. His experience of Dawn had been confined hitherto to witnessing her in his consulting room, closed in and cut off from others and from life, inarticulately suffering. He found the evidence of the recordings and transcripts utterly startling. He was particularly struck by the way in which the imagined life of the poem became a presence in the real life—in the very room—of the participants, enlarging their sense (hitherto isolated, precarious, fragmentary) of the possible. This evidence of the resonance between the depressed mind and poetry suggests the way out from the low has to be finer or more deeply touching than ordinary experience or the problem-solving methods of standard therapy. The change which poetry brings to Lorraine and Dawn here is as unforced as beauty itself, and that is its power.

Eleanor McCann, 'Reading Shakespeare's *Hamlet* with Psychiatry Inpatients'

Eleanor McCann was Reader in Residence with Mersey Care NHS Mental Health Trust for two years. Here, based on the log she kept[5] during that time, she describes her experience of reading Shakespeare with a group of patients on an acute psychiatric ward.

Some months into the reading group, at a request for some science-fiction from a group member, I found a short story by Isaac Asimov in which, among other wild things, Shakespeare is brought back from the dead.[6] It is not, perhaps, a 'great' story but what it led to was. The Asimov story gave me an ideal opportunity to slip in some *real-life* Shakespeare—a bit of one of his plays. To continue the theme of spirits, and to create some interplay between the prose and the play, I chose a section from the first act of *Hamlet*, the fifth scene. This is where Hamlet is visited by the ghost of his father, who tells his son that he was murdered by his brother, Claudius, now husband to the dead king's widow, Gertrude, Hamlet's mother. When the ghost departs, Hamlet vows to avenge his father's death: 'I have sworn't'.[7]

There were three group members whom I will refer to as Christine, Anya and Ian. There were also two members of hospital staff, Julie and Terry, whom I was training up to become reading group leaders: I encouraged their responses as much as those of the patients. We began at the opening of the scene: 'Where wilt thou lead me?' asks Hamlet, fearful, as the Ghost appears. The Ghost speaks:

> Ghost: My hour is almost come
> When I to sulph'rous and tormenting flames
> Must render up myself. …
> … I am thy father's spirit,
> Doomed for a certain term to walk the night,
> And for the day confined to fast in fires
> Till the foul crimes done in my days of nature
> Are burnt and purged away. But that I am forbid
> To tell the secrets of my prison-house

I could a tale unfold whose lightest word
Would harrow up thy soul, freeze thy young blood,
Make thy two eyes like stars start from their spheres,
Thy knotty and combined locks to part,
And each particular hair to stand on end
Like quills upon the fretful porcupine.
But this eternal blazon must not be
To ears of flesh and blood. (*Hamlet*, I. v. 3–22)

The effects of the untold secret feel almost as great as the telling itself could have been. There's a whole lot of stuff that happens after 'But that I am forbid/ I could a tale unfold', before the too-late censoring 'But this … must not be' ('I can't') at line 21. It is as if, as with the ghost, Shakespeare half-gives the thing which isn't there, before he takes it away again. Ian read this speech making gleeful 'ho ho ho' noises and rubbing his hands with relish. '"Thy two eyes like stars start from their spheres"! Your eyes are popping out of your head!' he exclaimed, widening his own eyes as he said it. Ian *did* what the ghost is forbidden to fully bring about. His reaction was a physical demonstration of Shakespeare making the words *do* what they say. Similarly, and usefully, Anya, who is from Eastern Europe and speaks limited English, asked what a porcupine is, and, in defining the word for her, the group members found themselves making spikes with their hands. They ended up *acting* by accident, forced into actualising what was happening in all our heads when we read that single word.

The physical 'doing' of the text could be heard, too, in Ian's rereading of a line or two: 'I could a tale unfold whose *lightest* word/ Would harrow up thy soul…'. I pointed out to Ian that he had stressed the word 'lightest' this time—an interesting variation on the first time he'd read it. He said, 'Well, yes, even a bit of the ghost's story would be enough. Lightest … So you know it's *heavy* stuff then. Really bad stuff'. Ian recognised the *weight* of the words, and in doing so he seemed to feel the weight moving around, transferred from the ghost on to Hamlet, and on to us, reading it aloud. Even such a tiny thing as a single stress tells me something about Ian's growing reading ability. It is a marker of more complex functioning than straightforward, left-to-right reading along the lines, as Douglas Oliver tells us in *Poetry and Narrative in Performance*: 'Within the linear experience of reading we carry out smaller acts of mental reflection in which we appreciate the developing form'. Although it might pass undetected as a mere milli-second in the act of reading, 'poetic stress is a small moment of comprehension of this kind':

> The developing meaning and emotional significance of the line must play a part … in deciding how heavy we think the stress is. We can tap an instant of stress with a finger but it is also a paradoxical moment, since an instant should have no content. By a sort of mental trick we 'give' this instant a tiny sonic, intellectual and emotional content from the past of the poetic line and from its future considered from the standpoint of that instant. Without this mental trick … the stress would be perceived as empty of content, and therefore neither heavy nor light.[8]

Even though Ian needed a little practice—it was at the second attempt that he was able to detect an appropriate place to lay the stress—he was able to perform this 'mental trick'. This showed that he was learning to hold the meaning of what he'd already read, along with the anticipation of what he was about to read, in his head. Reading, done well, requires some practice and experience, of course, especially in relation to Shakespeare's language: but it always demands that the reader performs a little bit of mental magic.

During the session, we revisited the first words of the ghost twice. In this respect, I notice that we read with greater oscillation than usual—with a greater feeling of things only making full sense when the scene was allowed to confer within itself, so to speak. The first time we turned back was when we got to Shakespeare's description of the effects of the poison on the King. 'Thy uncle', says the ghost

> … in the porches of mine ears did pour
> The leperous distilment, whose effect
> Holds such an enmity with blood of man
> That swift as quicksilver it courses through
> The natural gates and alleys of the body
> And with a sudden vigour it doth posset
> And curd, like eager droppings into milk,
> The thin and wholesome blood. So did it mine'
> And a most instant tetter barked about,
> Most lazar-like, with vile and loathsome crust,
> All my smooth body. (*Hamlet*, I. v. 63–73)

Ian pictured it, saying, 'He must look disgusting'; then added from his imagination, 'Maybe he's covered in scabs'; next he went back to the text to check, '"vile and loathsome crust" -Urgh!'. Then something clicked: 'Maybe that's why he [Hamlet] doesn't recognise him [his father], you know, at the start – if he [the father] had changed, looks really old and scabby, he'd look completely different'. I suspect we didn't register that we were even asking ourselves the question 'Why hasn't Hamlet recognised his own father?' until we had a possible answer. It is like the way we feel watching Edgar and Gloucester, son and father, on the cliff-top in *King Lear*, when Gloucester attempts suicide. It isn't until Edgar says 'Why I do trifle thus with his despair…?'[9] that we realise we have been wondering, desperately, 'Why are you doing this?' This must be one of the things Shakespeare is able to do—create uncertainties, but keep them simmering under the surface, until the question is later present, and swallowed up, in the answer.

Anya's response to the poisoned body seemed particularly significant. Anya enjoys learning new words in the reading sessions as well as practising her English by reading aloud. She shows signs of extreme Obsessive Compulsive Disorder (OCD), only touching the paper on which the piece is printed if it looks immaculate. She cannot bring herself to sit in the room unless the windows are open to let in fresh air. I anticipated that she may not be able to bear this kind of language of decay. And yet Anya comprehended and stayed calm, even volunteering to read the subsequent speech of Hamlet's—beginning, viscerally 'Hold, hold, my heart,/And you, my sinews, grow not instant old, But bear me stiffly up' (93–95). It was a sign, I felt, that she was somehow comfortable with what we were doing. It might seem extreme to over-value this instant in relation to a condition so complex and deep-set as acute OCD. But I have often felt that reading with a patient about something they can't cope with in the physical world might somehow help them to acclimatise or come to terms with that thing. I am always concerned to create a space in which readers are potentially able to get across the gap between the emotions triggered by reading and the thoughts which come only subsequently. These lines were the filter through which Anya could experience something which even those of the group without OCD found repulsive. The reading allowed them to visit the unsafe.

One prompt for reading the spirit's revelation a second time was that we got stuck understanding the lines immediately succeeding those describing the ravages wrought by poison':

> Thus was I, sleeping, by a brother's hand
> Of life, of crown, of queen at once despatched,
> Cut off even in the blossoms of my sin, unaneled,
> No reck'ning made, but sent to my account
> With all my imperfections on my head. (*Hamlet*, I. v. 74–79)

After we had discussed the basic meaning of the words, the staff member, Julie, surmised, 'Oh right, so if he has died too quickly, and hasn't had chance to repent or anything, then he must have gone to hell'. Ian continued in agreement, 'Yes, that would explain the fire at the start. "Sulph'rous and tormenting flames". There are fires in hell aren't there? He must have come from hell… and he's got to go back there again'. Here, Julie and Ian draw two parts of the scene together; so, next, they connect up separated parts of the Ghost's first speech, going back to it of their own accord. 'There seems to be some time-limit' (Julie again), 'when the ghost says "*Till* the foul crimes done in my days of nature/Are burnt and purged away" (lines 12–13). Is he in – what is it - purgatory?' 'A few lines later, though', says Ian, 'it's "But this eternal blazon" (line 21)'. We talked about how 'till' feels more fragile followed up by the ever-elongated 'eternal'; and about how within 'eternal blazon' are the words 'eternal *blaze*'—as though Shakespeare were making the words dangerously close to *saying* 'hell' because the spirit is dangerously close to *being* there. There's intense imaginative flexibility at work in this careful re-assembling of the scene and in this thinking which goes back before it and on beyond it. Soon the patients will be recalled to the ward's daily routine: right now, we are all bounded by the other-world of the text.

Ian had taken over reading this part of the ghost's speech from Christine. Christine was relatively well and attended the session immediately prior to leaving the hospital for an overnight stay at home. She was anxious about the outing, saying several times that she was 'dreading it'. In our sessions, she struggled to take in a basic sense of what was happening in the stories and poems but she would occasionally offer to read aloud, as she did at the beginning of this session. She seemed to find it far more appealing to be the ghost than Hamlet. Maybe the ghost had a certain glamour to it; or maybe the idea of being something unreal is pertinent to someone who knows they themselves are struggling to find their way back to some way of living. Reading aloud had a special function for Christine. When she was listening to someone else read, she zoned out, lost track and quietly panicked. When she was reading, she seemed to know she had the responsibility of bringing out the piece for everybody else and her concentration expanded to meet that demand. For the first time since I had read with her, Christine, this time, made the link between the literature and her life. She shook her head. 'It's hitting a nerve this is. Makes me think about my Dad'. She seemed very uncomfortable so I asked Christine whether she would prefer us to read something else, but she did not opt out, saying, 'No, I want to carry on'.

I always find this a moving thing for group members in mental health settings to say. Very often the reason they are in inpatient care in the first place is because they do not want to carry on, not with anything, not with life. If you can give someone in this position opportunity to want to carry on with something, even something so apparently small as a single story, is that not a start? a tiny sense of wanting to continue? It occurred to me that we often want to carry on reading because we want to know the end. Often we hope for a happier ending than what's going on mid-story. In this scene, however, there can be no completely happy ending—the ghost is a person who has already died, so it is what happens *after* an *unhappy* ending that mattered to Christine. It seemed that part of her whole struggle was that she was facing up to something, learning to live with her pain, and this was reflected in sticking with the Shakespeare, even though it hurt.

I asked the group whether they would, if they could, choose to come back in another time. Questions like this can be tricky for people with a limited sense of reality and/or a limited sense of there being a future, with or without them in the world. Ian offered a thought: 'It would be easier to go into the past because we know something about it, but in the future you don't know what you're going to find'. Christine picked up Ian's thought: 'Yes, if you came back into the future, you would be confused probably, and scared. You might go like dust, like particles… (a pause) I've got my Dad's ashes at home'. I can't immediately figure out why, but that was a powerful moment. I don't think it was one single thing. There's simply the fact that a real death has been mentioned—the ghost of Christine's father was in the room now, too. There's also the idea of the disintegration of the body in a hypothetical way turning into something very real: something that's never going to happen (returning in the future, like the Ghost) led Christine to something that's *already* happened. Then there's the fact that Christine is so anxious about going home after weeks in hospital, but she's just remembered that that's where her dad, or the memory of him, is. Maybe this was a real and practical comfort to her, for something she has got to be brave about. I do know that this is why reading in hospitals is not some 'soft', aesthetic thing to do: after the psychiatrists and nurses had treated her effectively, this last-minute bit of reading braced a patient for returning to her own home, a place where self-managed health independence and what we call 'mental health' can begin to be rebuilt.

Anne Line Dalsgård, 'Serving the Literary Experience: Librarians as Reading Guides in Danish Public Libraries'

Danish librarians were once experts in books. They would be the ones that children came to, when they wanted to read about the wider world, real or imagined; they were the ones adults consulted about practical problems ('Do you have a book about…?') or personal longings ('I like books about…'); and they were the ones who read, discussed and selected the books that should compose the comprehensive collections of the libraries. In many municipalities 'book buses' would visit marginal areas and be the local meeting point. As a study on the role of public libraries in small communities found:

> The book bus in [name] municipality also had a much clearer social function than the library itself. Both the driver and the librarian had been driving the route for a lot of years and knew almost all the borrowers, so there was no need to mention names […] Many of the adult borrowers were regulars, and several of them used the book bus visit to talk about the turns of life: unemployment, the spouse's disease, a lost cat, alcohol problems, etc. The librarian and driver listened patiently to what was said and did not hide the fact [to the interviewer] that social problems were many in some of the villages.[10]

Today the role of public libraries in Denmark is undergoing significant change. Recent decades have shown a move towards their integration into more hybrid cultural institutions,[11] and librarians have many different responsibilities and generally less contact with the public through books. Most libraries are centralised and digitalised, and book buses have been cut off the budget. Most users search, find and borrow books without assistance. Some Danish libraries even have self-service access outside opening hours. There is no longer a need among borrowers for help with the catalogue as search programmes on the computer are relatively easy to use, and there is less time for the librarians to read and discuss the purchase of books for the constantly shrunken collections. These changes, however, have happened along with an upsurge in social activities organised by the libraries, such as reading clubs and book evenings where librarians make short book presentations. They may also offer social and non-book offers, such as internet access, sofa-corners with board games and game consoles, and places to listen to music.[12] The project 'Time to Read' (see also Chapters 12 and 18), which I shall focus upon here, is one among many attempts to rethink the role of libraries. It constitutes a significant step into public libraries' engagement with social issues, as it is a collaboration between libraries in a specific geographic region of Denmark (RegionMidt), the NGO The Danish Reader Association, and the local psychiatry and municipal health centres.

'Time to Read' offers Shared Reading groups, which aim to promote mental health in a formally non-therapeutic way, and librarians have been educated specifically to facilitate the reading. As will be evident, these librarians have found it deeply meaningful to engage with people through Shared Reading. The following builds on ethnographic interviews (see Chapter 9) with 14 librarians, who were all involved in the 'Time to Read' project. Six had facilitated groups at the time of the interview, the others had gone through the training and looked forward to starting. All libraries were located in towns outside the big metropolitan areas.

Being a Public Librarian

The interviewed librarians had similar stories about why they became librarians. Listen to a few:

> I have always known that I wanted to become a librarian. I loved reading. That is how you often start. I felt that books could do something. And I liked the service part of the job, helping people. (female, 38)

> I have always liked books. Even though I am not very good at remembering them. What they are about. I have a feeling of the book. I remember 'Oh this book, it did something good to me'. (female, around age 55)

> I've always wanted to be a librarian. Since I was 10 or 11 years old, it was simply my desire. I knew a librarian, who had become a role model for me. […] I then went to an introductory meeting, and I sat and thought: 'If I get into the library school and am allowed to become a librarian, I will be the happiest person in the world'. (female, around 60)

> I liked to read. When I was aged 15-16, it was … books I found in my parents' bookshelves, I got completely euphoric, I read everything [—] And then, what could be more privileged than a job where I would have the possibility to convey, as you may say, the joy of literature at a library. (male, age 61)

A particular passion emerged in the interviews, i.e. the joy of sharing your love of reading with others:

> I like telling stories. When I have read a good book it is like experiencing it again, when I retell it. I get the atmosphere of it back. And it is also because I want others to have the same experience. (female, around age 60)

> I like to be the cream. I like to give people something extra, something they did not know they were missing. You sit down in a … you sit and read a good book, and when you come up again, you think 'Hey, you know what? That was really good!' (female, age 38)

> [It is] a magical world to get into. And you can convey it to others and find that they also think, well, that was amazing! Still, today I can be happy when I have recommended a book, and then they come and say to me: 'I am so happy you recommended it. It was so exciting to read'. Oh, it just warms you. (female, late 50s)

At the front desk, some borrowers still come and ask about books and recommendations. Some borrowers come when they know a specific librarian is at the front desk, and make sure to report back on the help they get. A woman had phoned one librarian on a recent shift to say that a book she had recommended was the best she had ever read. 'That is touching, isn't it? Then you have made a difference', she said, satisfied.

In their recommendations of books librarians might speak of their own reading experience, but they do so in general terms and often with reference to other people's responses to the book. However, in the reading groups it is different. You have to give more of yourself. Not all librarians joined 'Time to Read', and those who did emphasised in the interviews that they were not representative of the staff at their library. Other employees preferred the tasks with less contact with borrowers.

Giving of Oneself

The experience of being a reading guide in 'Time to Read' both challenged and satisfied the librarians—satisfied because the Shared Reading gave moments of the kind that they had always seen themselves providing. As one reading guide related (female, age 38):

> There were many who came regularly. I asked the last time what they felt about it. One with bipolar - she was looking forward to reading a group every Wednesday and she had not been looking forward to anything for 10 years since she got ill. It's that which makes me quiver, because Wow! That's why I'm doing what I'm doing. Imagine what that had meant to her. She did not

> miss out once. It is completely breath-taking that I make something that makes such a big difference to her. I'm not saving people's lives as a surgeon or a policeman does, but I do something else - and, wow, that is why you go to work. It is just so important to mental health that people not only consist of physical joints but also mental joints and that these should also be able to function. And many of them lack some pluses, they have really played a lot of matches, they have had a lot of minuses, many things they have not been able to do. Then it's really cool that I can give them a plus. I want them to contribute to those two hours when we sit here - nothing more than that! We may want to have all the good side effects, yes, but it's the time together that's important. Someone from the group took the text home and reflected on it, another smashed the text immediately - both are fine. One said she simply gets so much out of getting her thoughts out, another said 'I get a lot from taking in what others say,' and I think that's fantastic.

Some participants in the groups were regular readers, others had read before but could not concentrate on reading in their present state, and some were new to literature. But all seemed to find it valuable to come to the groups. One reading guide expressed what she gave like this:

> It is the feeling that you really experience something here that makes an impression. That, that … that somehow touches one. I can see it on them or sense it because they say 'thank you for today' or take … that's how small things are … take the text home or mention something about the text afterwards. Then I think … that's the way to present the literature to them at its best. That pure literature experience, isn't it? And the desire to read.

As reading guides the librarians were first of all professionals. As the reading-group leader, you are the one who guides the reading and gets the conversation back on track if it is drifting too far away from the text. You also have to facilitate a good atmosphere in the group. When someone has been away, you are the one who says 'Good to have you back again!', and two experienced reading guides found this specifically important in the 'Time to Read' groups, as participants here did not have strong social networks and appreciated the recognition of their presence. In their interaction with the groups the reading guides drew from their experience as librarians, because as a librarian you already have certain relevant skills:

> One has to be curious. And then you should also have a form of organizational talent or structure and so on. The whole library is a big system. So if you do not understand the system and do not respect the system, then you can really

> destroy it for many others. And then there is the questioning technique. We have the reference interview as it is called. It is a very systematic structure for how to ask [if someone asks for a kind of book but does not know the exact title]. It's such a bit of a curly curiosity.

However, to create the particular effects of the reading it is not enough to be a professional, you have to give of yourself. One guide found that her own positive mood and humour affected the group, another said that you cannot stay too professional but have to give 'a chunk of yourself'. As one said: 'There is a fine border between personal and private. You decide how much you wish to give. But it can become very personal and I have to open myself, because sometimes I do not understand the text myself'. The fact that the texts were not chosen by the reading guides at this particular project was something that had affected their position in the groups, mainly in a positive way they found. Somehow they were on equal standing with participants. And as one reading guide said: 'That's why, I think, when you facilitate a reading session, you basically do it as human being'.

Asked if these reading groups differed from other reading groups she had led, an experienced guide said:

> I got an impression of what they have tumbled with, they have given themselves and told about themselves, family, everyday life and interests. We've all given of ourselves. Little by little you get insight into their suffering. But that happens in other groups too, like with the 50+ ladies. You think to yourself 'What hasn't she been through in her life?' It hasn't been different here. I was nervous beforehand, but you meet a person not a diagnosis.

Summing Up

Not all librarians become librarians in order to share the joy of literature with others, but some do, and in the project 'Time to Read' some of these found the role as reading guide deeply fulfilling. Working with psychologically vulnerable people accentuated the need to care for the individual and create a good atmosphere, as the participants did not all have a strong social network. Beyond this, however, the groups were not particularly different from other Shared Reading groups led by the librarians. The emphasis they all put on the common humanity seems to be a general ethos in Shared Reading activities, but in this particular context it seemed extraordinarily manifest. Surely, there are critical debates to be taken about the role of public libraries if they continue to move closer to the health services, but in the present case the librarians did not feel out of their role as librarians. Rather, closer than ever.

Notes

1. Ethics approval was provided by Sefton NHS Research Ethics Committee. All names are pseudonymised.
2. J. Billington, C. Dowrick, J. Robinson, A. Hamer, and C. Williams, 'An Investigation into the Therapeutic Benefits of Reading in Relation to Depression and Well-Being' (University of Liverpool: Liverpool Institute for Health Inequalities Research, 2011), pp. 6, 26. https://sites.google.com/a/thereader.org.uk/get-in-to-reading-downloads/files/TherapeuticbenefitsofreadingfinalreportMarch2011.pdf?attredirects=0&d=1https://sites.google.com/a/thereader.org.uk/get-in-to-reading-downloads/files/TherapeuticbenefitsofreadingfinalreportMarch2011.pdf?attredirects=0&d=1.
3. C. Dowrick, J. Billington, J. Robinson, A. Hamer, and C. Williams, 'Get into Reading as an Intervention for Common Mental Health Problems: Exploring Catalysts for Change', *Journal of Medical Humanities*, 38.1 (2012), 15–20 (p. 17).
4. W. Shakespeare, *The Sonnets and a Lover's Complaint*, ed. by J. Kerrigan (Harmondsworth, Middlesex: Penguin Books, 1999), p. 91.
5. The log was a requirement of the Reader in Residence post (jointly funded by The Reader and Mersey Care NHS Mental Health Trust) and under the ethical auspices of Mersey Care NHS Trust Research and Development. The notes were first revised in this form for a postgraduate (Masters) degree which was subject to (generic) ethical approval by University of Liverpool Research Ethics committee. All names are pseudonyms.
6. I. Asimov, 'The Immortal Bard', in *The Complete Stories*, 2 vols (London: Harper Collins, 1997), vol. 1, pp. 193–97.
7. W. Shakespeare, 'Hamlet', in *The Oxford Shakespeare: The Complete Works* (2nd edn.), ed. by J. Jowett, W. Montgomery, G. Taylor, and S. Wells, pp. 681–718 (I. v. 1–113, pp. 689–690).
8. D. Oliver, *Poetry and Narrative in Performance* (Basingstoke: Macmillan, 1989), pp. ix–x.
9. W. Shakespeare, 'The History of King Lear', in *Complete Works*, pp. 909–41 (IV.vi. 33, p. 933).
10. N. Vaaben, *Små folkebibliotekers rolle i lokalsamfundet-en antropologisk undersøgelse* [The Role of Small Public Libraries in Local Communities—An Anthropological Study], Københavns Universitet, 2003. https://ckk.tors.ku.dk/afsluttedeprojekter/smaabiblioteker.pdf.

11. N. Dahlkild, 'Biblioteksrummet under forvandling' ['The Library Space Under Transformation'], in *Folkebiblioteket som forvandlingsrum* [The Public Library as Transformative Space], ed. by I. Emerek, Rasmussen, and Skot-Hansen (Danmarks Biblioteksforening, 2006), pp. 121–146 (p. 137).
12. For a thorough overview of the development of public libraries in Denmark, see N. D. Lund, 'Vistnok Uvurderlig! Folkebibliotekerne i det litterære liv i Danmark' [Probably Priceless! The Public Libraries in the Danish Literary Life], *Nordisk Tidsskrift for Informationsvidenskab og Kulturformidling*, 7.3 (2018), 42–58.

6

Reading for Dementia

Katie Clark, Charlotte Weber and Susan McLaine

Katie Clark and Charlotte Weber, 'Read to Care'

Since 2007, Katie Clark has pioneered the reading aloud of poetry in residential care groups for people living with dementia. Here, she and her co-worker, Charlotte Weber, write of their experience of delivering reading groups in a care home for older people with mild to moderate dementia in Cheshire, North-West England, over a period of three months.[1]

Katie Clark, *Triggering, Stimulating and Translating*

When I first started to read with older people I soon became aware of the obstacles that needed to be overcome to make the reading experience accessible and meaningful: residents often showed poor concentration, loss of short-term memory, difficulty in following conversation, confusion and

K. Clark (✉) · C. Weber
The Reader, Liverpool, UK
e-mail: katieclark@thereader.org.uk

C. Weber
e-mail: charlotteweber@thereader.org.uk

S. McLaine
Public Libraries Victoria Network and VicHealth,
State Library of Victoria, Melbourne, VIC, Australia
e-mail: smclaine@internode.on.net

J. Billington (ed.), *Reading and Mental Health*,
https://doi.org/10.1007/978-3-030-21762-4_6

disorientation. I learned that poems worked particularly well. They can be reproduced on a single page, making it less likely that group members lose their place. I always give a copy of the poem to each participant so that he or she can listen, or listen and read. People in these groups are often of the generation when poetry was learned by heart in schools, and it was frequently the case that group members with even the most severe level of dementia were able to recite poems learned at school word-perfect. More, rhyme and rhythm, the formal shapes, sounds and structures of the poem, helped to stimulate and maintain concentration, particularly at the level of personal emotion and autobiographical memory. The syntax of poetry is often more compressed and immediately striking than that found in extended narrative prose. 'Poetry constitutes what in neuropsychology is called an "engram", a representation of a whole experience analogous to one's own, thereby encoding a memory trace'.[2]

One word characteristically used by both the care staff leaders to describe the immediacy of the effect of poetry was the verb 'trigger'. What was triggered was often deeply, even hiddenly individual as well as specific. On one occasion, we were reading war poetry and as I read John McCrae's 'In Flanders Fields', Ivy shifted in her seat, and I could tell before I finished the poem that she wanted to speak.

> We are the Dead. Short days ago
> We lived, felt dawn, saw sunset glow,
> Loved and were loved, and now we lie
> In Flanders fields.

At the end I looked at her

> If ye break faith with us who die
> We shall not sleep, though poppies grow
> In Flanders fields.[3]

and she said, without any prompting, 'That was lovely that, my Dad went away in the war and people used to say to him "But what about your family?" and he would say "Family are one thing but so are your mates"'. She was clearly very proud of her father and remembered him in great detail. Much of her memory of him seemed connected with the war in which he served, the idea of missing him, and revering him when he returned home. One memory in particular, translated through the poetry, brought tears to her eyes as she shared it with the group:

> I remember once I walked in on my Father as he was changing his shirt ready to go out with Mother. He shouted 'Don't come in, I'll be down in a minute,' but it was too late, I had seen his side and there was a great hole there. I ran down the stairs to Mother crying and said 'What happened to Dad? Did he fall down the stairs?' And she said, 'No love, that is a war wound'. I remember I was so upset.

Her emotion at recalling the story of the wound demonstrated why, even though it took place when she was very young, this was an event which shaped her and has stayed with her over the years. I asked her if she was happy to continue reading the poems and she replied 'Oh yes, I like them'. When we read next 'Now to be still and rest, while the heart remembers' by P. H. B. Lyon, she smiled and nodded and was keen to point out, 'We celebrate every year, we never forget'.

Reminiscence therapy often works by offering participants a material stimulus, frequently an object (a ration card or photograph, for example). But I believe it is the *clarity* of the memories that spontaneously comes from the less material object called poetry—giving something of the feeling of the original life, no matter whether it was a pleasant feeling (conventionally called 'positive') or a painful one (usually thought of as 'negative'). In poetry's version of 'lest we forget', so-called negative emotions of sadness are given expression in a way that does not allow simple dissociation of the positive emotions (for example, of love) contained within them. Poetry, gently delivered and non-coercive, is more personally surprising and complex in the emotions it makes available than a single object related to a common, shared past might have power to be.

In another session we were reading Thomas Hood's poem 'I remember, I remember':

> I remember, I remember,
> The house where I was born,
> The little window where the sun
> Came peeping in at morn;
> He never came a wink too soon,
> Nor brought too long a day,
> But now, I often wish the night
> Had borne my breath away!
>
> I remember, I remember,
> The roses, red and white,
> The vi'lets, and the lily-cups,
> Those flowers made of light![4]

And a resident, John, suddenly said, 'They called it The Roses, and we drove them up with cameras to see it'. Often people come out with something abrupt, like that. Sometimes they seem to be looking for a very specific, tangible word or name, and when they do find it isn't always right, but it is descriptive and is like their version of poetry. Here it was 'The Red Roses' that John kept repeating. John's daughter was sitting in on the group and she realised it was, by rhyme, the Red Noses, rocks in New Brighton.

Some care staff have recommended the use of pictures in these sessions. But it is not so much the visual that has an effect here as the *translation* i*nto* the visual in the mind of the participant: 'The roses, red and white', the colours and the rhymes lighting up the brain. Perhaps by working through linguistic pathways, visual memories seem to be triggered more powerfully—more deeply and more individualistically—by non-visual means. That route seems at once more personal and the translation more holistic. Something very *bright* is brought into the mind.

There is growing research into this variation of mental structure, in terms of fragments, mosaics and quilting.[5] But the 'finding' here is that literature not only allows but also encourages this form of response, even among those readers who have no obstacles to immediate comprehension or articulation. In the group-experience of people living with dementia, the process requires a greater and more patient understanding of the role of apparently discontinuous silence. One Reader project worker comments:

> It is different from other groups, though there too silence is important. But more so here. First, because staff present don't like silences: sometimes their idea of an activity for these people is being jollied along; but it seems really important to allow them the silent gaps. Second, that dementia patients live in silence a lot of the time so I don't think it fazes them as much. Third, because it's important not to confuse (as a group-leader) silence for non-presence/non-engagement. Someone will say nothing, you think nothing is happening, then suddenly they may recite, or go exactly to the right place in the poem. It is as if there is a word or a feeling sort of floating around in the silence, and then suddenly it's there, it doesn't seem to need to be linear.

Charlotte Weber, *On Repetition: Triggers, Memory and the New*

The reading group I led took place every day, rather than weekly, a new model for this care home. In the early weeks, I tried to avoid repetition of poems. I wanted to create new conversations with residents by using new material at each session, and to keep myself fresh. However, after a few weeks, I noticed we were getting through fewer poems in the sessions and having more conversation around them. I decided to take advantage of the regularity of the daily sessions, and, as a sort of improvised experiment, to limit the poems to one or two (five to seven had been standard practice) and to repeat the same poem from time to time across different sessions. I chose for this purpose William Wordsworth's 'Daffodils', always a favourite in care home groups and the very first poem I read on Day 1 of the group.

> I wandered lonely as a Cloud
> That floats on high o'er vales and Hills
> When all at once I saw a crowd,
> A host, of golden Daffodils;
> Beside the Lake, beneath the trees,
> Fluttering and dancing in the breeze.
>
> Continuous as the stars that shine
> And twinkle on the milky way,
> They stretched in never-ending line
> Along the margin of a bay:
> Ten thousand saw I at a glance,
> Tossing their heads in sprightly dance.
>
> The waves beside them danced; but they
> Out-did the sparkling waves in glee:-
> A Poet could not but be gay
> In such a jocund company:
> I gazed - and gazed - but little thought
> What wealth the show to me had brought:
>
> For oft when on my couch I lie
> In vacant or in pensive mood,
> They flash upon that inward eye
> Which is the bliss of solitude,
> And then my heart with pleasurepleasure fills,
> And dances with the Daffodils.[6]

What I found, remarkably, was that regardless of whether residents seemed to remember and recognise the poem or not (from previous sessions or from memories of school), they kept coming up with different thoughts at different times, new thoughts, new places in the poem, or different formulations of old thoughts. There was no mere repetition of a default response.

I pick up from Day 35 (week 7) in my log, where I first read the poem again.

Day 35. I wanted to get conversation concentrated more tightly around the poem's language. I told the group that I loved the descriptions of the daffodils 'dancing' in the poem—that it made me happy, but I wasn't sure why. I pointed out that the word 'dancing' was repeated in each stanza of the poem (lines 6, 12, 13, 24, saving the variation at line 18) and asked what they thought about it. Joan came out with a lovely description of how if you were standing in a field watching daffodils moving in the wind, they wouldn't all go the same way—'some of them would be going this way, some that - so it *would* be like they were dancing'. Myra agreed, and for a few seconds, we were all swaying in our seats as we thought about the motion of the flowers.

Day 37. We read the poem for the second time this week. Myra recognised it (whether from Day 1, Day 35 or childhood was not clear) and the other members were all smiling during the first reading. Kenneth was initially very quiet during the discussion, though he continually looked back down at the words on the page and seemed to be mouthing some of the lines to himself. After I'd read the poem a second and third time, I asked Kenneth if there was anything in particular he liked. He felt the daffodils had their own particular character, saying 'they're funny, aren't they. Dancing around. They're like people'.

Encouraged, I tried, as I had tried at both previous sessions, to initiate discussion about the final stanza, where the poet has returned home and is remembering the vision of the daffodils:

> They flash upon that inward eye
> Which is the bliss of solitude.

In both previous attempts, none of the residents volunteered a response, and conversation moved on to more general topics. This time however, when I asked, 'What do you think the 'inward eye' is?', Myra immediately said, 'It's imagination!' I can't say exactly what produced this sudden verbalised, ecstatic thought, other than the atmosphere of excitement, energy, exploration, which the poem had created in the group that day, possibly building on the momentum of previous conversations. After this, we talked about how imagination helps us to see things that aren't necessarily there, or obvious.

Towards the end of the session, there was an even bigger breakthrough. Alice, a fairly regular attendee of the group, was at a far more advanced stage of dementia than the rest. Alice's symptoms presented themselves in an inability to form coherent sentences, or often even to pronounce words. Her communication mainly took the form of exaggerated facial expressions, or blowing her tongue, waving her hands, and, as it were, babbling. During this session, the activities coordinator at the home was sitting next to Alice, and sharing her copy of the text with her. She was tracing her fingers along the lines of the poem, which allowed Alice to follow my reading. As I was reading, I realised Alice was reading aloud, very slowly, along with me. Or rather, as she was a little way behind my own reading and seemed not to notice or mind, it was as though she were reading the poem one-to-one with the activities' coordinator. She read almost the whole poem through, losing the thread of it just before the final stanza. The coordinator looked up at me, visibly amazed, then praised Alice very highly, pointing out how much of it she had read, and asking had she enjoyed the poem. Alice said: 'There's something about it, I can't explain'. This identification of a vague, unverbalised 'something' in the poem, signalled to me the depth of thought and feeling the poem had prompted in Alice, even if, or perhaps especially because, she wasn't able to explain or say more about it. Poetry is good at creating that effect for any of us, whatever our supposed mental or cognitive ability or disability: poetry is content with making something present though not fully explicable. After the group, the coordinator told me that she had never heard Alice able to string so many words together, let alone read aloud words from a page, and in the right order. Alice now has a framed copy of 'Daffodils' on the wall in her room.

Day 38. This was the third time this week I read the poem. During an early conversation, we discussed the first lines of the poem and what it would feel like to 'wander lonely as a cloud'. Nina (a regular who had been present on days 1, 35 and 37) commented, 'It's a different type of thinking'. I asked her to elaborate, and she described something like getting in touch with a new kind of thought, which was like a cloud above you—or perhaps your previous way of thinking, your worries, being lifted like a cloud. She used lots of hand and facial gestures to try and get across what she wanted to say when the words weren't quite there.

We spoke for a while about what a shame it is that the countryside is neglected and people stay within the cities. Kenneth took our conversation back into the poem: 'It's like him here, I wandered lonely as a cloud'.

He read out the whole first stanza, stopped, and said, 'I suppose you would wander lonely as a cloud, wouldn't you?'Cause you are walking around, and looking around you, and you're sad that what you're seeing might not be there much longer'.

Day 43. Myra was still the only member to show explicitly that she remembered the poem. I again drew attention to the final stanza, and this time Nina commented that the 'inward eye' is 'a thought that comes from inside, not from the eye', and about seeing in a 'new way'. Myra, who in previous sessions had only ever expressed pleasure in hearing the poem and was delighted in being able to recite it from memory, today had a quieter and more troubled response to it. She said it made her feel sad. She related it to a 'longing' for something, which was different from her simply pleasant feelings and responses in previous sessions. Kenneth spoke about poems more generally at the end: 'They do make you feel emotion, these words. You can get all sorts of books out there now - adventure, mysteries or whatever. But this makes you feel emotion - I get all choked-up! And you can get your emotion out - give it to a friend and they know what to do with it. Be a friend… I like it'.

Day 44. There was a new floor being laid-down, which had caused a lot of re-organisation, noise, and clutter. The staff were very preoccupied, and the activities coordinator who normally brings the group together for the sessions was off sick. After eventually gathering the regular members of the group with help from other staff and settling them in their seats, there was a palpable feeling of unease and confusion within the group. I made a last-minute decision to use 'Daffodils' as I thought that hearing familiar words and rhythms might help to soothe the atmosphere. Nina had read the poem aloud in the group previously with great emphasis and eloquence. This time, after reading the poem aloud she independently linked the 'inward eye' to 'something that God has given us, in the mind—what brings us here, not just one, but all of us (she waved her hand around the table)—as a whole? It's so that we can see all around, like we can travel all around the country' (she gestured in a wide circle). I asked her if this was like being connected to other people in some way, and she said—'Yes, we see all around - we can all see and feel one another'. Kenneth again linked the poem to his love for nature and sadness at its being destroyed, but this time through a new memory that he had not spoken of before—of a small lake on the Wirral where he took his children: 'They want to put something more interesting there now - but what could be more interesting than water and ducks and kids playing?'

Day 56. Kenneth said of 'Daffodils', some time after we had turned from it to look at another poem, that it brought 'the outside in'.

Day 57. Kenneth arrived with a copy of 'Daffodils' from the previous day folded in his top pocket. He took it out when he sat down at the table, unfolded it and began to read it silently to himself. I suggested that we could all read it as a group, as I had some copies with me, which seemed to please him. We read it in the group, and Kenneth picked-up on the lines 'continuous as the stars that shine/And twinkle on the Milky Way'. He started speaking of his interest in astronomy, mentioning the cosmos, black holes and infinity, and we spoke about how un-knowable space is, how it goes beyond our thoughts and ideas about it.

Day 63. The penultimate reading session at the home. Another great moment with Alice, as she read the whole first verse through on her own, very well, without prompting. Myra recited the poem from memory along with me the whole time. After the first reading, Alice was the first to speak—her speech was very difficult to understand and many of the words were incomprehensible but I made out 'wander lonely as a cloud'. Myra said she wouldn't like to be like that, because you need company when you're on a walk. We spoke about the benefits of having someone to share things with. Then I pointed out the daffodils that are 'jocund company' in the poem—and Myra said, 'oh yes, jocund company - something to keep you happy and smiling and in good spirits … They are happy, the flowers'. We spoke about why flowers make us feel good: 'It's the colour, the smell', Myra said, 'they make you feel homely, like you've come home'.

Kenneth read aloud the first two stanzas, very quietly and slowly, without being asked, saying 'yeah' every now and then. Then he started remembering going out for walks in North Wales with his children and wife—the mountains and hills. He said of the person in the poem, 'It seems like he's trying to get away from some troubles'. I asked him what he meant by this, and he said, 'Like, it's all got a bit much, and he's not talking to people, so he's just gone out - and he's with the daffodils and he "floats on high over vales and hills" - he needed to go out'. I asked if sometimes it can help you deal with problems or difficulties if you go outside into the country. He nodded and said, 'Yes'.

The repeated slow readings did not actually result in repetitive discussion or in slow mental responses to which one might condescend. Conversations around the poem never felt formulaic, even when we were discussing similar matters. Perhaps this is because even when I recognised responses that individual members were having to the poem, they would express them in different ways. For example, Nina's enjoyment of the images of the flowers led her to describe the feeling they gave her in different sessions as 'dainty', 'homely' 'comely' and 'feminine'. Group members' responses to the poem could also change in what seemed like quite significant ways, for example Myra's wistful remarks in session 43. The poem suddenly was no longer just about a pleasurable experience and happy things, but also an expression of a sense of desire for something that was perhaps not attainable. Similarly, in a variation of Kenneth's repeated response to the poem as love of nature, his thought in session 63 about what had led the speaker to be out in this landscape and why he was 'lonely' before he arrived. Or Nina's different formulations across different session as to the deep meaning of 'the inward eye'.

By repeated readings of the poem and conversations with other residents—looking at the elements both of 'loneliness' and of 'pleasure'—the poem nearly always produced an uplifted, or at least a more peaceful or reflective mood than had previously existed. Whatever the failures of conventional memory (working memory, procedural memory implicit in the performance of task, semantic memory of general knowledge, short-term or long-term recall), the residents kept associating the poetry with core parts of their personal selves retrieved through careful and repeated attention to the poem's language. It seems important not to underrate what residents are capable of, in a context of safety and regularity which itself can provide through Shared Reading stimulating opportunities for something more than default responses or repeated phrases and stories in a continuous loop. What is vital is not complete autonoetic consciousness (the full and steady awareness of being aware), but the sudden episodic awareness itself. Transient though that awareness is, it is capable of being re-activated and, what is more, re-activated newly and freshly through the poetic stimulus, especially when repeated on a regular basis.

Here is a final example (from a related study of a reading group for older adults in London[7]) of the value of that sudden liveness and how poetry can be its 'trigger'. This group has been reading Wordsworth, too: the sonnet 'Composed Upon Westminster Bridge'. The session has ended and the group is about to disperse. Suddenly however, Ava says, 'It's a beautiful poem. Absolutely lovely' and begins to read it again, with wonderful relish and emphasis.

> This City now doth, like a garment wear
> The beauty of the morning; silent, bare,
> Ships, towers, domes, theatres, and temples lie

Open unto the fields, and to the sky;
All bright and glittering (Wordsworth, p. 285)

'I think it's beautiful', Ava repeats, smiling broadly, and the group bursts into applause. As part of the study, the reading group sessions were filmed and sound-recorded. At interview afterwards,[8] Ava looked at this moment but, to the interviewer's surprise, did not recognise that the person doing the reading was herself—though she was happy to read the poem aloud again, and again functioned beautifully in the present:

Earth has not anything to show more fair:
Dull would he be of soul who could pass by
A sight so touching in its majesty (Wordsworth, p. 285)

In the session itself, the poem had recalled to Carmella her first arrival in London from the Caribbean in the 1950s—the city cold, she said, yet 'glittering'. Following Ava's joyous reading, Carmella had said in what was itself extra time for the group: 'Sometimes you have something that you don't know you've got, and after other people come, you realize that this is precious, we have got it in our hands'. This is about not being 'dull of soul and passing by', as the group leader quickly points out, referring back to the text. Carmella is speaking of how literature captures and re-captures what too often is missed or taken for granted at the time of its happening. Recovery here, does not mean simply trying to get better by going forward but the capacity to get back something of what was lost or damaged, restoring a renewed continuity to a life. It is time recovered. It is surely no accident that the stimulus here is a sonnet, whose formal mission is to create perfection against the dark of time, the closure of final endings, the chaos of disordered mentality (see above, Chapter 3).

Susan McLaine, 'Reading for Wellbeing in Old Age'

Susan McLaine has travelled to the UK to undertake training in the field of bibliotherapy. Since 2009, she has been initiating Australian developments in bibliotherapy, including developing and coordinating State Library Victoria's Book Well program, a collaborative initiative of the State Library of Victoria, the Public Libraries Victoria Network and VicHealth. Currently, she is a PhD candidate at RMIT University, further investigating bibliotherapy through a research project aimed at establishing how facilitators from non-clinical backgrounds can effectively deliver bibliotherapy to support the general well-being of individuals and communities.

Introduction: The Development of Shared Reading for Older Australians

For many Australians, the idea of reading for health was first introduced by Blake Morrison's 2008 Guardian article 'The Reading Cure',[9] reprinted in *The Age*, a daily Melbourne newspaper. Morrison's source of inspiration were the stories collected from people involved with UK charity The Reader's community reading programme (then called 'Get Into Reading'), and its unique model of Shared Reading. His article incited the first training course offered outside the UK by The Reader. The Australian training was rebranded the Book Well program and was delivered through a collaboration between Victorian Health Promotion Foundation (VicHealth), State Library Victoria (SLV) and Public Libraries Victoria Network (PLVN). SLV coordinated the program. Support for the training came through VicHealth's 'Building health through arts and new media' action plan which lists among its objectives, the aims of increasing social connection for participants, increasing involvement in community and group activities and working in partnership across sectors.[10] An integral part of the Australian pilot programme was to develop community partnerships. Initial community contact showed that aged care providers were keen to provide a facilitated activity for their residents to complement other activities such as arts and crafts. Partner organisations looked to the reading groups to provide cognitive stimulation. Facility managers believed the 'literature used, and the relevance of the topics selected for the lives of persons with dementia made these materials a natural for eliciting engagement and a great way to communicate with them'[11] through offering a renewed sense of being present and paying attention.

The Programmes

Over two years, 23 groups and 180 sessions were conducted by 20 facilitators. Groups ran for eight weeks, with one 90-minute session per week. There were a variety of partner organisations, number of participants and the venues for the groups. Participation rates at each session varied, often dependent on the health of the participants in any week. 97% of the participants were aged over 65 years, and 82% of the cohort was female.

Data to evaluate the programme was collected through surveys, semi-structured face-to-face or telephone interviews with both partners and group members, group observations, journal entries, focus groups, and facilitator debriefing.[12]

The Residents: Alertness and Community

In the process of leading programme implementation, I developed a partnership with a low-care aged care residential facility of St Vincent's Care Services. Shared Reading aligned well with the organisation's commitment to providing social and health-focused activities, enabling the elderly residents to enjoy time with others and feel connected.

Initially, residents who had said they enjoyed reading were targeted. However, it was the residents who were isolated in their rooms in particular who accepted the invitation to take part in the group. The manager of the facility joined us occasionally to observe first-hand how the reading group reaches and touches those residents living with dementia.

Reading and listening stimulates both an inner and outer engagement—what I would call a companionship first with the words and with the images, and then with others. There was a sense from group members that they had connected with people on a deeper level than they would typically in life, creating a domino effect of shared participation. A group member described this experience as feeling a 'real sense of calm and this real sense that we'd all been uplifted in the room upon exit out the doors. And that every single member of that group had created that atmosphere – it wasn't just left up to the one person'.

A sense of community grows also from sharing the life experiences that members bring to the group. As well as listening to the texts being read, group members also listen to each other. Participants often have a desire to relate an experience; something that they are giving of themselves that allows others to be part of that journey with them. There is a willingness to give thought to another's story, empathetically. The manager believes the group helps to ease tensions between residents as they warm to each other.

The sharing of poetry in particular can assist people to retrieve core elements of their inner being through careful attention to the language. After listening to the poem at least once, group members each respond by individually reading the poem or lines from the poem, or perhaps just a single word to which they have felt drawn. Participants' feelings of accomplishment when they make meaning out of the poem can be seen in alert postures, expressive eyes, smiles and glances at each other. It is here that a sense of group members' attention and of being present is palpable.

The manager feared that one of the group members who had dementia had also lost his ability to use language and a move to a higher-level care facility with dementia-specific services was being considered. This resident was struggling for words, but after the reading of a poem, he said, 'Something sinister must have been coming there'. We straightaway saw that he was right—that the poem gave a metaphoric image of impending war. It was decided that he still had use of language and the move was averted.

Building Relationships: Residents, Staff and Family

As the groups offered the stimulus for new ways for participants to connect with one another, they also fostered a different connection within the staff and resident relationship, so often necessarily bound by the demanding routines of an institution.

An aged care coordinator found the reading groups created a 'therapeutic relationship in the sense of people being able to listen to each other, and understand their grief and their stresses and their joys. Our definition of success for this group was promoting the emotional independence of the group. In a residential unit you can quickly become institutionalised'. When 'Stewart', a ninety-four-year-old male participant, requested 'The Man from Snowy River' by Banjo Paterson, Stewart explained how he learned the poem as a boy and how he recited it to himself as 'a sort of comfort when he couldn't get to sleep when he was in the army'. He went on to explain how he had lost the book containing all his poems in a flood. He also recounted that he had lost nearly everything. The recreation coordinator later described how Stewart and his wife ended up as residents in the facility when they lost their house and all their possessions in the 2011 floods. What impressed her was the way that, when 'Stewart' stopped telling his story, the facilitator did not 'jump in' to comfort him. Instead, she waited and allowed the group to support him. (After a short silence, one of the group members had said 'Stewart, that's a real bummer' and at the end of the session, Stewart told the facilitator that attending the group had been 'priceless'.) This was one outcome this facility was seeking when it had agreed to the programme—to try to develop relationships between the residents that would be autonomous and independent of the staff, and to make their overall experience of the facility 'less institutional, more like home'.

Barbara has dementia and vision impairment. In the first week of the reading group, Barbara listened to the whole session then retorted: 'I don't know about any of this – I lived my whole life on a horse'. The facilitator decided to present the group the next week with a story about a horse. During the following week's session, Barbara seemed chuffed that such a story had been chosen. As the discussion developed around nature and animals she shared several personal reflections of her childhood. Living on a remote station as an only child she was tutored and then went to boarding school. She recalled that she 'lived on the back of a horse' and they were her 'only real friends'. At the conclusion of the group, another participant commented that: 'This group provides an opportunity to talk to others and find out about their lives and experiences'. Another said: 'I've been so lonely, living beside you all but not knowing you'. The facility manager commented that she had gained an increased insight into Barbara—understanding her history explained something of her sense of isolation and withdrawal. Staff in other facilities also spoke of how the reading groups 'helped us to get to know the residents in a different way, when the residents shared more of themselves through the memories the stories brought up'.

Loss of vision affects many older people. Robin, a blind participant in a different group, stated: 'I enjoyed the group because of the intermingling with others. I'm blind. When the story is read out loud, we've all heard the same story. It makes you feel part of things. It's great. I can join in, even though I can't see. I can listen to [audio] books – but it's by yourself. You can't discuss it, I'm the only one who has heard it'. According to staff, due to her vision impairment, Robin had not previously left her room for any activity.

One manager observed how the reading group assisted in not only building but sustaining a sense of community, outside of the group itself and beyond its duration. She noted that 'residents going in for dinner on Friday were still discussing the group, which was on Tuesday morning. They were talking about the literature, saying, "I think in that poem…" That was quite surprising to me, to notice that they were still talking about the material'. The manager added that this was lovely because the residents had tended to keep to themselves over the course of the week but now had a different way of relating to each other. These people live side-by-side but there is often very little interaction, and what there is can sometimes be tense. A facilitator noted how the tension she noted between two group members seemed to dissolve when one of them, relating his personal experiences to the story being read, started speaking about growing up in a large family of 17 children, and the other person really seemed to warm to him. Staff were surprised that those two people had stayed in the same room together, and had positively interacted, given the tension that habitually existed between them.

In a dementia-specific day centre group, family carers attend the reading group with participants. The group has proved valuable to the carers, not only in easing their own isolation and often reduced wellbeing, but in offering a renewed sense of emotional attunement between the carer and person with dementia.

> Mum had always been a great reader. She inspired my love of reading. Now she shows little interest – when I get the newspaper she just flicks through one or two pages. Now, since Book Well, she is really showing interest again. We talk about reading and coming to hear the stories. I notice when she looks at the newspaper now she will really read, and talks about some things in detail. This has given me hope for the future – I am just so grateful. For us it has been a blessing.

Practical Lessons Learnt

The early data collected provided evidence as to what was successfully working in the reading groups. Feedback from the facilitators, partners and participants in the initial pilot programme was used to design an optimum reading model for the second round of pilot programmes. The attributes of the facilitator were critical to the success of the group, including their ability to build partnerships and their expertise and skill in reading aloud, developing discussion and managing group dynamics.

Partnerships

Developing alliances and partnerships to run groups required facilitators to review potential organisations' objectives and ensure the reading group aims were aligned with those of the potential partner.

Setting up the Space

Although public libraries offer a safe community environment for vulnerable groups, making them an ideal location for holding reading groups,[13] problems arose when aged care facilities were unable to supply a staff member to drive the residents to a library when groups were held outside the facility. Most groups were held within aged care facilities, where taking the time to set up the room before the group members arrive itself creates a sense that the participants are having an outing and a different experience where each person's presence and thoughts are valued.

Selecting Materials

Consulting on the literature to be used in the groups is an essential stage of partnership development. Facilitators found partners were anxious about the content of the texts. Shorter, stand-alone texts and poems are selected for the relevance of their topics to the participants and their ability as a medium of communication, which has a therapeutic power of its own.[14] Over time, facilitators get to know their participants and can choose texts to which individual participants will relate. This offers the group members an opportunity to get to know each other in a more intimate way, and for deeper relationships to form. By the end of the pilot programme, over 83 per cent of participants said they had made at least one or two new friends.

Validation

Many of the participants are from a generation where poetry was learned by heart, and they can often recite a poem, word-for-word. One aged care facility manager perceived a participant, after reciting a poem, to be 'walking taller. It was a validation of her memory, her life experiences. Others in the group were mouthing along'. The facilitator noted that 'this was a lovely moment of connection for the group; after the resident finished reciting, another member thanked her, saying it was "beautiful" and brought tears to his eyes'.

Reading Aloud and Developing Discussion

After a text has been selected, facilitators need to read aloud expressively to make the literature come alive in the room and create the atmosphere of attentiveness.[15] Rhythm, intonation and pauses assist the group members in recognising the intention of the writer. Guiding participants in a discussion, through capturing the broad concepts of participants' contributions, comments and questions as well as holding open key concepts in the text, is an essential skill which provides a 'forum for discussing personal concerns without having to recount personal experiences'.[16]

Knowledge and Skills with Group Dynamics

Upholding the essential pleasurable aspect of being read to requires facilitators to manage the needs of the group together with the needs of the individual. Broadly, it was observed quite quickly that even though there was no pressure in the group for anyone to interact or reveal more than they were comfortable with, group members often felt personally compelled to share. However, often aged care workers were also compelled to share which necessitates guidelines as part of partnership development to ensure the discussion focuses on the participants, not the facilitator or staff involved in delivering the reading group.

Expectations of Success (Facilitators)

When setting outcomes, the expectations for measuring success for elderly group members requires thinking differently about what success means—not active participation in discussions, for example, but agreement to take part and regular group attendance. Not all older people can communicate in familiar ways, and non-verbal communication such as body language and eye contact can be indicators of engagement. Group members may not share in discussions until a text resonates with them. Even if group members do not share often, it means a lot to other group members to hear them if they haven't shared stories of their lives before, and one comment is enough to change the residents' perception of each other.

Sustainability

Preparation time constraints resulted in the programme being unsustainable for many facilitators due to the amount of time that was required to source weekly texts for use in the groups. For library staff to be given the time to plan for a session, organisational performance measures of success need to change. Rather than focusing only on collecting quantitative data, achievement could also focus on qualitative outcomes. In improving wellbeing, the quality of the interaction is as important a consideration as the number of people who have been interacted with.

Conclusive Testimonials

The final word comes from the older Australians who took part in the groups: 'I didn't want to get up this morning. But then I remembered it was reading group. It was the only reason I got out of bed'. The reading group gave participants something pleasurable to anticipate in the days immediately ahead of them: 'I've felt happier in myself having something to look forward to. Even on Sunday, I start looking forward to the group'. Aged care workers observed that some residents' moods were agitated or low before leaving their rooms to attend and their moods were improved and enhanced as they were 'buoyed enormously by the social sense of belonging to the group'. One group member commented 'How wonderful it was to have a conversation'. Shared Reading offers a practical route—at levels both of *doing* something meaningful (for participants) and (for care staff) and of being a manageable care home activity—to nourish social and emotional wellbeing in old age.

Notes

1. 'Read to Care: An Investigation into Quality of Life Benefits of Shared Reading Groups for People Living with Dementia' (Centre for Research into Reading, Literature and Society, University of Liverpool, 2015). The project was approved by the local NHS Trust Research and Development office. All names are pseudonyms.
2. E. Longden, P. Davis, J. Carroll, and J. Billington, 'An Evaluation of Shared Reading Groups for Adults Living with Dementia: Preliminary Findings', *Journal of Public Health*, 15.2 (2016), 75–82 (p. 91).
3. L. Pirandello (ed.), *Poems of the Great War: 1914–1918* (London: Penguin Books Ltd., 1998), p. 1.
4. T. Hood (1799–1845), *Selected Poems*, ed. by J. Flint (Manchester: Carcanet Press Ltd., 1992), p. 64.
5. H. Arendt, *The Life of the Mind*, 2 vols. (New York: Harcourt, 1978), vol. 1, pp. 205, 208.
6. W. Wordsworth, 'Daffodils' (*Poems*, 1807), in *The Major Works*, ed. by Stephen Gill (Oxford: Oxford University Press, 2000), pp. 303–04.

7. P. Davis, F., Magee, K. Koleva, and T. M. Tangeras, 'What Literature Can Do: An Investigation into the Effectiveness of Shared Reading as a Whole Population Health Intervention' (Centre for Research into Reading, Literature and Society, University of Liverpool, 2016). Commissioned by Guy's and St Thomas NHS Trust. Participants (whose contributions have been video-recorded and transcribed in accordance with NHS/RCUK ethical guidelines in respect of informed consent) are referred to using pseudonyms. https://www.liverpool.ac.uk/media/livacuk/instituteofpsychology/researchgroups/CRIxLSWhatLiteratureCanDo.pdf.
8. This methodology is described in detail in Chapter 10.
9. B. Morrison, 'The Reading Cure', *The Guardian,* UK, 5 January 2008.
10. VicHealth. 2010. 'Building Health Through Arts and New Media', VicHealth action plan 2010–13, viewed 29 January 2018, file:///C:/Users/Susan/Downloads/VH_building_health_through_arts_and_new_media_WEB_FA%20(1).pdf.
11. S. McLaine, 'Bibliotherapy: Reading for Wellbeing in Old Age', *Alzheimer's Australia Dementia Forum*, p. 4.
12. Informed consent was obtained from all participants in keeping with the Book Well Evaluation Framework. All names are pseudonyms (see Chapters 9 and 10 for extended discussion of qualitative interview methods).
13. L. Brewster, 'The Public Library as Therapeutic Landscape: A Qualitative Case Study', *Health & Place*, 26 (2014), 94–99.
14. S. Hodge, J. Robinson, and P. Davis, 'Reading Between the Lines: The Experiences of Taking Part in a Community Reading Project', *Journal of Medical Humanities*, 33.2 (2007), 100–104.
15. J. Billington, C. Dowrick, A. Hamer, J. Robinson, and C. Williams, 'An Investigation into the Therapeutic Benefits of Reading in Relation to Depression and Wellbeing' (Liverpool Health Inequalities Research Institute, University of Liverpool, 2010).
16. G. R. Jarjoura and S. T. Krumholz, 'Combining Bibliotherapy and Positive Role Modeling as an Alternative to Incarceration', *Journal of Offender Rehabilitation*, 28.1 (1998), 127–139.

7

Reading in Prisons

Alexis McNay, Charles Darby-Villis and Ann Walmsley in interview with Josie Billington

Alexis McNay, Charles Darby-Villis, Josie Billington and Ann Walmsley

Alexis McNay, 'Getting the Inside Out'

Alexis McNay co-ordinated the 'Read and Relax' programme at HMP Walton, Liverpool, UK. What follows is based on the report for the programme commissioners.

If someone were to ask me to point out the importance of the Read and Relax Shared Reading group at HMP Liverpool, I could do little better than have them accompany me through the wings towards it. They would see individuals and small huddles of men, all caught in a real mixed-up message of a posture, standing with hands down the front of their regulation grey jogging sweats. It is an attitude unsettling and inscrutable. It seems both

A. McNay (✉) · C. Darby-Villis
The Reader, Liverpool, UK
e-mail: alexis.mcnay969@btinternet.com

J. Billington
Centre for Research into Reading, Literature and Society,
University of Liverpool, Liverpool, UK
e-mail: jbilling@liverpool.ac.uk

A. Walmsley
Author and Journalist, Toronto, ON, Canada

J. Billington (ed.), *Reading and Mental Health*,
https://doi.org/10.1007/978-3-030-21762-4_7

brazen and insecure, a stand-off between statement and question—'I AM a MAN' and '*am* I a man?'—positions between which most men may find themselves negotiating their presence in the prison.

I have witnessed these negotiations in verbal altercations between men in the reading group, and in fists flying just outside, and the razor's edge between positions of brazenness and insecurity was demonstrated in a recent group. A very quiet young man attending his third session was asked by another member of the group what he thought of the opening of *The Pearl* by John Steinbeck. 'It's shit,' he replied. When I asked him to elaborate, he said, 'It's just about some little Mexicans and their baby… It's boring, I'm not interested'. A little piqued, I let my own guard down momentarily: 'Would it be better if it was about you?' I ask. 'No, it would be worse,' comes the immediate reply. Even in the relative calm of the reading room, there's still an atmosphere of sufficient hubbub that this little subconscious distress flare fizzles out largely unnoticed. Yet it's registered with me, and increasingly others are becoming more receptive, and there is an appreciation among those men who have become regulars that the Read and Relax group can provide opportunities for a sensitivity not perceived as weakness. At the end of this session, Michael,[1] who with thirty sessions under his belt, and a perceptive intelligence, is a valuable asset and sometimes advisor, says, 'Persevere with this'. He means, I think, both the book and the young man in question: 'There's a lot of front out there; they have to present it. But they see after a while that they don't need to bring it in here: they can leave it out there'.

'In here' and 'out there' *are* very different places, though only a nine-inch wall apart. The room we use for our reading group is actually just two cells knocked together. I can't help seeing this as symbolic, given the opportunities for open communication that the room and the reading enable. On one occasion, I go to speak to Michael, who has not turned up for the group—unusual, for him. For the first time I see him in his cell—barely see him through a central narrow slab of glass misted by thickness and age. I ask him why he hasn't come. I want to make eye-contact, but Michael knows that the best way to be heard is to speak through the side of the door, through a chink left hinge-side. There's a disconnect for a while as I try to see him while he tries to be heard, and something strikes me as profound about our inability to do both.

The men who attend the Read and Relax group see and hear each other in a way that marks a major demarcation between 'in here' and 'out there'. One afternoon we're reading Raymond Carver's poem *Happiness*, which describes the simple beauty of the companionship between two boys delivering papers, appreciated at a remove by an onlooker. There's a new man in the room, and when we read the line 'I think if they could they would take/ each other's arm',[2] John, uninitiated, and testing the water in mischief more than malice, says, with a nudge and a wink: 'Sounds a bit gay, doesn't it?' I'm scrabbling for a response suitably diplomatic—this is his first contribution, after all—and corrective. Before I can sort my Ps from my Qs, Michael raises his own point of order: 'What are you saying that for? This is a serious group, this; we take it seriously—it's not for dickheads'. John, surprised, amused *and* slightly wounded, says defensively, 'I'm not a dickhead!', and Michael completes the exchange: 'Well, don't say dickhead things, then'.

It is all taken in good spirits, and we segue directly into some really good discussion, but it's been a revelatory moment for me. Not only is it moving to see such a vehement protection of this space valued for a different kind of interaction, but there's a bigger and more significant implication in the wording of the exchange; that any distinction between the said and the sayer doesn't hold, here. In prison, as in society generally, where a lot of people 'speak their mind' without much thought as to what they're saying, the idea that one is inseparable from what one says, and should take responsibility for it; the idea that what you say represents you in a fundamental and important way; the potential for this rigour to refine thought itself; and the fact that a group member is demanding it: this makes me realise what a great thing we have going here. With the increased opportunities—or, more truly, obligations—for thought, as well as for discussion shaped by thought, come enhanced opportunities (and responsibilities) for listening, and men are revealed in different lights.

Later in the same discussion we address the line 'They are so happy/ they aren't saying anything, these boys' (Carver, p. 65) and a young man, unfettered, is able to say: 'Sometimes you can feel so close to someone that you don't need to talk, or be so happy in understanding that talking could spoil it'. Such thoughts want the opportunity to be brought out into the light sometimes, to remind us not only that it's OK to have them, but that they are there at all. I cannot imagine this utterance coming out of any other of the day-to-day opportunities for interaction offered by prison life. In an environment where the dominant look is askance, where much communication is banter mediated by front, the way we can talk in our Read and Relax groups seems momentous.

We read James Thurber's short story *The Greatest Man in the World*, followed by Kipling's famous poem about the model man ('that's a lot of "ifs"' says one man; 'yeah—big "ifs"', adds another), and I ask 'what is a man?'—just like that—in this room swampy with testosterone. It's a question that 'out there', on the landing, might have men rummaging down the front of their joggers. But it's safe in here—for me to ask and for us all to reflect upon—and there is not so much as a snigger, the impulse doesn't occur. Some of the responses seem indigenous enough; ideas about 'standing your ground', because 'a bloody nose costs less than being seen to back down'. This meets with widespread approval. But then, from the biggest, burliest man in the room, a qualification: 'It depends whose opinion you're asking, though. If you asked a woman, she'd say what's important is a good father, a good husband, who's caring and responsible'. It's John speaking, the man who had, a couple of weeks before, initially reacted against the sensitivity in Carver's poem.

Reading on the vulnerable prisoners' wing of a prison has prompted a lot of introspection on my part about the aims and limitations of our work. Of course, the watchword for any intervention into the life and mind of prisoners is 'reform', and, behind this, the urgent social and political goal of reducing re-offending. I'm as wary as anyone about making claims for Shared Reading in this direction. But reform—let's call it 'positive change'—is a process achieved in small increments, starting with appreciation of the need and belief in the possibility, two perceptual shifts that I believe are assisted by Read and Relax. If prison is the site of masculinity in crisis, then 'what is a man?' is a question that wants thrashing out in a more productive way than the frequent violent flashpoints on the wings provide. Communication is key here. The literature—our engagement with it, responses to it, responses to each other in relation to it—offers a different model. On a personal and physical level it's about address; mine is frank and direct and trusting to every man, looking them in the eye and offering them my belief, even if they're cagey, scowling, apparently mocking. Mindful that brazenness and insecurity are one and the same, I persist with this look until, sometimes, I see it coming back. It's when you see men realise and inhabit and enjoy versions of themselves that have always been there, but have perhaps been buried away for whatever reason, that Shared Reading quietly reveals its value.

We've been grappling with a line of *Macbeth* for ten minutes, and a man suddenly twigs both his meaning of it and that good literature is accessible to him. Four hundred years collapse as he sits erect and says, 'Clever stuff this Shakespeare!', tapping his own forehead. Reading Frank Cottrell Boyce's story *Accelerate*, a gamble given its theme of the perceived relative value of time, the danger of wasting it, the choice is rewarded by the men's intelligence and sensitivity. They talk of how their present situation makes them value time and the minutiae of experience; one talks of going to the beach to feel the sand between his toes, another speaks of the sun on his face, the rain on his head. We read *Korea*, a short story by John McGahern, a dark, poignant story about a son forced to confront the fact that a father traumatised by war and hardened by economic worries would gamble the life of his son.

It is beautifully written and we're trying to decide if and why this makes it less sad. One man tries to articulate a difficult idea he has in his head, that 'there can be a kind of beauty in hardship and pain'. He's struggling, and it's good to see. The other men give him the time to try.

This type of interaction—this way of being a man—becomes a norm in our room, but what are the chances of it being replicated 'out there'? I read with six to eight men at a time, usually, once a week, on a wing of up to 150, in a prison of up to 1500. That they value it is certain. One sign of positive change is knowing what's good for you and fighting to keep it. When I had to tell the group earlier this year that repeat funding for the programme looked uncertain, they readily put something of themselves back into Read and Relax, organising to get together during their Information Technology sessions to produce a PowerPoint presentation to which each man contributed his own testimony to the impact of Shared Reading. The result was very moving, and was critical in securing renewed funding.

If anyone were to doubt the importance of Read and Relax at HMP Liverpool, I would like to lead them through the wings, where they could see for themselves some of the men who fought to keep it. They would see what we do in our room is little more than express ourselves in a humane atmosphere which the literature we read has helped to create. Yet that little allows these men, whose day-to-day experience of exclusion, alienation, and disenfranchisement raises that defensive front, to leave it 'out there', come in and be themselves. That little is how, in the words of Michael, 'this group can take difficult people and give them a sense of belonging'.

Charles Darby-Villis, 'Reading in a Women's Prison'

Charles Darby-Villis records and reflects on the experience of delivering two weekly reading groups at HMP Low Newton, an all-female maximum security prison in the North of England, where he was Reader in Residence. What follows is based on the journal Charlie kept while facilitating the groups as part of a 12-month research study (see below, Part III, Chapter 9).[3] *Participation in the group was voluntary and the reading groups took place in different settings within the prison: one on a wing of the prison specializing in therapeutic care as an intervention for women diagnosed with severe personality disorder, the other in the Library. The practice report is divided into three. Part I charts the progress of a single group (the Library group) over a course of a year. Part II compares two groups reading the same work, John Steinbeck's The Pearl. Part III offers case studies in relation to two women serving long-term sentences.*

Practice Example 1: The Library Group—'A Time to Stop'

The journal extracts below take up from a month or so after the group had become firmly established (with around six core members), following three months of 'taster' sessions to encourage recruitment. During this time, the stable composition of the group had been unsettled by the transfer of two group members to other prisons, and the severely disruptive attention difficulties of one participant, whom I was obliged to ask to take a break from the group. I recount these experiences as examples of the 'teething' problems which can affect the setting up of a group, especially in the specialised environment of a prison. It is also worth noting that I made a point each week of personally reminding the participants (and potential participants) when and where the group was taking place. A week is a very long time in prison; many women are suffering depression and are medicated, so that motivation to attend can lapse very quickly even in very committed group members.

This is the first session after the departures. Up to this point we had read modern short fiction and poetry (Joanne Harris, Frank Cottrell Boyce, Jeanette Winterson, Carol Anne Duffy) as well as selections of Romantic poetry (Blake, Shelley, Coleridge). Elizabeth joined the group for the first time formally even though she had been present in the learning workshop and had listened from the sidelines for weeks.

Month Five

> The difference in the group today was remarkable. We read Ray Carver's short story 'Cathedral' and the women perceptively related the narrator's prejudices [in relation to another's blindness] to their own experiences of small-mindedness. Mary Oliver's poem 'Wild Geese' was a huge success. Elizabeth offered to read the poem aloud, always itself a significant moment.[4] 'Whoever you are, no matter how lonely' the world calls to the imagination 'like the wild geese'.[5] Elizabeth said how the poem spoke directly to her of the difficulties of living with remorse and the importance of always trying to be part of the world. This broadened out to a discussion about the importance of imagination to sustain people, particularly when in prison. Dawn linked this to the reading group (perhaps influenced by the final lines, 'announcing your place/in the family of things' Astley, p. 28)—how the group helped sustain imaginative life in prison. There was a general nodding of agreement. Hannah, who had been quiet but very thoughtful, told us that she shared everything we read with her husband and would be sending him a letter with this poem, telling him how it made

her feel. At the end of the session, Elizabeth said she'd found the group good but hard, that for the first time for a while she had sat and concentrated on something, given it focus. She said that her life was distracted and chaotic and that this was so different.

This 'difference' was what mattered to the women who regularly attended. Many spoke of the 'relaxation' they experienced in the reading group, the feeling of 'leaving the prison behind', with its day-to-day pressures and hazards, as well as of release from hopes and fears about their custodial sentence or the constant worry over what was happening to their children which would beset them when 'relaxing' in a locked room—bored and lacking occupation.[6] This, by contrast, as Elizabeth put it, was 'hard', 'concentrated'.

In the final third of the reading group, we took on a classic nineteenth-century text. I had been concerned about tackling a novel from so long ago, the content and characters of which might seem remote or irrelevant, and which would demand a lot of commitment from the women for the immediate future. My worries proved unfounded.

Month Eight (second week of reading Charles Dickens's *Great Expectations*)

I was impressed by how quickly and how strongly the story gripped the group. The drama was heightened by the setting; the women really liked the penal references. The hints of domestic abuse were discussed, in a thoughtful and sensitive way, and there was an intense discussion about conscience and the importance of truth-telling. There were lots of non-verbalised nods and sighs, for example, when Pip wrestled with the idea of telling Joe about what he had done [stealing food for a convict]. Bernie declared, 'but we all feel better when we tell the truth'. She talked about how perceptive Pip could be on reflection, yet couldn't 'act it out', and how this was very much like experiences in her teens. Zoe wanted to take the book back to her cell and finish it tonight.

If anything, the moral-psychological depth of this classic work made them more open and responsive to older (nineteenth-century) poetry also. Robert Browning's 'One Way of Love' brought to life fond reminiscences of adolescence, the unrequited love of the poem being related to teenage crushes and the lute substituted by an electric guitar.

Paula's last group (she's being transferred): she asked about groups like this at other establishments and the possibility of carrying on. Hannah is leaving this week so this was her last group. She said she is going to read the book aloud with her husband! She also thanked me for the group saying that it was the only thing that has kept her sane during her time in prison.

Month Ten

Zoe related Miss Havisham's condition to modern understandings of mental illness and trauma. She spoke of how strong the sense of embarrassment and denial can be. Elizabeth disclosed that she had not left the house herself for four years, and movingly talked about a shrinking world and how it gets harder and harder to change. At the end of the session, in response to Mark Strand's 'Lines for Winter'—beginning 'Tell yourself', when it grows cold that 'you will go on'[7]—Bernie said 'Everything isn't always all right, but it is possible to keep going, and to remain true to oneself even when you cannot continue as you had expected or hoped'.

Dawn had heard from Paula: she'd taken *Great Expectations* out of the library as soon as she'd arrived at her new prison and had since finished it. Bernie told how 'her 10 year old daughter has started *Great Expectations* because she wants to be reading the same thing as her mother' and the mother's sister is helping her daughter to work through the book. Dawn spoke of the ways she, too, shares the poems with her husband, writing to him a synopsis of the group. Caroline said Mark Strand's poem reminded her of her grandad and she took a copy to send to him. The possibility was enthusiastically discussed of holding a reading group during family visit days—all agreed that this would be a great idea.

The fact that the women engaged so fully with a 'classic' novel changed staff's perceptions of their capabilities and talents.[8] It also changed staff's perceptions (including my own) of what reading could do—enable the women to consider scenarios of action or reaction, trace effects over time, look at the consequences and impact of behaviour on others. Literature offered a broader view—philosophical, moral, humanitarian—of issues which the staff themselves could only deal with as matters of discipline when rules were breached: 'Some things are difficult to tackle head-on, formally; in books, the women can have insights into how things can change or be done differently' (Robinson and Billington, pp. 61–63: see also Chapter 9). One compelling example of this happened in one of the final sessions.

Month Twelve

As we concluded Sherman Alexie's short story, 'What You Pawn I Will Redeem', Dawn opened up about her homeless past, and both she and

Elizabeth spoke of their alcohol and drug use. The issue of trust and being trusted when you have nothing, resonated with the whole group. When the story described an offender spending a year trying to work out why he'd offended, Zoe immediately responded, saying, 'You know, lots of us are like this - I did bad things, and now I'm here and I spend my time trying to work out why I did them and I don't know'. Alexie's poem, 'Poverty of Mirrors', produced a strong reaction as the women talked about self-reflection, self-image and ageing. Zoe and Elizabeth spoke of their dislike of mirrors in prisons, admitting to avoiding them at all costs.

This level of honesty from Zoe, a serious offender, felt like a wholly new departure, a personal breakthrough. The openness at every level was a measure of how the reading group had overcome the distrust of human relationships which often destroyed any possibility of authentic or meaningful contact within day-to-day prison life.

There were strong signs too of the reading group offering a space for reflection which did not end with the group experience. Reading Henry Davies's poem 'Leisure' before her transfer ('What is this world if, full of care,/We have no time to stop and stare'[9]), Hannah had talked about 'prison time' and using its space to think. She spoke of how she had looked at a bunch of flowers with a focus and concentration here, inside, in a way that she had never done outside prison. Bernie reminisced about the 'time to stop and stare' her father had had, and sounded a note of regret that she has not always done this. She also looked forward to an imagined future where she could take more time. Before leaving the group to transfer, Paula read Ted Hughes' poem 'The Horses': 'going among the years, the faces,/May I still meet my memory in so lonely a place'.[10] She spoke movingly of how 'whatever you've done, there are beautiful moments in your past that can't be taken from you'. These are small signs that the place or space made possible by the reading-group could also be personally recreated in mind, anywhere and everywhere, as a thinking space.

Practice Example 2: Reading John Steinbeck's the Pearl

Group 1 took place on Mondays, Group 2 (see section above) on Tuesdays, and we read *The Pearl* in Months 6–7. I had begun by reading the same material with both groups. This habit was to change after the experience recounted below, where I display the responses of the group in successive weeks side by side.

Week	Group 1 (specialised wing)	Group 2 (library)
1	Both myself and the group were a little unsettled at first as the room was noisier than usual. But the story was so involving, the noise mattered less and less. The women, at first intrigued by the setting, and by the idea of traditional medicine and folk culture and music, became vocally impassioned at the injustice of the doctor's actions	The story went down very well. There was great deal of indignation about the behaviour of the doctor. The problem of money also really struck a chord with the group. Hannah read, which is unusual for her
2	An intense discussion about the dangers of money. One participant was firmly of the opinion that it corrupts all and that the pearl should be thrown away. There was some discussion about trust and how you can know who your friends are. Another group member related it to her own experience: she said prison had taught her that material goods were less important, that as long as she had family she was going to be all right	The story continued to attract the complete attention of the group. The details of the pearl fishing—and the collusion and cheating of the pearl's sellers—were fascinating to the group. There was full and flowing discussion about the value of money and the idea that riches made you a better person. Dawn, in particular, had very vocal and heartfelt views about friendship and what that might mean in the prison context
	This group was slow to start, but once it was going it was difficult to stop the extensive discussion about the morality of greed, money and the class system. Gaynor in particular was adamant that Kino should not give into the poor offer of the sellers. Other were less sure particularly because of the disempowered situation of Kino and his family. It was difficult to get people speaking today not because they were uninterested but because their attention was so rapt. One participant drew parallels between Juana's reaction to Kino's violence, and her own life. Another was moved by the change in Kino, thinking he'd 'sold his soul' but that it was important for him to keep on fighting	A very difficult group that was saved by the poem. The group have really become attached to Kino and the characters but could not cope with the way events spiral out of control. Bernie was very tearful and Dawn and Caroline very withdrawn. Both started crying, saying the writing was too close, and reminded them too much of their own lives and in particular their offending. I was particularly concerned about Caroline, a prolific self-harmer. Hannah disengaged but was still obviously finding the story hard. This was all within the first twenty minutes of the group. I took the decision to stop reading the book. We then had a frank and open conversation about the power of writing while people calmed down

Week	Group 1 (specialised wing)	Group 2 (library)
3 (Chapter 3)		The poem, William Henley's 'Invictus' proved ideal for the mood. All were visibly moved by the final stanza. Dawn said that for all the darkness she felt she kept her 'unconquerable soul'.[11] The anecdote about Nelson Mandela [who prized the poem during his incarceration] really stuck a chord with the women. Caroline spoke very affectingly about six months she had spent in segregation, her self-harm and suicide attempts. She then looked up and smiled and said 'you know, through it all, I remained, I'm still here - I'm alive, "I am the master of my fate: I am the captain of my soul"' (Henley, 1, p. 125). To finish, Caroline stood and read the whole poem again, to applause from the group. She announced she was going to type it out so everyone could have a copy to stick on their walls I'm not going to continue with *The Pearl* with this group particularly because of what happens to the baby, but have lent copies to those members that want to finish it
4	The 'wrapped-up' quietness of this group was even more pronounced this week as we reached the end of *The Pearl*. The tragic end really got to us all, but the sense of achievement in reaching the end was palpable. One participant, who doesn't read much independently, and is normally very quiet, shook her head and said 'that was really, really good. Really, really sad but in a good way'. All members were keen to impress how much the story had meant to them	

Practice Example 3: 'Gaynor' (Case Study)

Gaynor, diagnosed with severe Personality Disorder, resides on Primrose, the specialist psychiatric/therapeutic wing at Low Newton. Gaynor presented some challenges, especially in her highly individual responses to the poetry. The other group participants, for example, had found George Herbert's 'Affliction' a 'powerful' poem about inward pain and trouble, and—in ways akin to Group 2's moved response (see Practice Example 2 above)—had connected William Henley's poem 'Invictus' with aspects of their own situation of imprisonment. This participant described these interpretations as 'misreadings', or dismissed the poems as unnecessarily difficult, or blamed me, as group leader, for failing to read the poems in a way that made them accessible. These views were often steadfastly retained by Gaynor, who was resistant to any modification of them by myself or by other group-members' views. Conversely, when the group struggled with the meaning of Shakespeare's Sonnet 116, this participant claimed the poem was both beautiful and easy to understand and came close to saying that other's failure to 'get' the poem was because of personal defects. A similarly absorbed concentration was often shown in relation to the prose works. When group members were very moved by Raymond Carver's 'Cathedral', Gaynor found the story's conclusion 'disappointing' having found the darkness of the story quite funny, arguing it was a 'black comedy'. When she started to read aloud she wanted to keep reading and when she reluctantly stopped and another prisoner began to read, she sometimes became belligerent, correcting them when they read. Gaynor would also unreasonably expect the group to restart the reading for her benefit if she were delayed. These behaviours were very hard to manage at times and irritated the rest of the group though other group-members were remarkably tolerant.

Though aspects of these behaviours were markedly present during the reading of *The Pearl* (see Group 1, Weeks 1 and 3), Gaynor progressively and demonstrably becomes 'part of' the group response to the book, the collective rapt attention, not resistant to it. Perhaps it's significant that these shifts occurred in relation to prose narrative, where a sustained imaginative attention and sympathetic engagement with other views and worlds is demanded, in contrast to poetry's often briefer intensity. (Notably, Gaynor responded very positively to Helen Hunt Jackson's poem 'October's Bright Blue Weather', liking its 'narrative nature'.)

At any rate, the experience of reading *The Pearl* seemed to 'prime' Gaynor for a key shift which came in relation to *Great Expectations*, several weeks into the book (Month Nine):

A fascinating group in all sorts of ways. A breakthrough with Gaynor. She tried to start the group, wanting to bypass me altogether. I firmly asked her to stop. She said 'I can do your job just as well as you'. The rest of the group laughed out loud at this, forcing Gaynor to take it as a joke, after which she backed off and was content to participate in the group.

The discussion turned to Mrs Joe. The casual domestic violence was regarded as shocking by most of the group, who found Mrs Joe unsympathetic and irredeemable. Gaynor asserted how strong and admirable she was. She tried again to make it an 'I'm right, you're wrong issue', but I was more explicit in stating the expectation that we should be able to hold contradictory views, and there doesn't have to be one right answer. This seemed a genuinely new idea to her! From this point we were able to have a fascinating discussion, particularly focussing on whether Joe was weak in letting Mrs Joe dominate the household. Gaynor was able to contribute fully without demanding everyone agree with her. Afterwards I spoke to her briefly in private, diplomatically reinforcing the group expectations while making sure she was still happy.

Significantly, in the group discussion of Miss Havisham a few weeks later, I noted that Gaynor '*thoughtfully* commented that Miss Havisham was too feeble and this led onto an important discussion of the latter's character and the steely malice at her core'.

Progress of this kind is especially significant for women in the personality disorder unit, in whom inflexible thought patterns and processes are characteristic. Reading, as witnessed here, is a practice of inhabiting a range of imagined positions and understanding from alternative viewpoints, represented by the thinking-feeling presences within the book and within the group. It offers a potentially powerful model for shifting ingrained mental habits and galvanising new ones.[12]

Practice Example 4: 'Two Steps Forward, One Step Back' ('Vicky': Case Study)

Vicky is a young woman near the beginning of a very long sentence. At first it seemed that her chaotic lifestyle and poor mental health meant that her isolated life before coming to prison would continue on the inside. Yet, slowly but surely, with the support of staff and prisoners, things began to get better for her and after protracted negotiations over logistical and security issues, she was able to join the reading group (Group 1). From the beginning, she was a quiet and thoughtful group member who was very dependent on the support of close friends from the wing.

As, over the next two years, the reading group continued beyond the research study which had initiated it, Vicky was to become a stalwart of the group. She relished the challenging literature we read together, including (in the second year of the group) *Frankenstein, Silas Marner* and the whole of Homer's *Odyssey* in verse, which she particularly enjoyed, seeing parallels between Odysseus's journey and her own struggle. By now she had settled down significantly and had worked her way to enhanced status [i.e. the highest privilege level, above basic and standard].

Then things went wrong. She was involved in a violent incident with another prisoner, was segregated for a number of days and downgraded to basic regime. It is a testament to the support of the prison and her own dedication to Shared Reading that she was allowed to come to the group the following week. We were nearing the end of Somerset Maugham's novel *The Painted Veil*. Throughout the novel, Vicky's attitude to the main protagonist, Kitty, had shifted between sympathy and exasperation at her very human failings. At this point in the novel the seemingly changed Kitty weakens, makes a poor choice, and has a temporary return to old patterns of behaviour. Understandably most of the group, including Vicky, were disappointed and angry with the character. In the book, after her relapse, Kitty is disgusted with herself and resolves to continue moving forward:

> What had happened seemed to have happened in another world. She was like a person who has been stricken with sudden madness and recovering is distressed and ashamed at the grotesque things he vaguely remembers to have done when he was not himself. But because he knows he was not himself he feels that in his own eyes at least he can claim indulgence. Kitty thought that perhaps a generous heart might pity rather than condemn her. But she sighed as she thought how woefully her self-confidence had been shattered. The way had seemed to stretch before her straight and easy and now she saw that it was a tortuous way and that pitfalls awaited her. The vast spaces and the tragic and beautiful sunsets of the Indian Ocean rested her. She seemed borne then to some country where she might in freedom possess her soul. If she could only regain her self-respect at the cost of a bitter conflict, well, she must find the courage to affront it.[13]

Vicky said:

> She's vacillating – moving between self-pity and self-loathing. And neither position is right, they're both dangerous, but it's a necessary process. When we do something really bad you've got to go through that self-pity and the self-loathing, don't I know it, to be in that place in the middle where you can

move forward again. And it's by this temporary setback that Kitty can see how far she's come.

This is a language emerging out of saturated thinking inside 'hard' complexity—'moving between ... neither position is right ... that place in the middle'. I had no doubt that while talking about Kitty she was thinking about herself. This middle ground between herself and the book seemed to help Vicky find, like Kitty, a 'generous heart' *within* herself towards the wrong she did when '*not* herself' while acknowledging those actions as *part of* herself. She was seeing clearly, through the text, that, despite temporary setbacks, she had not returned to the beginning of her journey.[14]

Interview with Ann Walmsley, 'Reading Groups on the Inside and on the Outside'

Canadian author and journalist Ann Walmsley talked to Josie Billington in February 2018 about her book, The Prison Book Club, published in 2015. The book recounts Ann's experience of monthly book discussion groups inside secure federal men's institutions in Canada (Collins Bay and Beaver Creek Institutions) while continuing her involvement with a women's book club in Toronto. (Page numbers refer to the Oneworld edition, 2015. When referencing individual prisoners, she uses the pseudonyms she gave them in her book.)

JB: You mention in your book that the men liked non-fiction [for example Greg Mortenson, *Three Cups of Tea: One Man's Mission to Promote Peace... One School at a Time*; Ian Brown, *The Boy in the Moon: A Father's Search for His Disabled Son;* Jeannette Walls, *The Glass Castle: A Memoir*] and enjoyed the sense of participating in something 'timely' and newsworthy. Yet the group-leader Carol—in relation to reading Hemingway at a book club meeting—'wanted more classics for the book list' (p. 239). I wondered whether you became aware of any particular differences in the men's responses to classic literature or literary fiction as opposed to, say, memoir or autobiography?

AW: Relevant books were appreciated because the men felt they were reading something that other people were talking about on the outside. You can't plan for that, you can't predict where the news will go, but you can generally think, well, books about migration at this point in history would resonate. I observed that both contemporary books and classics could feel of the moment. Among classics, John Steinbeck's *The Grapes of Wrath* is about massive migration in America in the 30s but it feels like Europe right now—people looking for work, people leaving areas where they could no longer sustain their families. And when we read it in the prison in 2011, it had echoes of the Occupy Movement that was happening everywhere, which resonated for the men. So, relevance was important.

I do certainly think that classic literary fiction produced a greater richness of thinking. I don't have more than anecdotal evidence, but it's as though the language in those books became a 'feedstock'—a sort of a model for the men's own greater facility with language and more abstract thought. And it got me thinking, what were the mechanisms for this: could it have been the cadence of the language; was it the use of metaphor; was it the silences in better literature that allowed the men to engage more imaginatively with the text?

I do think (not scientifically but anecdotally) that their responses to literary fiction and classic literature moved me the most. I was thinking about the inmate I call Ben responding to the Joad family in *The Grapes of Wrath* and his great appreciation of Rose of Sharon's breast-feeding of a starving man at the end, and how he pointed that out to me and to the other men as an example of humanity. Wow, where did that come from? That's a beautiful moment. And Peter reading O. Henry's short story, 'The Gift of the Magi', and saying the author was thinking about how it's not the value of the gifts that we give, it's the intent, and the love. That blew me away. I was still reflecting at a more superficial level, appreciating the story's irony and the humour. But here he was digging deeper into the text, philosophically. Would that have happened in a discussion about a non-fiction book or a work of autobiography? I don't think so. I think literature invites us to dig a little deeper.

As for autobiographies or memoirs, the men sometimes had a view of those books' authors as being opportunistic and were often harsh in their criticisms. If the authors had a tale of woe, they'd say well, you know, their tale isn't anything compared to what I've been through and what I've seen and known. They were more dismissive of those stories I found, more suspicious of the author, so it was a different kind of engagement.

JB: Perhaps that's the advantage of literary narratives. Though it's not entirely true that all memoirs are misery memoirs, there is a sense in which personal experience is only interesting if it's got suffering in it.

AW: (laughing) You nailed it! A writer can't go to a literary agent with a memoir that isn't a struggle against great adversity, like 'I had a great life'.

Classic literary fiction, by contrast, has the whole range of human experience.

JB: I noticed that you loved it when the guys noted page numbers or read passages out loud.

AW: Yes, I think the alchemy happened most often when the men read aloud, or when one of us read aloud, a passage they had flagged: that meant it was immediately in their heads. I'm thinking of *The Cellist of Sarajevo*, which we read at Beaver Creek, where an inmate I call Richard selected this passage for the men to read:

> If this city is to die, it won't be because of the men on the hills, it will be because of the people in the valley. When they're content to live with death, to become what the men on the hills want them to be, then Sarajevo will die.[15]

Richard said he had written it down because he thought it was the essence of the book. And we all agreed with him. In a prison you might expect that fighting back would be the men's natural response to the idea of being content to live with death. Certainly, they were reluctant to agree with Carol's hypothesis that greater humanity, putting ourselves out for another, was needed to fight this kind of surrender.

But shortly afterwards, an inmate who served as the prison librarian, a book club member I call Bookman, pointed out that one person in the book had dodged sniper bullets every day to get water for his family. And of course, there were others: the baker who dragged the man off the street where he had been shot so that a camera-man couldn't take a photograph of him for the evening news, because that would suggest that civilisation had completely been abandoned, that they would leave their dead in the street. So even though the book club members were resistant to broadening the discussion to humanity and kindness, they were finding their own humane language. Bookman found it in the language of self-sacrifice. I think that wouldn't have happened if Richard hadn't read the passage out loud.

At the Collins Bay Book Club, the medium-security prison where there was a slightly different literacy level (quite a number of them said they hadn't read anything since their last class in high school), we read aloud in the second half of the meeting, after coffee, for half an hour or so. This was part of introducing them to the new book and a way of breaking the inertia towards opening the cover. Because we were demanding a fairly high level of commitment from them—an entire book in one month. And not all styles or genres worked for them.

I'm remembering the example of *Such a Long Journey*, a novel by Rohinton Mistry, where they had such a difficult response to the passages of descriptive narrative. Several complained about how there were 25 pages about a chicken! And of course, we wanted to challenge that response. So Carol read the passage about Crawford Market in Mumbai to them, saying 'What does it make you feel?'—the viscera on the floor, the butcher's full of sweat and flies. It was very smart of her to give them a passage that was gritty and not flowery. They wouldn't perhaps connect with a flowery passage, they couldn't sink their teeth into it, but a gritty passage made them feel something. And then they allowed, after she read the passage, yeah, it's very visual, it's very 3D. That was one way they grew. They didn't naturally love narrative description. But they could be shown the value of it. One inmate, Gaston, said that experience had persuaded him (this is in the book, p. 89): he wasn't going for 'flashy bang and cool story' in a book any more. He was looking for what the writer was thinking or the words the writer was using: and he recognised that he was now looking for different kinds of books instead of fantasies and spy stories: he was looking for books that dealt with real life.

JB: [alluding to the prison reading experiences recounted in Chapters Seven i and Seven ii (above), where the groups do not read the book in advance but read it aloud together in real time] What would you say are the gains (or losses?) of reading the book in advance?

AW: I guess I feel that the gains of reading in advance are that readers get their private time with the book. That lost feeling—of being immersed in the author's imagination, and creating their own visual images. They're creating the world in their mind. I just imagine they would always feel a little bit more self-conscious if they were reading aloud in a group. And reading in advance gives the guys time to mark passages and re-read, go back, check against something else. Those are the gains for reading in advance. Losses? I guess you would lose those who had dyslexia and other reading impediments who maybe month after month would read just 20 pages and then come in feeling self-conscious, only able to participate in the latter half of the meeting when we're raising broader issues. I do think *this* is true of all book groups—read-aloud, or read in advance—that when you're sitting in a circle with other people and responding to a book, you're actually making history. You and the characters and your observations are all being exchanged and remembered. So that later on when you think back about your life, you remember where you were, what room you were in, what the room smelt like, who was sitting across from you and that gets layered on top of the literature that you're talking about—as a third narrative, a shared history; almost like a memory.

JB: Perhaps it's all the more important for people who wouldn't be reading outside of the book group that this kind of imprint or deposit is laid down mentally, imaginatively, emotionally in Shared Reading.

AW: Yes, yes, I agree with that completely.

JB: Do you have a sense of what was most important in engaging the men in reading?

AW: A key element was that the group was volunteer-led, by people from outside the prison, and that it was secular. As most of the volunteers in Canadian federal prisons are from faith groups and there to facilitate hymn-singing and other forms of spiritual practice, the inmates initially couldn't understand why we would bother to come hear what they had to say about books without being paid and without a religious agenda. In my view it contributed to an atmosphere of openness and trust.

Institutional support was also important in providing a safe place both for the volunteers and the inmates—a place of recreation that wasn't right next to the basketball gym; a less chaotic, quiet place, so that people could really cocoon. Also a place without guards, a place of refuge, where the inmates felt safe and could express themselves.

The ambassador programme was a help. Carol invited several of the more dedicated readers in each book club to be ambassadors for the club—recruiting new members when prisoners got transferred out, or making sure people were getting the book read.

We discovered that giving the club members the books to keep was a big motivation. Inmates had so few possessions, each book became a precious object. It could be read and given to other family members or a cellmate. Some inmates donated their books to the prison library when they left. According to the prison librarian those books were circulated more frequently than other books.

So word got out even though we're talking about a prison population of 450 men and a book club of only 15–18. There was a sort of privilege attached to the books. And privileges in prison are so rare. To have a bookshelf set aside of donated books that are reserved just for the book club—that was very obvious to the rest of the prison population. All this was certainly reinforced by author visits. When a famous author like Lawrence Hill (author of *The Book of Negroes*) visited the Collins Bay Book Club, suddenly everyone wanted to be in the book club!

Another great thing was exchanging comments with a book club on the outside. In doing so, the men were not just talking about books in the prison bubble. They were actually establishing a lifeline for themselves to the outside world.

JB: Yes, your description of passing on the men's comments to the women who are reading the same book, and who are stunned into silence by the idea (coming out of a house of correction) that 'goodness was more contagious than evil', is very powerful (Chapter 18, p. 228). I notice, at the very end, you say that you would choose the prison book club over the Toronto women's club. It reminded me of what you record Lawrence Hill saying after his visit to Collins Bay, when he describes the conversation there as the 'most intimate' he'd ever had about his work: these guys 'have more need', he says (pp. 42, 46).

AW: Yes. That need. And I think my scribbling away frantically during the book club when insightful things were said must also have been reinforcing for the men. When I wrote notes, they realised they were saying something important. They could see when they had impressed me.

JB: In addition to the interviews, you encouraged the men to keep journals. It's clear from the book that the journals allowed the men to reflect on their reading experiences and even extend, in both time and 'inner' reach, the affective influence of the books. Was this an unexpected outcome of the journal writing?

AW: Yes, I was stunned by the quality of what they wrote and the self-awareness that came about through sitting with the book and then sitting with the journal. In my instruction to the guys I said, respond to the book, tell me about your life. There were two strands. The book is happening and your life is happening. I was encouraging them to look at the connections.

At author readings, I often read this passage that Peter wrote in response to Diane Ackerman's *The Zookeeper's Wife* about the animals that appeared inside the walls of his prison: 'I came to realise that the resident bird population here is not unlike the resident and employed human population here. Predator, preyed upon, and scavenger. But, among the human element it is difficult to discern which is which' (p. 224). When I read that passage to an audience, almost every time I hear a sigh of amazement. The interviewer will say 'That's publishable'. Peter went on to write his journals even after he left Collins Bay. He kept going and, as I understand it, he has enough for a book now.

And you know they could see me writing all the time. When they wrote and reflected and observed changes in themselves, we were writers together.

JB: Throughout you speak of Carol's mission to offer, via fiction, reading models 'worth emulating' (p. 25) and 'to rally the men's moral selves' (p. 21). Her message is often very direct and explicit. Where Carol's urgent mission is to change the men, yours seems (more patiently) to see how the book club helps to unfold who they are.

AW: I did come at it differently, from the point of view of being a writer and wanting to understand these men as they were, only knowing that in my book choices I was hoping to make them love literature. What I discovered along the way was that I felt like I was a character in a novel myself. I went in thinking I wanted one thing, to help these men love literature, and I came out realising I haven't changed them, they've changed me; they've expanded my humanity. When I asked Ben what was his favourite book, he said 'Oh I don't have a favourite book, each of these books becomes a new window in my life'. I loved that response. When Gaston was reading *The Book of Negroes* and saw that Aminata had survived slavery by reading Jonathan Swift's *Gulliver's Travels*, he chose Swift for his own summer reading. That inspired me to read a book that was prized by a character in another novel we read. The generosity of these fellows—the time they gave me, working hard at their journals. For me it was really—friendship. I was the one who was privileged to be there.

JB: For me the most deeply affecting moment in the book is when, after reading T. S. Eliot's 'The Journey of the Magi', Carol gives the men lamb-shaped Christmas ornaments made of wool. 'They cradled the balls of fluff in their hand. No-one joked that the gifts were silly or useless, at least not in front of us' (p. 151). It seems really important that you value these smaller moments, for what they are, whether or not they can be replicated or lead to personal transformation. I suppose this is related to your sense that 'the men were bringing their best selves to the book club and trying to live a different life for a couple of hours' (p. 17).

AW: I absolutely agree with that and I love that you observed it. That's how I felt. I did ask Frank, one of the most avid readers, much later, 'Did the book club change you?' And he said, 'No, it was just a good way to pass the time'. This was the day I visited his house to give him a copy of the book. But he did take me up to the second floor to show me, along his bed, the display of all the books he'd been reading—a rich array. He was showing me that he wasn't going back to his true crime books.

JB: In the book, you relate your journey with the men very movingly to a literal journey you took with your late father to Little Gidding and to the T. S. Eliot poem which bears that name [from *Four Quartets,* 1944]. There is a 'web of meaning', you say, that connects 'the men to me, me to my father' (p. 150). It has to do with what Eliot says in 'Little Gidding': what you came for is a purpose 'beyond the end you figured', one which 'is altered in fulfilment'.[16]

AW: The passage is right in the middle of the book. While I was sort of aware of the memory in my consciousness when we read 'The Journey of the Magi', it wasn't until much later that I wrote it. I woke up one morning and I just sat down and put it all together—the stuff that was happening in my unconscious. And I ended up crying as I wrote it and I've never cried while writing anything before.

It was just so unexpected, it was just so beautiful. The two journeys that we were on—and the discovery that I was not doing what I thought I was doing at the beginning.

JB: It's several years since you wrote the book. How does the journey strike you now?

AW: It still feels like a period when I was living more fully. I was living the examined life with these men. Sometimes I get emotional because I think, how will I ever have as rich an experience again? I was so very lucky.

Notes

1. Pseudonyms are used throughout the chapter.
2. R. Carver, *All of Us: The Collected Poems* (London: The Harvill Press, 1997), p. 65.
3. The research was approved by North and Yorkshire National Health Service Research Ethics Committee.
4. J. Robinson and J. Billington, 'An Evaluation of a Pilot Study of a Literature-Based Intervention with Women in Prison' (Centre for Research into Reading, Literature and Society, University of Liverpool, 2013), pp. 27–29. https://www.liverpool.ac.uk/media/livacuk/instituteofpsychology/FullPrisonReportJBMarch52013,.pdf.
5. M. Oliver, 'Wild Geese', in *Staying Alive*, ed. by N. Astley (Hexham: Bloodaxe Books, 2002), p. 28.
6. Robinson and Billington, p. 31; see also below, Chapter 9.

7. M. Strand, *Collected Poems* (New York: Knopf Publishing, 2016), p. 185.
8. Robinson and Billington, p. 35 and see Chapter 9, below.
9. W. H. Davies, *Collected Poems* (London: A. C. Fifield, 1916), p. 19.
10. T. Hughes, *The Hawk in the Rain* (London: Faber & Faber, 1957), p. 17.
11. W. Henley, *Works: Poems*, 2 vols. (London: David Nutt, 1901), vol. I, p. 125.
12. J. Billington, E. Longden, and J. Robinson, 'A Literature-Based Intervention for Women Prisoners: Preliminary Findings', *International Journal of Prisoner Health*, 12.4 (2016), 230–243.
13. S. Maugham, *The Painted Veil* (Harmondsworth: Penguin Books Ltd., 1953), pp. 226–27.
14. 'Evaluation of Shared Reading Groups in Psychologically Informed Planned Environments (PIPEs) at HMP Frankland and HMP Low Newton', The Reader Organisation, 2015. See also Chapter 20, below.
15. S. Galloway, *The Cellist of Sarajevo* (London: Atlantic Books, 2008), p. 206.
16. T. S. Eliot, 'Little Gidding', in *Four Quartets* (London: Faber & Faber, 1959), p. 36.

8

Reading in Clinical Contexts

Grace Farrington, Kate McDonnell and Helen Cook

Grace Farrington, 'Reading and Mental Illness'

Grace Farrington writes of her experience of reading with patients suffering severe and protracted mental ill health at an in-patient facility.[1] *'Nigel', diagnosed with personality disorder, is a long-term resident of a high secure hospital supporting the provision of specialist care to forensic psychiatric patients. 'Angela' hears voices and has spent many years in psychiatric care.*

Nigel

The particular focus of this ward is rehabilitation. It is where patients are assessed before being transferred out of the hospital, although patients can still be on the ward for several years. A reading group had been running on the ward for the past two years, promoted by a ward psychiatrist and,

G. Farrington (✉) · K. McDonnell
The Reader, Liverpool, UK
e-mail: graceframe@thereader.org.uk

K. McDonnell
e-mail: katemcdonnell@thereader.org.uk

H. Cook
NHS Service User, Royal Liverpool Hospital, Liverpool, UK

J. Billington (ed.), *Reading and Mental Health*,
https://doi.org/10.1007/978-3-030-21762-4_8

latterly, delivered by myself. The group had got into, I realised, a routine of steadily reading through a book rather than regularly breaking for discussion, settling for a manageable level of stimulation and group interaction. What had not been tried for a while were shorter stories or poems. The psychiatrist suggests that starting off with these might help revitalise the group.

Nigel first drew my attention by the way he kept his eyes fixed on the book (the group was reading *David Copperfield*) almost throughout the session, responding very little to the other people in the room. I wondered what he felt in relation to the book, whether he was moved by it, and whether he and I were both engaged in the same mutual experience of reading as we followed Dickens's thoughts down the page. It was only as I began to learn more about some of the characteristics of the patients on the ward that my expectations of how they might be affected by the literature began to change. It would not be possible to use my own feeling about the text as an accurate measure of what the rest of the group were feeling. I was coming up against the challenge that mental illness represents to the ideal of a sharable human experience. As the ward staff member who sat in on the sessions put it, personality disorder patients tend to 'break away' from normality; the lengthy programme of rehabilitation is designed to try to help them to get 'back to' it.

Nigel's apparent lack of emotional response might be viewed negatively as a symptom; an indication of what Nigel *cannot* do. Yet Nigel was at the same time the most committed member of the reading group. There were occasions when he would be waiting near the door of the ward for me to arrive. It was clearly an event that he anticipated and valued as a significant part of his week. This factor alone suggests the problem was not to do with what was lacking in Nigel, in terms of feeling or interest. As I found out, it was more that he struggled to know how to *read* what was going on around him—to make a connection between what he saw and the feeling that ought to accompany that experience.

Nigel would sometimes try almost to talk himself through this process, wondering aloud what the real purpose of an emotional language might be. The short poem 'Boy at the Window' by Richard Wilbur (1957), first inhabits, in stanza 1, a child's perspective as he looks at a snowman and 'weeps to hear the wind prepare/A night of gnashings and enormous moan'; then shifts, in stanza 2, to the viewpoint of the 'man of snow' who is 'content/Having no wish to go inside and die', but is nonetheless 'moved to see the youngster cry … surrounded by/Such warmth, such light, such love, and so much fear'.[2] After a pause, Nigel returned to the last line:

I wonder what 'fear' is being spoken of there at the end of the poem. Any ideas? Are people afraid for, you know, the welfare of small boys, or is he talking about the small boy's fear?

'Are people afraid for …' places the feeling as something to be interrogated, something that belongs to 'people' but not individually to Nigel, and yet it also acknowledges the possibility of having such a feeling. He goes on to ask another question:

It's saying 'the small boy weeps to hear the wind prepare'. Now why do, why is the boy weeping. Weeping 'cause the snowman is standing alone in the 'dusk and cold'. So he's very sympathetic to Mr Snowman. But the snowman's quite happy where he is thank you.

Nigel is concerned about the superfluous expression of emotion in any setting, unsure of what to make of it if there are no apparent grounds for its expression. For him, the poem seems to inherit this more general difficulty from a world that he does not quite understand or even feel a part of. Yet the poem itself offers a turnaround of conventional worldly expectations in the break between the two stanzas, and the alteration of position that follows. The 'normal' thing would be for the snowman to feel pity for his *own* condition, as the apparently forsaken one who is about to melt away. But instead of staying stuck within himself he is 'moved' beyond his own 'frozen element' to drop a melting tear for the child on the other side of the window pane. This very act of reciprocal mirroring and reflecting back is itself beyond the norms of possibility—overcoming the rational separation between the human and the non-human, the inanimate cold and the warm tears. It is a way of representing the human in a form which is alien to it, 'the man of snow', in order that the feeling can be translated back into life. This is the area that Nigel is (and needs to be) interested in, even if the way he has to express such interest is through a kind of objection to the poem.

For Nigel is almost stuck with the one single position: the snowman's contentment makes sense to him, but he cannot then occupy that additional position of the boy who feels for the snowman.

I keep coming back to this 'so much fear' thing at the end, with the child 'surrounded' by 'so much fear'. I suppose the child is fearful that the snowman's gonna get cold out there. That's a strange thing to think of but that seems to be just about the only problem somebody has in the cold. You know cold climate is – that somebody's going to be damaged by it.

Nigel often needs others who are also in the room to help him to grasp possible alternatives. But here he grapples for himself with that 'strange' reciprocity and how it might be reached or achieved. When the problem of the 'fear' is exchanged for a problem of the natural—that of literally surviving in the cold—Nigel is still trying to make it more manageable for himself. But the ungrounded part of him keeps coming back to the 'fear thing', and it is the same instinct which allows him to pull out that word 'damage' in connection with the fear. 'Somebody' is one indicator that there is a potential translation of the poem into thought which is deeper and more personal than the ostensible subject of the poem: that of a child and a snowman.

In one of my final sessions on the ward, we read a sonnet by Keats, beginning:

> Four seasons fill the measure of the year;
> There are four seasons in the mind of man.

Nigel focussed on the part which refers to Autumn:

> Quiet coves
> His soul has in its Autumn, when his wings
> He furleth close[3]
>
> *Nigel:* I was just thinking about the ducks, who can fly, but don't do very much of it.
> They are busy furling their wings …

He is referring to the ducks that are often to be seen in the hospital grounds in the area onto which each ward, housed in its own separate building, opens out. Certain patients who are based in the rehabilitation wards can ask to take a walk here, and Nigel does this quite regularly. He has taken an interest in the ducks, and the issue of their safety, realising the threat of 'damage' posed by other birds. Yet he also seems aware of how he has begun to identify with the ducks as with another kind of non-human living thing:

> But I think they perform a very useful function here reminding us that, you know, the seasons are going round and that kind of social living that they enjoy is also enjoyed by us. Last year, I was on an R&R [Reasoning and Rehabilitation] course and the teacher gave us a big sheet of paper on a flip chart and said put down all the emotions you can think of. And all the emotions came down, starting with hate, and they came down and down different emotions being written in and suggested. But at the end of it nobody

suggested love or friendship at all. You know they were just not there, in the list. So I think the ducks are quite a beneficial aspect of our stay here.

It is a 'useful function' that the hospital authorities, who have arranged for the provision of the R&R course, would not tend to encourage: the ducks are in fact treated as a pest. But what Nigel is seeing here is the restoration of a natural order even from within the boundaries of that highly regulated institutional framework. The ducks are for him a vital reminder of what the environment itself seems to argue against: that at some level he does still play a part in this community of living things, however isolated he often appears to be in relation to other people on the ward. It is the word 'furleth' which has caught Nigel's imagination. The physical action of a bird folding its wings triggers his imagination almost to feel what that is like, in a way that Nigel could not quite feel the child's fear in the Wilbur poem. This reminder of what Nigel does know or might be able to access is the more significant given that Nigel knows how big the gaps are in his own personal experience. He understands that 'love' and 'friendship' ought to have a place in the list, when recalling the workshop on emotions, and that they stand for something to which he ought to be able to relate. But what he notices is how this is profoundly missing, from his own life, as well as from the lives, or at least the mentality, of his fellow-patients.

In this context, it is significant that Nigel, always rather a lone figure, began to find a particular role for himself, in helping another member of the group, Rick, with pronouncing unknown or difficult words. Nigel had been educated to degree level and admitted to enjoying the opportunity that reading aloud gave him to 'show off'. But his approach towards Rick, who, now in his fifties, learned to read only since coming into hospital, was careful and considered, first giving Rick time to attempt the word, before slowly pronouncing it himself, marking each syllable to make sense of the word. He later did the same with another group member who struggled to read because of a stammer. In this demonstration of an attentiveness not just to the reading but to the fellow reader, it was as if reading aloud became for Nigel a medium for kindly human contact.

Angela

The reading group that Angela attended took place in the early afternoon. There were usually a number of patients dozing, and often a drowsy lull in the atmosphere. Angela told me that the television, which was always on in the lounge area, could feel 'hypnotising' after a while. There were rarely any signs of communication between patients. Angela was often seated on her own, sometimes after having taken refuge in a smaller sitting room which she liked to call 'the parlour'. Angela suffered from very low moods. I would sometimes find her crying and talking to herself distractedly. 'They'—she told me more than once—had 'wiped her memory'; it was 'empty', 'wiped clean'. Whether an effect of the medication, or a kind of persecutory delusion, this thought represented something traumatic that Angela felt had happened to her. Often she was caught up in what to another person would sound like a strange, otherworldly narrative of events. She talked of being 'burned to cinders' during the night, of having died over and over again, and of there being some kind of requirement that she should fulfil the role of a saviour.

One early discovery was that the psychotic symptoms did not necessarily have the effect of distorting the reading, and need not stop Angela from reading. When a poem by Emily Brontë was introduced, prefixed on the page by the title and the name of the poet, Angela, as if recognising it or quickly identifying with the poem, said: 'Oh, I wrote this'. She said the same of Wordsworth's 'I wandered lonely as a cloud', which reminded her of a personally known, beneficent voice: that of her father, whom she remembered reciting the poem. On at least three occasions she said that she would save the poem we had been reading to give to her father (whom I doubt she now sees, if indeed he is still alive). She was quite clear about the poems that he would have liked.

As well as identifying sometimes with multiple people at a time ('I'm x, I'm y'), Angela was also regularly affected by the voices she heard. In the reading group these voices would sometimes add to the competing claims upon Angela's attention, including that of the text itself and the other people in the room, thus involving her in multiple conversations at a time. At other times her gaze would become fixed and her eyes would glaze over a little, as if the internal voices that she was hearing had become suddenly louder or more insistent. I was often conscious when reading aloud to this group of the need to use my own voice, and make eye contact with individual people, to create a kind of invisible net of support, to carry people with me. It was a way of using my eyes to try to interest them in what I was saying with my voice, and of staying with them long enough that they might begin to stay with the text. I noted down after one session the 'lifting of Angela's gaze until she is looking at me as I am reading'. At the end she had commented: 'it holds you doesn't it'. And on another occasion she told me: 'You hold a person when you read a book, you know'. It is an instance of Frost's 'momentary stay against confusion' (see Chapter 3). To find this temporary hold, and indeed to be held as an adult, is like having one's own strength reinforced; feeling held together; finding a foothold.

Yet there was a difference between welcome and unwelcome voices; between voices that often threatened or seemed to inflict death and those that might speak of the 'secret' of life. At best, poems seemed able to offer the latter. Reading, like being spoken to, when it works well, can allow a person to hear thoughts 'spoken' that they seem to have had inwardly themselves. This makes reading a quite different activity to the dreaming mind's evocation of fantasy. Imaginary thoughts become a vessel for a kind of shared reality. Angela was sometimes particularly attuned to hearing those thoughts.

On a day when Angela had been particularly unwell, I was told by the staff that she had needed to be given extra medication an hour beforehand to calm her. It was only when we had come to the final poem, 'The Flower of Mending' (1917) by the troubadour poet Vachel Lindsay, that Angela for the first time that day seemed 'held' by what we were reading. Only Angela and myself were left in the room and Angela was keen to continue:

> When Dragon-fly would fix his wings,
> When Snail would patch his house,
> When moths have marred the overcoat
> Of tender Mister Mouse,
>
> The pretty creatures go with haste
> To the sunlit blue-grass hills
> Where the Flower of Mending yields the wax
> And webs to help their ills.
>
> The hour the coats are waxed and webbed
> They fall into a dream,
> And when they wake the ragged robes
> Are joined without a seam.
>
> My heart is but a dragon-fly,
> My heart is but a mouse,
> My heart is but a haughty snail
> In a little stony house.
>
> Your hand was honey-comb to heal,
> Your voice a web to bind.
> You were a Mending Flower to me
> To cure my heart and mind.[4]

The poet addresses this to 'Cousin Eudora', to whom he paid a visit during a time when he was out of favour with other family and struggling to find enough money to live on. He later wrote, 'it was the kind hearts around me in that particular spot that made me want to live'.[5] I thought the poem might make Angela think of people in her own life whose 'hand' or 'voice' had been dear to her. (I knew she had a husband who still visited her, and that she was a mother to several children.) Yet Angela focused initially on the non-human—the dragonfly and the snail, and the suggestion of a bee given the presence of the 'honey-comb'. There was then a long pause (half a minute at least). Gradually, Angela began to wonder about the flower itself.

> Odd isn't it. It's a strange flower: heals, makes honey. And heals the dragonfly; and the snail, when they go on it. Strange flower isn't it. I've never heard of a, a mending, mending flower - flower of mending. It's one that heals, a flower that heals – a dragonfly if it's hurt its wings or anything, or a snail's hurt himself, or that's hurt himself, that heals it.

There is something much more vulnerable about Angela's statement than even Nigel's word 'damage' might have indicated. It is her openness to the idea of 'a flower that heals' which has disclosed the sensitivity, even at the level of the nerve endings, of 'hurt'. This is the emotional area that the poem is actually working in, even through those tiny representatives, the fly and the snail. It is as though Angela finds the poem's hidden hurt (which is not made explicit in the poem—the closest word is 'ills', line 8) by imaginatively recreating the poem in her own human terms. The poetic indicator is in the shift from 'hurts *its* wings' to 'hurts *himself*'; from the creaturely illustration to the personal depth of human feeling.

It was during this session that Angela said of poetry 'It makes your feeling come out'. Trying to describe the way it brought relief without blunting feeling, she added: 'It makes you feel inside true'. At the beginning Angela had a heavy look about her—her head resting on her hand. By the end she was smiling—grinning; making eye contact, sitting back against the chair and resting her hands on her stomach, contentedly.

* * *

During one reading session, Nigel read a piece he had written at the creative writing class he had begun to attend, in which he remembered being a child of eight or nine, going down to the local river with his sister to play. It was the first time he made reference to anyone he had known or been close to. The reading had helped to show him a way he might do that, and perhaps a reason for doing it too. Significantly, on this first occasion of relating something of himself and his own story to others, he began with an early memory, from before his adult troubles began.

Back with Angela, at one point, we read Henry Van Dyke's 'A Child in the Garden' (1903) together:

> ... I dared to tread that garden loved of yore,
> That Eden lost unknown and found unsought.
>
> Then just within the gate I saw a child, –
> A stranger-child, yet to my heart most dear;
> He held his hands to me, and softly smiled
> With eyes that knew no shade of sin or fear:
> 'Come in,' he said, 'and play awhile with me;
> 'I am the little child you used to be.'[6]

Angela tried to imagine the motive for this poem:

> He could be an old gentleman, and he's wishing to have, wishing it could happen again I think, to him. Or what he saw – saw then, he can see now. Realize it now.

At its most profound, literary reading can make available a 'now' that is not simply felt as damaged, but which contains the good of the past ('used to be'), *together with* the hurt of the present.

Kate McDonnell and Helen Cook, 'Reading and Chronic Pain'

Kate McDonnell has been running a Shared Reading group for people living with chronic pain at the weekly pain clinic of a city hospital (see Chapters 10–12 *for research findings connected to this group). She has lived with rheumatoid arthritis herself over the past three decades. Helen, a pain patient, has been attending the reading group for two years, and has recently completed a volunteer training course to become a group leader herself.*

Kate

As I prepared reading material for the first session with this group (the first time I had worked with chronic pain sufferers) I was very conscious of the particular difficulties which Shared Reading might present. Chronic pain affects every aspect of a person's daily life, from physical mobility and inclination for everyday tasks, to sheer energy for life. I anticipated that group members may have trouble sitting for any length of time and might struggle to attend sessions, given that walking any distance or accessing public transport would often be out of the question. I was also well aware that it is common for people with pain to experience anxiety and low mood and that the analgesic and anti-depressant drugs administered to alleviate these very symptoms can often lead to excessive tiredness and poor motivation. I decided to adapt the Shared Reading model accordingly. As attendance was likely to be more fractured than with a standard group, I chose to focus exclusively on short stories, extracts and poems, so that each session could be 'stand-alone'. I also opted to use stories with a strong plot line or with a strong focus on 'feeling' or emotional response, sensing that these would work best in terms of distracting people from their pain where the concentration levels required for more difficult texts would be too great and pain would intrude.

The first early surprise for me was that participants universally showed a preference for more challenging texts—works which were intellectually as well as emotionally demanding—as the 'difficult' stories and poems made them think more deeply. All group members agreed that reading and puzzling together over meaning produced closer concentration and absorbed attention to details of language, and reduced awareness of pain. It appeared the more participants were focused on thinking in a literary way about the stories or poems, reading closely and carefully, the less they were affected by their pain or the more distanced from it they became: 'the extra mental effort helped shift immersion to another level and blocked out the pain more successfully'.[7] The mental challenge of reading seemed to create a state of 'flow'.[8] People lost awareness of their physical needs and bodily state, 'becoming more fully themselves – more fulfilled and absorbed, more vitally alive – in forgetting the self, whilst engaged in meaningful activity' (Billington et al. 2014, p. 24).

One particular session stands out for me, some months into the reading group, when the group of around ten members had become well-established.[9] We were reading Edith Wharton's short story, 'Mrs Manstey's View', in which the protagonist has only the back view from her New York apartment to live for, until the development of a neighbouring building obscures it. The story is a sad one, and I had some worries about my choice when I realised that one particular group member, Janet, was there. Her presence was unexpected as Janet was dealing with a lot of problems at that time—family illnesses, hospital tests, her mother's growing infirmity and reluctance to accept help—and she had indicated that she might struggle to attend. She was feeling quite overwhelmed by the sense that everything was going wrong, and I was concerned that the story could tap into currents of feeling very close to the surface. I was mindful of what had happened a few weeks before when we were reading Elizabeth Bowen's story 'The Visitor', in which a young boy tries to know, before anyone can tell him, the news he awaits of his mother's death. 'I can't let them tell me. It would be as though they saw me see her being killed!'[10] 'He wants to be alone for the first wave of the shock – where no one can see him', said Janet and, quickly becoming emotional, recounted how she had told her own child of his grandfather's death. "I'll always remember, he just turned away, he just took a few steps away from me. Just for a few seconds. It was a horrible experience that. This just reminded me'. As the session ended she said, 'I can honestly say that's the only story I haven't enjoyed. I don't know what it was'.

In fact, in relation to the Edith Wharton story ('Mrs Manstey's View') that I had worried about reading for Janet's sake, it was another group member, Susan, who was the first to relate it to her personal experience:

> This upsets me, you know,'cause my dad can't, my dad doesn't go out. But he knows, you know, the people going to church, he says to me Mrs So and So passes every day. It quite upsets me thinking – Is that all there is for him? That he's content like that?

A general discussion followed about whether 'living our life through everyone else' could really be called a life, and about the need for 'connection'. But there was recognition also that, while Mrs Manstey's range of vision and experience was severely restricted, what she did see was 'lovely'. The view from her window is a 'whole world' as Susan put it. Helen (Cook, see below) took up this idea of contraction and how it can be more intense than limitless opportunity.

> The garden is alive. It's growing. That's how she connects with the world, by watching these processes. She notices things in tiny detail that would bypass us – we'd take things for granted. I've kind of noticed it myself as my circumstances have changed. Things I'd always aspired to and wanted have totally

> changed. I think you learn what you can't do. Rather than struggling you learn to enjoy doing other things. I remember enjoying some things – camping for example - but I don't want to do it anymore. I don't know where the desire goes or how the shift happens.

Janet now spoke at length for the first time:

> I can understand that because my mum hasn't been out for a few years now and she's got accustomed to it. My mum's only got me, I'm an only child. It gets frustrating sometimes. But - she's … content. She's got her garden and she enjoys her gardening. What I'm trying to say is I can understand this woman through the way my mum has her own little set thing.

At the end of the story, Mrs Manstey dies at the window, the view as yet 'undisturbed':[11]

> Susan: Her whole world had gone. Oh it's so sad. But it was nice the way it says at the end 'Her head fell back and smiling she died'.
>
> Helen: Yes, the building wasn't continued for her; the building had stopped and for her it never happened.
>
> Susan: The view was still there when she died. Her world was still there. I think that's lovely.

Janet did become upset at this point, crying a little, involuntarily. This time, however, she said how much she had enjoyed the session, that it 'had brought out a lot of things' especially in relation to the struggle she was having with her mother—wanting to do things for her and thinking she knew what was best, while being constantly pushed away. It was as though by tuning into what made Mrs Manstey contented, she saw from her mother's perspective that small things, which might look like nothing to someone else, might be important to her. As Helen had pointed out, reading from the text, 'a view in which the most optimistic eye would at first have failed to discover anything admirable', was to Mrs Manstey herself, 'radiant' (Wharton, pp. 2, 5).

I have since used this story in an annotated anthology for volunteer group leaders as an example of how Shared Reading can help people acknowledge or occupy those 'shifts' of perspective which Helen spoke about. Mrs Manstey's death prompted Susan, for example, to talk of when she had trained as a counsellor in palliative care and the difficulty of 'trying to explain to families that it's not really what *they* want that counts when a person is dying'. She related this to a discussion she had had in a pain therapy group about 'how people were taking our choices away'. In the course of this session, Susan had been first a grieving daughter, then the counsellor who could understand the daughter's sorrow and help modify it, and then the pain sufferer herself, able to reflect on the therapy she had received. These flexible shifts of position come from a person who habitually describes her brain 'as spongy' following a stroke. Significantly, Susan sent a text to me the following day saying how good the group had been and how much she and others had brought their lives into the session. Susan also referred to this story months later, saying of Mrs Manstey, 'I love her' and adding that the stories 'make me think about things beyond things'.

The session was memorable also for the response to the poem which followed the story, Norman Nicholson's 'A Pot Geranium'. I focus here on Andrew, who had joined the group in only the last few weeks. 'Mrs Manstey's View' had recalled to him the elderly woman living on her own with whom he used to lodge when he was a long-distance lorry-driver. 'She used to expect me and watch for my wagon. She always knew when I was late.' When a young couple moved in next door and built an extension, 'she couldn't see any more so she didn't know when I was coming'. This was Andrew's first contribution of length in the group: it is 'about' his own former life and also a poignant tale of somebody else's pain. This was also the first time he read aloud. The lines from the poem read by Andrew concern a person confined to a hospital bed (thighs and spine 'clamped', 'looping strings' twined round the chest) seeing a crimson kite flying in wind outside, and regretting that 'wind and sun/Are mine no longer, nor have I kite to claim them'. 'But', the poem goes on,

> there on a shelf
> In the warm corner of my dormer window
> A pot geranium flies its red balloon[12]

Susan: This is like when you're in pain, this little bit here isn't it. The doctor always says to me, if you're in really bad pain, think, it's not going to last forever. There will be a bright light at the end. So you've got to think about that.

Helen: That there is still life.

Janet: That's what gets me about the geranium, you know, 'Contains the pattern, the prod and the pulse of life'. I think that's lovely that.

Andrew: And the joy of seeing the kite has been assimilated into the geranium. I like that.

Towards the close of the poem, the speaker compares his 'circumscribed' situation to that of a limpet 'confined .../To one small radius of rock'. Yet, he says, 'I eat the equator, breathe the sky' (Nicholson, p. 32).

> Helen: It's got – wider. Now it's gone to the breadth of existence, anything and everything is all there for you.
> Kate: How do you get that when your ways are circumscribed, confined?
> Andrew: Those two last lines, that's me [re-reads]... that just takes me back to what I used to do. I used to love driving. As I came off the ferry at Dover, and I got onto the A16, and I'd just do what I do in the wheelchair now: sheer relaxation, and sheer sort of 'Look what I've got in front of me. That's where I breathe the sky'.
> Helen: I access it by reading.

Momentarily, Andrew's wheelchair is emotionally connected to his past, rather than being the most visible symptom of his disadvantaged present: more it is, for a second, a *means* to peace in the here and now—suddenly itself an *advantage*. These shifts away from default attitude and usual language—'I breathe the sky'—are involuntary happenings, not intended outcome, as they might be in more formal therapy.

Witnessing this moment for himself at interview, Andrew said:

> The poem is saying everything is there combined for life. The geranium starts off as a small thing and then its life goes on and on doesn't it?

He added, later:

> Helen had been so quiet, and then suddenly she sort of came alive. There are little moments like that where you are just quite subdued and then bing, it is like the light comes on. And you can feel that happening inside like a connection.

These vital inner happenings are especially important in relation to chronic pain, as the pain consultant at the clinic always explains to patients as part of a pain management course. There are specialised cells in your body, he says, whose job it is to detect and transmit pain and nothing else. Usually pain is picked up by one of these receptors, and impulses are sent through the nervous system to the brain. What happens in people with chronic pain, however, is that other nerves are recruited into this 'pain' pathway which start to fire off messages to the brain when there is no physical stimulus or damage.

'When we look back through case notes for people who have been coming for a long time, we often see that we're treating a different area to the one we were concerned with originally, and that's because the pain wiring system has set itself up and the body's joined in with it'. But the body can 'unjoin' again. Nerve blockers (drugs) are one way; reading might be another.[13]

Andrew's very language—came alive, bing, the light comes on—is a kind of testimony that the inner connections which happen in reading can galvanise the over-rigidity of nervous impulses or 'pain pathways' by firing new messages or producing a mental 're-wiring' of kinds.

Andrew's quasi-physical language also resonates with my own experience of this group. The bond of intimacy, always strong in Shared Reading, is especially palpable in this group compared with others I run. Perhaps it has to do with the intuitive and implicit shared experience of suffering, living and thinking with pain. The connection between us all is itself bodily, occurring almost at cellular level. This is curious insofar as group members rarely talk about their pain directly. It is as though the story or poem acts as a carrier for our shared pain, holding us together as one body, one mind.

I asked Helen whether she had felt this too, when I invited her to reflect on her experience of Shared Reading.

Helen

It is like a collaboration of thoughts. It is very different to normal chat with someone. And I think it is because, as we talk through different stories and poems, we all at different times open ourselves. We share very personal stuff—not every week, but we all have done so at some point—and it is not very often about pain. Funnily enough it is very rarely about pain. But we open ourselves to the group and say look I am vulnerable and this is how I am feeling. And everyone is accepting of that. I think there's an unspoken bond between us because of that—because we have said, you know, this is the real me. You don't do that when you are just having a cup of tea or you bump into someone at Sainsbury's. You don't bare your soul. The only people you do that with are very close friends, partners and therapists but there is always a comeback to whatever you say: in this there isn't.

There is never any judgement. When you read something or say something there's no return to the therapist. There's no why, what, when, where, who—'Well, why don't you', 'how did you feel', 'why did you do that'. There is none of that. There is just, in this moment, I feel this and I am thinking about this. This relates to my life at this point because of … And that's it. People listen but they don't—'therapise' isn't a word is it. But they don't make it feel like therapy. You don't get a grilling on it, or told what to do next time. Instead you are given that time to explore whatever you are going through at that time. You are not asked to relate personally to it: you just do.

And there is comfort there if you need it. I mean there have been times when people have cried or have got upset. The reading gets out thoughts that would otherwise stay inside. But it is not made a 'thing'. You won't necessarily talk about it ever again, because it won't be pertinent to whatever you are reading next. It is given freely and it is accepted freely, with silent understanding. We are all experiencing pain, and to be in that group kind of normalises our abnormality if you like.

Maybe that is why we pick up on each other's cues. Andrew, for example, is often very quiet. I have seen him going to speak, but hesitating. He doesn't necessarily speak straight away. He takes a breath and a pause, and in that breath and a pause, other people have spoken: he can be 'over-spoken' quite easily. I've been aware that I want to give him space to think. So, now when Andrew wants to say something, I try to draw on it so that what he's trying to say can become a thought and stay in the room.

When I did the Read to Lead course [The Reader training programme][14] and learned how to listen carefully to group members and pay attention to even slight utterances, I was kind of aware that I had sort of learned that from being in the group anyway.[15]

Notes

1. Originally part of a PhD research study (funded by an Arts and Humanities Collaborative Doctoral Award) this project was approved by the Liverpool East Research Ethics Committee.
2. R. Wilbur, *Poems 1943–1956* (London: Faber & Faber, 1957), p. 124.
3. J. Keats, 'The Human Seasons' (1829), in *The Complete Poems*, ed. by John Barnard (London: Penguin, 1988), p. 232.
4. V. Lindsay, *Collected Poems* (New York: Macmillan, 1955), pp. 329–30.
5. M. Chénetier, ed., *Letters of Vachel Lindsay* (New York: Burt Franklin & Co., 1979), p. 386.
6. H. Van Dyke, *Music and Other Poems* (London: Hodder and Stoughton, 1921), p. 52.

7. J. Billington, A. Jones, A.-L. Humphreys, and K. McDonnell, 'A Literature-Based Intervention for People with Chronic Pain', *Arts and Health: An International Journal for Research, Policy and Practice*, 8.1 (2014), 13–31 (p. 24).
8. M. Csikszentmihalyi, *Flow: The Psychology of Optimal Experience* (New York: Harper and Row, 1990).
9. All examples which follow are derived from a published research study, J. Billington, G. Farrington, S. Lampropoulou, K. McDonnell, A. Jones, J. Ledson, A. L. Humphreys, J. Lingwood, and N. Duirs, 'A Comparative Study of Cognitive Behavioural Therapy and Shared Reading for Chronic Pain' (Centre for Research into Reading, Literature and Society, University of Liverpool, 2016). The project was approved by the Liverpool Central NHS Research Ethics Committee. https://www.liverpool.ac.uk/media/livacuk/instituteofpsychology/Comparing,Shared,Reading,and,CBT,for,Chronic,Pain.pdf.
10. E. Bowen, 'The Visitor', in *Collected Stories* (London: Vintage 1999), pp. 128–40 (p. 139).
11. E.Wharton, 'Mrs Manstey's View' (New York: Literary Classics of the United States, 2001), pp. 1–12 (p. 11). (The transcript of this reading group session is the subject of detailed linguistic analysis in Chapter 11.)
12. N. Nicholson, *Selected Poems: 1940–1982* (London: Faber & Faber, 2003), pp. 31–32.
13. Adapted from J. Billington, *Is Literature Healthy?* (Oxford: Oxford University Press, 2016), pp. 95–96.
14. For information on *The Reader*'s Read to Lead training courses and a suite of online training films, developed by CRILS and funded by AHRC, see: www.thereader.org.uk.
15. See also, J. Billington, G. Farrington, K. McDonnell, S. Lampropoulou, J. Lingwood, A. Jones, J. Ledson, A. L. Humphreys, and N. Duirs, 'A Comparative Study of Cognitive Behavioural Therapy and Shared Reading for Chronic Pain', *Journal of Medical Humanities*, 43.3 (2016), 155–65 (p. 163).

Part III

Research Methodologies

9

Qualitative Methodologies I: Using Established Qualitative Methods in Research on Reading and Health

Jude Robinson, Josie Billington, Ellie Gray and Melissa Chapple

Jude Robinson and Josie Billington, 'Drawing on Ethnography (Prison Reading Groups)'

The method and findings outlined here relate to the prison reading groups established as part of the research at HMP Low Newton, Durham which are described by Charles Darby-Villis in Chapter 7.[1] *Jude Robinson is a social anthropologist and Professor of Health and Wellbeing at the University of Glasgow. Her collaboratively and interdisciplinary research focuses on gendered health inequalities and on the development of participatory research methods in different settings.*

The aim of this study was to assess whether a literature-based intervention developed in non-custodial mental health settings[2] could be successfully transposed to a women's prison. Two, weekly reading groups, each lasting two hours, were established by the Reader in Residence (Charles Darby-Villis) and were delivered in the prison library and in a specialist therapeutic

J. Robinson (✉)
University of Glasgow, Glasgow, Scotland, UK
e-mail: Jude.Robinson@glasgow.ac.uk

J. Billington
Centre for Research into Reading, Literature and Society,
University of Liverpool, Liverpool, UK
e-mail: jbilling@liverpool.ac.uk

J. Billington (ed.), *Reading and Mental Health*,
https://doi.org/10.1007/978-3-030-21762-4_9

wing developed to address the needs of women as part of the Dangerous and Severe Personality Disorder Programme in England and Wales. As women entered and left the prison over time, the opportunity to take part in the research study was offered to women who participated in the reading group during the twelve-month data collection period.[3] All participation was voluntary and followed the principles of informed consent.

Method

Drawing on ethnographic methods, the research was designed to observe people's verbal and non-verbal interaction within the groups and in the setting of some aspects of wider prison life, and to elicit understandings as to how they and others believed their participation shaped their experiences.[4] Ethnographic inquiry involves inductive and participatory practices and is concerned with the interaction of structure and agency.[5] While there was not the scope for a full ethnographic study, the researchers engaged within the necessary limitations they experienced in terms of time and access to produce closely observed and reflexive accounts of the participants' engagement with reading aloud.[6] Digital recording was not permitted within the prison, and observations and notes of informal conversations were collected in the form of contemporaneous fieldnotes.[7] The researchers, an anthropologist and a literature specialist, observed both reading groups over a total of seven visits at intervals throughout the research period. These occasions included not only observing the women in the reading groups, but also the wider environment. Particular attention was paid to the ways in which the women engaged with the group-reading experience, such as their attentiveness and involvement with the text, and their levels of participation in the activities (reading aloud, speaking). Note was also made of non-verbal communication; for example, each group member's position relative to others in the group and the level of eye contact, evidence of enjoyment (laughter, smiling).[8] A parallel record was made of the researchers' emotional response and any interpretations of reactions or happenings in the groups.

E. Gray
Cumbria Partnership NHS Foundation Trust, Cumbria, UK
e-mail: ellie.gray@cumbria.nhs.uk

M. Chapple
Department of Psychology, University of Liverpool, Liverpool, UK
e-mail: melissa.chapple@liverpool.ac.uk

Interviews and Focus Group Discussions with Women Participants

As the women participants were required to return to their rooms after the reading group, maximum use was made of the limited opportunities available to talk to the women, either one to one, or in the group: sometimes immediately after the groups; or in association rooms on the Wings with the Reader in Residence within sight; or in the specialist therapeutic wing with a member of staff monitoring a video (only) link to the room. These conversations took place at different time points across the research study and invited the women to describe their experiences of the reading group, why they chose to engage with it and how their participation may have influenced other aspects of their life. We also wished to know about any past experiences the women may have had around reading, or being read to.[9] Using a biographical and narrative approach, we suggested participants start by telling something of their earliest memory of reading, or being read to, moving on to further memories of personal significance, and finishing with their experience of taking part in the reading group.[10] It was made clear to participants that they could begin wherever they liked, and could take as much time as they needed.

Interviews and Focus Groups with Staff Working at the Prison

At the end of the project individual interviews and two group discussions were carried out with custodial, clinical, learning and Library staff.[11] Participants were asked to talk about and discuss any observed and reported outcomes for women prisoners taking part in the research study, and about their own engagement and attitudes towards the effectiveness and sustainability of reading groups at HMP Low Newton. Interviews and focus group discussions were audio-recorded outside the prison and later transcribed verbatim. Other informal conversations with library and prison staff took place on each of the seven visits, which spanned at least two days, both inside and outside the prison and were recorded as fieldnotes.

Findings (Abbreviated)

Shared Reading Aloud

Taking part in a reading group was described as representing a big step by around half the people interviewed for this study, many of whom had not read for a long time, and some of whom experienced difficulty reading. Staff commented that taking part in such a group was outside the previous experience of many of the women. Some women remembered being read to at school, but, for the majority, reading aloud in secondary school had been an ordeal, and something they had sought to avoid. While these women still found reading aloud a challenge, many had started to do so, some weeks or months into attending the groups. Staff in the focus group discussion reflected on their observation of this phenomenon:

Staff Member 1: If somebody isn't a very good reader they can go along and listen to the book: they're being read to without having to say, 'I can't read'. There doesn't seem to be pressure. One lady has come from the very beginning and she continues to go now religiously, without being made to: she hasn't missed. She's got quite a serious speech impediment and when she first came to us, there was not a hope you would have got her to read out anything, even a sentence, in front of anybody else. And yet now she gets up and speaks in front of people, she'll do role play, she'll read out from books. That's an immense change.

Uniformly, the women found the reading group environment supportive and inspirational. The enthusiasm of the Reader in Residence was commented on by all the women, who said it helped them engage with texts they would otherwise have given up on. The fact that the Reader really believed that they *could* understand something made them try harder, which added to their enjoyment and sense of achievement. As one staff member commented:

> The Reader is very, very keen for everyone to take part, everyone to be comfortable and he'll not let anybody kind of disrespect anybody else. That creates a wider ethos in the group, which at the end of the day is created by women and the Reader together. Like ripples in a pond but ripples both ways! One feeds the other.

A member of the Library staff, who had observed many of the groups and knew the women who took part, commented on how open the women seemed to be to reading books they may never even have heard of before.

> Nobody seems to complain about the books. I've never heard anybody say, 'oh we're reading this' [makes a sad face]. It's 'oh we're reading this next' as if to say, 'Let's try everything, let's just see'. The title doesn't matter - it's the telling and the tale; they're going on a journey of discovery.

Prison staff were 'amazed' by what the women were reading as this challenged their ideas of what could be achieved by the project and by the women themselves:

Staff Member 1: Some of the women will never, ever have read anything like Charles Dickens or shown any interest in it before, and yet now they want to talk to you about it. It gives them a real broader view about things.

'Disciplined Relaxation'

The staff were struck by how participants viewed their engagement with reading as 'totally separate' from other things they were required to do in the prison:

Staff Member 2: Most of the work that they have to do is behaviour-led, a task to complete, the carrot and stick of getting through their [prison] sentence. The reading group is voluntary. Women especially tend to not know what they're interested in because they've been so busy outside being ten other things. When they get in here, they've got time to sit down and think, what is it that I really want to do with my life and what am I interested in?

Staff Member 4: It's almost like narrative therapy. I'm tempted to say maybe it takes them subconsciously back to childhood when maybe your parent read a story. But I'm sure there's a lot of women in here who have never had a story read, who have never had that type of parental love. So maybe it just takes them to a place they didn't even know existed.

All the women described their experience in the group as 'relaxing', variously saying that it was the sound of the Reader's voice, or the story itself, or the fact that they were sitting down in the Library talking about books that helped them forget about any other worries or issues and helped their experience of prison life recede for that moment. They reflected on the pressures of living in the prison, how every day there were events and people to endure or negotiate, the possibility of fresh challenges or dangers. Far from being safe and predicable, for many women prison was a hazardous place, and the physical and mental strain of living there caused stress and tension. Lack of occupation when they were locked in their room was also a real problem, heightening worries and making the time pass slowly. Two women referred directly at interview to their history of self-harm. The staff, too, recognised how the reading group enabled the women to forget these concerns.

Staff Member 1: What's going on in your mind in response to the story or characters, takes you away from the other rubbish you'd been thinking about.
Staff Member 2: Another major factor is there's no white shirts in there, there's no discipline staff in there.
Staff Member 3: The difference in the environment is what they liked; it's an escape from the mundane ordeal of prison life.

The 'relaxing' dimension of the women's participation was further evidenced by their physical behaviour. They were not nervous at the start of each reading group session and took their preferred seats in an unhurried and sociable way. Often there was hardly any movement during the entire session.

'Something We Do for Ourselves'

One participant described the reading group as '*something the prison couldn't touch*' and another reflected how, because the prison didn't 'regulate' the reading group in the same way as other activities, taking part was a form of freedom and self-expression. This sense of personal freedom seemed a key motivational element. The women did not go expecting to get anything out of the groups, and the staff reflected that this could be the secret of its success. Therapies with very specific targets made the women less motivated to attend. 'They all want to be there. It's a choice. And it's serious to them' (Staff Member 1). The issue of 'choice' was clearly important to the women: the activity was described as '*my choice*', and 'something we do for ourselves'. The voluntary nature of their participation—the fact that the women attended without needing persuading, and returned happy and willing to talk—was appreciated by staff. 'It's good for us that they've got things they want to do, that they're not forced to go to' (Staff Member 1).

The staff were also aware that the women did not expect to receive anything from their participation. Many activities the women engaged with were in order to obtain their work allowance or educational qualifications and certificates, or activities that were a compulsory part of their sentence. The fact that taking part in the reading group did not offer them any material reward, was, for the staff, further indication of the women's intrinsic motivation:

P1: They're getting something out of it without wanting something from it.
P3: They're finding a self-satisfaction or enjoyment. Whatever they get, it is enough. (Focus Group Staff)

A 'Bubble' or 'Invisible Shield'

Staff commented on the phenomenon of reasoned discussion that characterised all sessions, and contrasted this favourably with what went on in other parts of the prison where people were less tolerant of opposition:

P1: They're more able to sit and listen to somebody else. That's something that doesn't happen very often! The women don't listen to what you or others have to say, they have something *they* want to say. Trying to explain or give advice or reassurance to women if they can't listen to you effectively is torture. If they're able to spend time taking in what you say, that can only be beneficial.
P2: And they're actually patient; they're respectful of each other.
P3: It increases their tolerance. (Focus Group Staff)

Shared Reading did appear to create a special social and emotional space. Reading aloud created an effect between the readers and listeners, resulting in complete mutual absorption and concentration. One staff member commented that an atmosphere seemed to envelop the group and set them outside of whatever else was going on in the Library.

> I see them sitting there, relaxing, the Reader's voice very soothing, gentle. I can see how it works – a sort of bubble. I'm thinking of one woman who goes into a kind of trance and just listens and absorbs it all. They're really concentrating. You can see people working very hard, listening to what's being said.

Another member of staff commented on the same phenomenon, calling it an 'invisible shield' that not only appeared to protect the women from the noise of their immediate environment, but also from any feelings of self-consciousness.

> People not only sit and concentrate; they also read aloud as if no-one but the other group members could hear them. They all give each other you know that space and that time. They just exist in that time and that space.

The unique atmosphere seems to be created by an intense concentration and focus not always associated with relaxation. The women contrasted the atmosphere in the group and the Library with elsewhere in the prison, and feeling 'safe' was an important dimension to their experience. Safety was more than shutting out the wider prison, it was about regulating behaviours within the group so that no-one felt physically or emotionally vulnerable. The women appeared to be working very hard to regulate their bodies, so to not fiddle, or twitch or walk around; to discipline their minds not to shout out, complain, interrupt or argue; and to concentrate so completely on the text that they could imagine the story. The reading group was an experience of total embodiment.

'A Lifeline … Keeping Going'

While staff commented on how important the reading group was in widening the scope of the women's lives (attending the reading group was still the only reading that some women did), the women themselves described reading not only as an activity of pleasure and enjoyment, but an important form of meaningful occupation. The anticipation of the weekly groups was an important point of reference. One woman said the thought of the next week's reading group 'kept her going' over the long periods of lock-up over the weekend, a time when she was likely to self-harm. Another spoke of reading as a form of 'release' that led to increased self-esteem. Where once she had tended only to read magazines in her room, now she had started to read books, the library staff helping her to find ones she liked. One woman loved reading the poems and took them back to her room to put on the wall. Most of the women folded the sheets of poetry carefully at the end of the session and took them away with them, suggesting that they may be read again, or stored, or even passed on within the prison. The potential of the literature to offer a sense of continuity not only thus within the prison but between institutions was powerfully suggested when one participant, who was being transferred to another secure establishment, asked about the possibility of joining an equivalent group there.

The group leader reported how one striking aspect of the prison reading groups was participants' use of the literature as a link to continuing and ongoing life outside of prison and a means of renewing connection to loved ones (see Chapter 7). The possibility was enthusiastically discussed 'of holding a reading group during family visit days - all agreed that this would be a great idea'.

Seeing Afresh

The women were very clear that the reading group was unlike anything else they did in prison. It had the power to 'take them away from being themselves and being in the prison'. The staff, rather differently, were aware of the potential to use literature to discuss issues from a philosophical and humanitarian point of view that they themselves could only deal with as issues of discipline, a breach of rules rather than of morality:

> The stuff that is very difficult to tackle from a discipline point of view – cultural or racial difference for example - can be explored within a reading group. The formal means of trying to tackle some things is quite draconian really and not likely to succeed. A perpetrator is more likely to address offending behaviour in that environment than with the wing manager. (Focus Group Staff)

While some of the women were undergoing multiple interventions to support their personal development, staff acknowledged the contribution of the reading group in supporting these initiatives. The social and emotional development of the women was reinforced, enabling them to deal more effectively with emotions outside the group and to express their feelings to avoid conflict, anger, violence and self-harm.

P1: It runs side by side with what we're encouraging. They're taking notice of what is being recommended and taking part in other treatments and activities as they would never have done before—not just for one or two weeks but actually staying and getting something back from it.

P2: We've definitely noticed a difference. They've been able to explain themselves and communicate with us better. It's helped massively with confidence, with self-esteem. (Focus Group Staff)

The staff were aware of the potential for literature to enable the women to discuss scenarios of action and reaction and to trace actions over time—to look at the effects and consequences of behaviours, including the impact on others. The fact that the human situations were presented within engaging, imaginative fiction, said one staff member, meant that the women were more likely to respond and internalise the possibilities of alternative patterns of behaviour than if they were simply given scenarios, or asked to reflect on their own actions:

> The hope is that when the women start their more in-depth treatment, some of the things they recognise from books will link over as well – the idea of things not always being as you think they're going to be, for example, or the recognition that things can change. That can be used in treatment - 'Do you remember, when we read about this?' - to underline an idea, once they start to realise that things can be dealt with in different ways, especially with people who are really rigid or don't have much insight into their own behaviour.

The reading group dovetailed with existing therapies and programmes, offering a unique alternative that enabled women to consider the 'big issues' of life in a non-directive, non-goal-orientated way. Staff were acutely aware that the success of the reading group was linked to the fact that the women were not required to take part, and that it was not specifically labelled as a 'therapy':

> With activities classed a therapy, there's that added pressure, 'am I here for this reason, am I supposed to be doing this, should I be doing that'? whereas the women get real therapeutic benefit from the reading group without having to consider whether it benefits them or not.

Conclusions and Recommendations

The study concluded that Shared Reading is sufficiently flexible, adaptive and fluid to transfer to custodial settings, and that women engage voluntarily with reading groups given the right support and assurances and appropriate reading material. Identifying which books and poems 'work' with different groups of women and why is one area for future study. Shared Reading helps to improve well-being for women for whom little else can. It was reported to enhance self-esteem, and encouraged a sense of achievement and self-worth, and of social participation and even friendship. Shared Reading gave participants something to think about that they carried with them back to the wings, and supported their participation in other activities under the momentum and energy provided by the reading groups. Group composition and recruitment may be challenging, however (see Chapter 7). In view of this, how to engage women from a wider range of backgrounds, histories and cultures, particularly those serving shorter sentences, and how to integrate older women and young offenders within the groups, are further areas for future research.

Ellie Gray and Gundi Kiemle, 'Interpretative Phenomenological Analysis (Community Mental Health)'

This study was conducted by Ellie Gray (now a Clinical Psychologist in a community-based adult mental health service in Cumbria) as part of her doctoral studies in Clinical Psychology at the University of Liverpool, and was supervised by Gundi Kiemle (Clinical Psychologist and Academic Director, Doctorate in Clinical Psychology, University of Liverpool).[12]

The aim of the study was to explore participants' experiences of being in a community reading group, and the impact of participation upon how people made sense of their lives and relationships, in the context of their past and present experience of mental health problems. Data were collected via individual semi-structured interviews and analysed using Interpretative Phenomenological Analysis (IPA).

Rationale for Using IPA

IPA draws on the long-established philosophies of phenomenology and hermeneutics[13] to understand how people attach meaning to lived experience.[14] Phenomenology posits that reality cannot be separated from subjective experience, because reality *is* experience, thus the meaning people attach to their experience is key to understanding how humans make sense of the world. A series of inter-related meanings—the product of an individual's 'practical engagement with things and others' in the world[15]—become bound together in what Husserl termed the 'lifeworld'. Understanding the lifeworld requires going 'back to the things themselves'[16] or exploring the subjective lived experience from which such meaning is derived. Because there is no 'direct' route to experience, phenomenology employs the expertise of individuals in their own experience[17] to provide an 'experience-close' account of a particular phenomenon, from which the researcher interprets meaning.[18]

It is this 'meaning-making' process that constitutes the 'interpretative' aspect of IPA. Drawing on hermeneutics, Heidegger proposed that it is through our state of 'being in the world' that we make sense of ourselves (Eatough & Smith, 2008), so we cannot meaningfully exist outside a temporal/geographical context (Larkin et al., 2006). Our perception and understanding of objects/events is influenced by existing knowledge and beliefs, derived from experience (Eatough & Smith, 2008). In IPA, the researcher and participant engage in a joint meaning-making process, using a 'double hermeneutic'; seeking out the participant's perception of their experience ('first hermeneutic'), while also critically analysing aspects of experience which the participant may be unaware of, or unwilling to acknowledge ('critical hermeneutic'[19]).

IPA is also idiographic, with in-depth analysis occurring at the individual level (Larkin et al., 2006). Accordingly, IPA involves detailed analysis on a case-by-case basis (Smith, 2011). Data are analysed in an iterative process from initial coding through increasing levels of abstraction to the identification and organisation of themes (Smith et al., 2009). The final narrative moves between the two levels of interpretation outlined earlier ('double hermeneutic'); 'from rich description through to abstract and more conceptual interpretations' (Eatough & Smith, 2008, p. 187), to capture the totality and complexity of individual experience (Smith & Osborn, 2008).

In the study by Gray et al. (2015), IPA enabled a fine-grained understanding of the lived experience of being in a reading group from the perspective of individuals with mental health problems. Because IPA seeks to uncover a chain of connection between what participants say and their thoughts and emotion states (Smith & Osborn, 2008), this approach helped shed light on the underlying cognitive and affective processes involved in reading group participation, and associated meaning-making (Eatough & Smith, 2008).

Design/Method

Sample sizes in IPA vary between studies, but tend to be relatively small due to the homogeneity of samples and other factors, including ease of recruitment, depth of analysis, and data quality (Eatough & Smith, 2008). The current study opted for four to ten participants, to enable strong investment in the analytic procedure for each individual (Smith, 2011). Eight participants—over 18 years old and sufficiently fluent in English to participate in a one hour interview—were recruited from existing reading groups (i.e. using purposive rather than random sampling). Each participant: (1) had been regularly attending a reading group for six months or more (long/frequently enough for the group to have some impact on their life/psychological state); and (2) was experiencing mental health issues (from formal clinical diagnosis, through contact with mental health services, to self-identified psychological distress). Groups were located in urban areas with high levels of deprivation (Table 9.1).

Semi-structured interviews were used to accommodate the variability of subjective experience and enable the flexible probing of areas of interest (Eatough & Smith, 2008), as well as to establish rapport with the participant and elicit a more natural account (Reid et al., 2005). Open-ended interview questions covered the following areas: inter- and intra-personal experience of being in a reading group and the meaning attached to participation; the relationship between participants' experience of the reading group and their life outside the group, both past and present, including

Table 9.1 Participant demographics

Participant number	Pseudonym	Age	Mental health problem
1	Olivia	30	Depression, low self-esteem
2	Nadia	42	Bipolar disorder
3	Alfie	53	Depression
4	Liz	56	Depression
5	Jim	58	Depression
6	Ian	44	Anxiety, depression, substance misuse
7	Hassan	42	Anxiety, depression, Asperger's syndrome
8	Richard	44	Anxiety, depression

mental health issues; the perceived impact of participation on how people related to themselves and others, and made sense of their own lives and relationships; experience of Shared Reading relative to other group activities and reading alone. Participants also provided demographic data. Most interviews took place at the reading group locations (public library, mental health drop-in centre). Interviews ranged from around 30 to 120 minutes, with a mean of 66.5 minutes. All interviews were audio-recorded and transcribed verbatim.

Because interpretation and experience are inextricably linked, IPA researchers explicitly examine their own backgrounds, priorities, and interests, and consider their potential influence on the research process, especially the interpretation of participant accounts.[20] The primary researcher in this study (Ellie Gray) kept a reflective journal throughout the research process. To outline my position (at the time the research was undertaken): I am a 29-year-old white British female, and I have worked in the field of clinical psychology for five years with a range of client groups. In both clinical and research contexts, I am an advocate of viewing the client/participant as a 'person-in-context', and I am critical of a purely diagnostic/symptom-based approach to mental health, which I believe overlooks contexts and experiences. I have a strong interest in exploring alternative or additional means by which activities with therapeutic effect may be made accessible to people with mental health difficulties, particularly those for whom traditional services are unsuitable.

Analysis

Immersive readings and self-contained analysis of each interview transcript involved increasing levels of abstraction from initial noting to emergent themes as illustrated in Table 9.2.

Table 9.2 Initial noting and emergent themes (participant 1)

Emergent Theme	Transcript	Initial Notes (descriptive, *linguistic,* conceptual
Attention to detail valued	The fact that you can discuss	*'fact'* – truth, known (trust?)
Significance of small details Optional personal/emotional focus	how a line in the book made you feel, not just how the book as a whole made you feel and the	Importance in single line (vs whole book) deconstructing into small parts *'not just'* – focus on whole book missing something? *'can' – option, not obligation*
Book doing to: eliciting emotions	book groups I've gone to want to discuss the books in depth	*'book made you feel' – book as active subject, you as object* group exerting influence Focus on feelings (relate to internal state)
Distinctness of reading group model?	and I suppose I don't know if they're…more in an educational	Contrast to 'classic' book group *'want to' – expressing different ethos*
Educational focus as pressured/unsafe?	sense like 'you must understand the book', you must…and it	Educational, in-depth, academic understanding *'you must' (repetition) – obligation,* emphasising pressure/expectation Academic focus more pressurised?
No pressure to perform/meet intellectual standard	feels like a bit more pressure whereas in the reader group there's no pressure to participate	obliged to meet standards Too much academic focus is unsafe? Pressure (*repeated for emphasis?)* *'whereas' – direct contrast*
Optional participation (passivity is accepted)	at all, you can sit there and just listen to other people's opinions.	*'at all' – totally* pressure free *'can' – choice/freedom,* *'sit there' 'just listen' passivity?*

Emergent themes were then clustered together to develop superordinate themes, followed by sub-themes and master themes. Connections were made between themes using processes of abstraction (identifying shared relationships), polarization (identifying oppositional relationships), and subsumption (emergent theme acquiring superordinate status). Table 9.3 provides an example of emergent themes clustering into a superordinate theme.

Table 9.3 Emergent themes clustered into superordinate theme (participant 2)

Superordinate theme	Emergent themes
Developing interpersonal self-efficacy: learning how to relate to others	Generalisability of interpersonal learning to everyday life Developing ways of relating to others Learning skills to counteract ostracism Developing self-awareness Confidence in forming relationships Improving communication self-efficacy Not obliged to relate in a certain way

Table 9.4 Master themes and sub-themes

Master theme	Sub-themes
1. Literature as an intermediary object	• Attunement to text, self, other • Literature eliciting self-reflection in safe environment • Testing ground for new ways of being
2. Boundaries and rules of engagement	• Reading group as separate (protected) space • Structure and unplanned happenings • Reading group as unpressured/failure-free • Acceptance and non-judgement
3. Self as valued, worthy, capable	• Fulfilment of otherwise unaccomplished endeavours • Sense of potential through (enjoyable) learning and achievement • Opportunity for contribution/involvement
4. Community and togetherness in relational space	• Interpersonal self-efficacy counteracting social difficulty • Attachment to others fosters trust and belonging • Reading group as a collective experience/venture
5. Changing view of self, world, other	• Re-appraising self as normal • Psychological flexibility • Connecting past and present self

This process was repeated independently for all interviews, before comparing theme clusters across the whole sample. The latter involved looking for patterns between cases, paying attention to convergence and divergence within the data to identify shared higher order categories as well as unique idiosyncrasies. The analysis moved between the two levels of descriptive and critical interpretation ('double hermeneutic') and sometimes led to the renaming or reconfiguring of themes. The end product was a series of master themes and subthemes (Table 9.4).

Literature as an Intermediary Object

The text is positioned between participants and the wider group, between intra-psychic and interpersonal experience. All participants spoke of a heightened awareness internally and interpersonally ('attunement to text, self, other'). Of reading Charles Dickens's *Great Expectations* and Willy Russell's *Blood Brothers*, Jim said: 'I looked at my own life, and I thought to myself "you're very good at loving other people, putting other people on a pedestal. But you're no bloody good at putting yourself on a pedestal. I could see myself as a doormat to be honest with you. In relationships"'. Through exposure to similar situations in literature, Jim made sense of self-other (idealising/pleasing) and self-self (critical/rejecting) relationships in his 'own life', attuned both to his own thoughts/feelings and himself in relation to others.

Safe, guided engagement with literature enabled exploration, understanding and expression of thoughts and feelings hitherto unexplored or undisclosed ('eliciting self-reflection in safe environment'). 'It's things in life, especially with Dickens, very traumatic things. But we can talk about it because it's happening in the book' (Richard). The text modelled exploration of difficult experiences, reassuring Richard that this was manageable and allowed, while maintaining a safe distance between him and his own difficulties. Literature also acted as a secure base to return to when group discussion strayed too far from the text.

Through discussion and exploration, reading groups provided participants with opportunities to relate to themselves and others differently ('testing ground for new ways of being'), both inside and outside the group. Some were able to evaluate and alter perpetuating default emotional responses in favour of adaptive alternatives.

Boundaries and Rules of Engagement

Reading groups were experienced as 'a separate (protected) space', qualitatively distinct from the outside world: Hassan describes going 'back into the normal world' after the group. Relationships changed on crossing the threshold: there was a temporary level of intimacy that was absent outside. 'You talk about something you never thought you'd talk about to a group of strangers' (Olivia).

'Separateness' and a sense of protection was experienced as being reinforced by unspoken rules occurring within semi-structured boundaries. 'You can't really have an agenda because something will come up and you'll discuss all kinds of things' (Olivia) suggesting discussion emerges naturally and spontaneously: 'We can go on anything all of a sudden' (Alfie). Where Olivia and Alfie contrasted this 'free will' to their experience of more controlling/prescriptive therapy, Jim commented 'there's a structure to the reader group' which he contrasted to groups in which 'just anything goes, chaos, anarchy'. Structure is differently construed by participants such that the balance of planned to unplanned happenings allows the level of perceived structure or containment to be tailored to individual needs.

All participants experienced the reading group environment as unpressured. In contrast to academic environments, the reading group allowed engagement with literature without 'fear of failure' or 'appearing stupid'

(Jim) while also offering protection from expectations of disclosure: 'If you don't want to say nothing, you can just sit there' (Richard). Patience also characterised the reading group: 'the pace of communicating is more eased' (Hassan) than the pace experienced outside, enabling more manageable interactions.

Safety was enhanced by trust and lack of judgement. 'It's one of the few places I can go and not have people say "who you are is not right"' (Olivia); 'They don't feel as if they're insecure or people are pointing the finger at them' (Nadia). Interestingly, Nadia uses the third person to distance herself from internalised self-stigma, where she uses the first person in relation to the reading group—'I feel very secure there'—connecting with the experience as her own.

Self as Valued, Worthy, Capable

All narratives conveyed a sense of worth, value and capability. Participants actively experienced learning and achievement ('fulfilment of unaccomplished endeavours')—'I'm doing something constructive in life' (Nadia)—in ways which challenged their sense of intellectual inferiority: 'I don't think I'm thick, you see, and yet that's the impression I give' (Jim).

Participants also experienced personal growth ('sense of potential'). 'People, I think, are developing themselves' (Ian); 'I've stopped feeling that I can't read' (Nadia). Jim conveyed a cumulative sense of achievement, through reading novels over several sessions: 'being able to say to yourself "yeah, week after week after week after week we ploughed through that"', suggests continued perseverance and ongoing accomplishment, while saying this 'to himself' indicates an internalised sense of achievement. The facilitator's trust in group members to succeed fostered growth potential; 'she always had great faith in our ability to understand' (Richard). Vital to the learning process was its being experienced as enjoyable. All participants shared Olivia's sentiment that reading groups 'can be a lot of fun' and Jim's statement 'you're there to enjoy the literature in front of you'.

Reading groups provided 'opportunity for contribution/involvement'—'I've put a few ideas in, you know, that have been taken up' (Ian)—partly through offering alternative access to literature to those who struggled with 'traditional' lone reading. 'Reading aloud gives me the freedom to take a piece of paper and, as the person is reading, I can map, visually, the storyline where we are [draws diagram]. And that's more adaptable for me to understand' (Hassan). The Shared Reading aloud model accommodates such idiosyncratic ways of engaging with text, maintaining inclusion in the reading process for those otherwise excluded. This suggests a sense of equality and an important protection against power imbalances, given the sense of inferiority/inadequacy that many participants expressed.

Community and Togetherness in Relational Space

Most participants experienced enhanced capacity to relate to others ('interpersonal self-efficacy'), important given their sense of social ineffectiveness: 'you're learning how to react to people without feeling that you have to be coy or egoistic or arrogant' (Nadia). Manipulating or disguising one's true self as a protective strategy is not replicated in the reading group, perhaps because of its in-the-moment nature and accepting atmosphere. Olivia transferred her relational experiences of genuineness and naturalness outside the group: 'with my husband I can say "I'm not feeling too good today, so if I do lose patience or I am upset, it's because I've not been feeling very well"'. For Alfie, the group provided an alternative interpersonal culture to that experienced outside, nurturing openness: 'I don't converse with my family. Outside I don't talk to people. The only people I talk to is in here' (Alfie).

The group promoted a sense of 'attachment to others' which counteracted feelings of isolation and alienation in an outer world perceived as threatening: 'The world can do things to you and you think you have no bond with the world at all. And then you come back. That's why the regularity of the group helps as well, cos I think it gives you that thing going back week after week. You can go back and you can get that same sense of community again' (Richard). This intimate emotional attachment, emerging as a function of sharing internal states via the literature, also requires time and patience: 'I suppose it would be hard for someone new to join the group, because we've had quite a while to bond' (Olivia). Connection was experienced even when members were physically absent. Alfie's 'when one person's not there you miss them' suggests absent members still occupied mental space in the group.

Most participants experienced the group as a 'collective experience/venture': 'we're all joining together as a total participation group' (Nadia). 'Joining', 'together', 'total', and 'all' emphasise holistic operation. Alfie contrasted this joint experience to other group activities: 'in the relaxation group, although you're with a group of people, you're on your own. In this one you're actually integrated'. Collective function is also valued for exposure to multiple perspectives: 'being able to get other people's opinions'

(Jim), 'feeding off other people's thoughts' (Ian). 'Feeding' suggests thriving off one another (resonant of early developmental attachment), implying that interaction between members sustains the group. Yet individual idiosyncrasies are nonetheless retained: 'the group would understand it in one particular way but ever so subtly there was a slightly different angle on how each one of us understood it' (Richard). The 'subtle' discrepancies within collective understanding ensure individual worth/value is not eclipsed and may enable greater tolerance of uncertainty in thinking.

Changing View of Self, World, Other

All participants commented on how sharing experiences of mental health problems, both with the literature and with the group, created a sense of themselves as normal. 'If this person experiences these forms of differences then it's quite normal for me also to express those differences' (Hassan). Hassan saw himself as 'different', but through identifying with similar 'differences' in others, he redefined his sense of 'normal'. 'Express' suggests he feels permitted not only to experience, but also to externalise these differences. The literature encourages the 'normalising' process both directly, through describing events with which participants identify, and indirectly, through discussion, leading others to disclose similar experiences. One book 'had a lot about not feeling significant in the world and because there were more people sharing how they felt about the book, it made you feel I'm not the only person that feels this way' (Olivia). 'More people' creates a shift from being 'alone' to 'one of many', perhaps enabling Olivia to challenge previous ideas of herself as different.

Psychological flexibility was influenced through exposure to multiple perspectives. 'You'll read a storyline, and you'll think, right, this is gonna happen but a statement can be ambiguous, can't it?' (Nadia); 'I was a lot more insistent that I had the correct way when everybody else's is just as valid as mine' (Richard). Engaging with others' ideas did not mean that participants adopted a different viewpoint, but that alternative opinions were considered, and challenged where appropriate: 'Some people have very strong opinions that I disagree with. But I find that it seems comfortable to be able to tell them "I disagree with this, and this is why"' (Olivia). 'Comfortable' (in contrast to Olivia's lack of assertiveness outside the group), resonates with comments on the reading group as a place of trust and safety.

Most participants make connections between their past and present selves: 'I used to be an avid reader: there was never, never not a book in my hand. But, I had a bit of a breakdown: now the only reading I do is here. It's helping me to have the ability, and the want and the desire to read' (Alfie). The reading group serves as a gateway for re-discovering important aspects of himself, not only to revive reading as an activity, but also its emotional aspects (drive, desire). Liz, too, was re-connected to a time when literature was an integral part of her daily life: 'The past when I was normal, I liked books, so every day I would read for at least a half an hour or an hour for example in bed' (Liz). Reading connects Liz with pre-illness 'normality' providing a bridge to her former healthy/whole self. The reading group also elicited more difficult memories—'it reminds me of a very dark period of my life, that's kind of returning, something that I've been hiding from myself all this time' (Ian)—re-claiming aspects of self previously concealed, or too painful to address or articulate. By assimilating these 'lost' parts of self, reading may help to process difficult experiences and restore a sense of functionality and wellness.

Conclusions and Recommendations

The study confirmed the findings of previous research that reading groups can bring about positive therapeutic effects and identified the literature as a key mediator in specific psychological processes, enabling and eliciting self-reflection and externalisation of internal states. Participants experienced greater attunement to the internal states of self and others, perhaps enhancing their capacity for mentalisation (the ability to understand our own and others' behaviour in terms of mental/emotional processes).[21] Like the secure base in attachment theory,[22] the literature and/or reading group enabled safe exploration in a boundaried environment, and permitted participants to experiment with novel ways of relating, leading to development and self-transformation. Many of these processes mirror those operating in psychological therapies, but in a less formalised manner.

Future research could consider whether prolonged participation in reading groups impacts upon positive attachment-related behaviours, such as those associated with mentalising ability. It may be fruitful to examine the development of mentalisation over time, by assessing members' ability to mentalise at different time points across group participation. Further research could also investigate reading group participation at earlier developmental stages, with children or adolescents, to study the potential preventative value for younger people with disrupted attachments.

Melissa Chapple, 'Framework Analysis: Reading and Autism'

Melissa Chapple holds an Economic and Social Research Council Ph.D. studentship in the Department of Psychology at the University of Liverpool and is working with autism organisations to study reading habits and impacts in respect of people living with autism. She was diagnosed with autism at the age of eighteen.

Introduction

Autism is a neurological condition that impacts on the way individuals interact with others and the world around them; it is often defined by repetitive behaviour, highly specialised interests and specific barriers in social and communicative understanding.[23] Previously, it was largely assumed that autistic individuals preferred to be alone[24] but more recent findings have challenged this idea, demonstrating that autistic individuals long for intimacy,[25] and experience more loneliness than neuro-typical (NT) peers.[26]

Research has, therefore, highlighted the need to facilitate social understanding in autistic individuals desiring social contact. Specifically, White and Roberson-Nay[27] found anxiety in autistic individuals to be associated with increased loneliness and argued that autistic individuals can have an awareness of their social disability in relation to NTs, leading to resulting anxiety over social misinterpretation, further exacerbating anxiety. Loneliness in autism is also associated with decreased life satisfaction, and worsened anxiety.[28]

A specific social skill that is argued to be difficult for autistic individuals is theory of mind (ToM), the ability to take perspectives with others, also known as 'cognitive empathy'.[29] Lombardo and Baron-Cohen[30] further argue that understanding of self is crucial to comparatively understanding others, a skill they found also to be difficult for autistic individuals. They maintain that approaches aiming to facilitate social skills in autism should, therefore, take a relational approach, focussing on self-other relations to understand self-other perspectives (ToM understanding). Good autism interventions should also provide tools to aid social understanding without causing distress or imposing NT values that conflict with the differential cognitive profile seen in autistic individuals.[31]

One such mode of facilitation is fiction-reading. Mar and Oatley[32] argue that fiction is a simulation of the real social world, facilitating communication and social understanding and improving both cognitive empathy and social inferences (see Chapter 15). Fiction allows readers to make predictions while uncovering processes throughout the book that model real-world constructs; indeed, fiction is at times more relatable than the real world, due to projection of the self into the events described. In this way fiction interventions may help support autistic individuals, as they simulate a complex system of the social world, encouraging predictions and the practice of understanding social systems and perspectives during ambiguous situations.

The facilitation of ToM through reading has been supported empirically with NT participants. Kidd and Castano[33] used multiple ToM tests in relation to literary and popular fiction and non-fiction, finding that literary extracts elicited higher ToM scores than other extract types (see Chapter 13). Furthermore, specific research on ASC and reading found that during reading ASC participants were able to make implicit emotional inferences about characters, but struggled to explicitly report inferences.[34] Koopman and Hakemulder[35] also theorise that fiction, via the same simulated social experience, should improve self-reflection, by permitting experimentation with boundaries between self and other to understand perspectives. Furthermore, fiction potentially serves as an autism-friendly intervention due to the ability to practice social situations in environments controlled by the individual to reduce social and environmental stressors.

Currently, however, little is known about the relationship between fiction and autism, partly due to the assumption that fiction is generally disliked by autistic individuals.[36] It is assumed that the complex social situations which fiction tends to be interested in are too abstract and unpredictable for autistic adults, while the more system-based nature of non-fiction is believed to complement the skills associated with autistic cognition.[37] Furthermore, the drawing of inferences[38] and the exercise of social imagination[39] which aid comprehension of fictional narrative[40] have been demonstrated to be problematic for people with autism. However, research showing that reality-based imagination is intact in autistic individuals (Craig & Baron-Cohen, 1999) bodes well for fiction-reading given fiction's grounding in reality (even fantasy novels carry parallels to the real social world, Mar & Oatley, 2008). Although fiction does not enable facial expression reading, it does allow for the understanding of complex emotional processes and contextual triggers for understanding broader emotional experiences, as well as understanding social interactive processes (Mar & Oatley, 2008). Moreover, Barnes' study[41] on text preferences in autistic adults found no avoidance of fiction and an ability to engage with fictional texts.

Using qualitative methods, specifically framework analysis, we have been able to explore the general reading habits of adults on the autism spectrum with a view to understanding the potential benefits and drawbacks of engaging with different genres.

Rationale for Using Framework Analysis

Framework analysis is a qualitative method that is 'not aligned with a particular epistemological viewpoint or theoretical approach and therefore can be adapted for use in inductive or deductive analysis or a combination of the two'.[42] For example, it can be used to examine pre-existing theoretical constructs deductively, then to revise the theory with inductive aspects, or it can be used inductively to identify themes in the data, before returning to the literature and using theories deductively for further explanation. Thus, Framework Analysis is not necessarily concerned with inductively generating theory. Rather, it permits researchers to develop a pre-conceived framework from theory, relevant research findings, pilot findings or other justifiable resources that lead to specific assumptions about the qualitative nature of the data.

The analytic procedure of Framework Analysis (modelled step by step in what follows) produces a highly structured output of summarised data—the matrix—offering a holistic overview of the entire data set. Yet the matrix is so constructed that the views of each research participant remain connected to other aspects of their account within the matrix so that the context of the individual's views is retained. This allows in-depth analyses and comparison/contrast across participant responses as well as within individual cases, providing case-by-case as well as over-arching understanding. By encouraging the use of as much data as possible, framework analysis reduces data loss. In areas of relatively new enquiry but where established, dominant theory exists which cannot reasonably be ignored or unknown, framework analysis presents a good way forward for looking afresh at data.

Project Design

This small-scale pilot study involved five participants, four attending a focus group and the fifth taking part in a single one-to-one interview. All participants were over 18 years of age, fluent in English, and were current or past students at the University of Liverpool in order to reduce ethical issues around intellectual vulnerability. The sample included three participants formally diagnosed with autism, and two who had been referred for professional assessment. All were current or previous higher education students, four of the five participants identified as female. Interviews took place in person on the university campus, and were semi-structured, with allowance for follow-up on interesting points. As allowed by framework analysis, there were some pre-conceived questions based on previous relevant research findings and theoretical assumptions. The first half of the interview elicited responses about current reading habits and preferences, metacognition, comprehension and (self-)reflection/contemplation. The second half of the interview assessed responses to specific extracts from Charles Dickens' *Great Expectations*. The first was primarily descriptive, while the other was a primarily social dialogue (see sample extract at the close of this section). These were followed by text-specific questions and questions inviting participants to compare the extracts.

Analysis

The five key stages of Framework Analysis were used to analyse the data.[43] As recommended, the process was not linear, but involved going back and forth between stages as necessary to extract the best resulting framework. A reflective diary of the entire process was kept in order to track and compare emerging ideas at different stages of the process, and ensure important ideas were ingrained in the final framework.

1. Data Immersion

Like all qualitative approaches, this stage involves becoming as familiar as possible with the transcribed interviews, noting emergent ideas for potential inclusion into the later analytical framework. Although designated Stage One, data immersion is a feature of all four stages, making the reflective diary (recorded in Table 9.5 as 'case notes') essential in monitoring data interpretation and ensuring preliminary ideas are not lost, and subsequent changes justified. Emerging themes—'social learning', in our analysis for example—can be identified at this stage but they are typically restructured throughout the process. Table 9.5 shows how social learning emerged early, in the stage of data immersion, in our study but evolved as the structured analysis continued. However, most themes do not emerge at this stage, and themes should not yet be the focus of the process.

2. Organising Data

The intention of this stage is to order the data in a structured way to make it easier for later analysis, while reducing data loss. Data was line-by-line coded with the purpose of *organising*, not analysing, data, into sub-themes, with themes *describing*, rather than explaining, the data. Codes were participant specific, but the same code was sometimes used for multiple participants within a sub-theme. Returning to stage one to re-immerse in the data is necessary to ensure that the data is organised in a maximally inclusive way. Though, it is important to resist the urge to begin analysing data for the final framework here, during creation of the organisational framework, ideas for a final framework do naturally emerge and should be noted. For example, in our analysis, 'Reading Preferences' which contained data around accessing books, and drawbacks and motivators for reading, was later turned into 'Factors Impacting Reading' with sub-themes of (1) Book Access Factors, (2) Commitment Issues, (3) Personal Barriers and Drawbacks, (4) Personal Motivators, and (5) Special Interest Influence.[44]

3. Indexing

Stage three is the process of coding the data for the final analysis. As codes developed in stage two should be used to describe the data, the codes developed in this stage should be more explanatory. As in stage two, codes are participant specific. Codes from stage two will often be re-imagined, broken down into smaller codes, collapsed into a larger codes, or sometimes completely new codes will be generated at the indexing stage. Reflection and going back to earlier stages is most beneficial here to ensure that the new codes are comprehensive for the final analysis. In our analysis, for example as shown in Table 9.5, the sub-theme of 'emotions' was useful for stage two as it categorised all of the data relating to emotion. However, this did not really say anything meaningful or useful about the data and it did not specifically capture how autistic individuals dealt with emotions in text. Therefore, reflective notes were reviewed to re-code the data within this sub-theme. As a result the sub-theme was broken into two sub-themes (1) Altered Emotional Inference, and (2) Difficulty with Emotion, which were

Table 9.5 Progression of social learning framework

Case notes	Organisational framework	Final framework
'All participants discuss social learning from texts to some extent, with participants experiencing real world benefits to varying degrees. The participants who report reading the most also report the most real world social benefits.' 'Participants also show varying levels of emotional understanding difficulties, with most reporting sympathy rather than empathy; but for some this appears to be more of a confidence issue. Some participants show empathic inference using alternative cues such as sentence length rather than explicit description of character emotions.'	**Theme**: Social skills **Sub-themes**: 1. Social communication 2. Theory of mind 3. Emotions	**Theme**: Social inductive learning **Sub-themes**: 1. Altered emotional inference 2. Difficulty with emotion 3. Perspective taking 4. Self-other awareness 5. Social skill facilitation

more relevant for the final framework in telling us about the challenges and differences autistic individuals had when assessing in-text emotions.

4. Charting

Stages three and four tend to co-occur, as the change from descriptive to analytical codes at stage three results in changing sub-themes, and eventually themes, which is the ultimate objective of stage four.[45] Immersion, and re-immersion in previous stages, is especially important to ensure that stage three and four are maximally informative and reflective of the data in contrast to the descriptive framework of stage two. These stages involve continually re-assessing the framework and seeing whether codes and sub-themes need expanding or collapsing to produce a pragmatic, manageable and useful framework.

5. Mapping and Interpretation

The final stage of the analysis is to produce a framework matrix, showing the codes within sub-themes and across cases for each theme. Each theme should have its own framework table, showing codes across sub-themes within participant codes horizontally, and codes within each sub-theme vertically. For illustrative purposes, Table 9.6 shows two participants in the framework matrix from our research. Ordinarily, all participants, or groups, will be presented in the matrix. If, after the themes have been entered into the framework table, part of the framework seems to require reframing, then previous stages should be returned to and reframing should be carried out until the framework tables are maximally representative of both the data and any pre-conceived framework ideas from prior understandings that the data has supported.

Across this pilot study, six main themes were identified, briefly outlined here.

1. 'Inductive Social Learning' (see above).
2. Visualisation (i.e. of aspects of the text): sub-themes include 'Varied Internal Representations', 'Difficulty with Faces'.
3. Relatability: sub-themes include 'Relatability to Character', 'Relatability to Situation'.
4. 'Factors Impacting Reading': sub-themes include 'Personal Barriers and Drawbacks' 'Personal Motivators' (see also above).

Table 9.6 Framework matrix example: Theme 'Inductive Social Learning', participants 2 and 3

Inductive social learning	(1) Altered emotional inference	(2) Difficulty with emotion	(3) Perspective taking	(4) Self-other awareness	(5) Social skill facilitation
P2		**Sympathy not empathy**: **P2**: 'I can sympathise with him but I don't really empathise.'	**Outside perspective**: (After being asked about which is easier internal or external) **P2**: 'Outside perspective for me.'	**Comparisons**: **P2**: 'I like it if there's something aspirational about the character as well.'	**Enjoyment**: (Talking about a non-social extract compared to social) **P2**: 'I found it easier because it was a bit more descriptive, but it wasn't as interesting.'
P3	**Maturity focus**: **P3**: 'How old is Pip?' **R**: 'In the novel he's a teenager at this point in the story.' **P3**: 'Ah alright, I wondered why he was getting teary eyed and crying at a girl not looking at him.'	**Sympathy not empathy**: **P3**: 'I can see what they're getting at, why he's upset I just don't relate to it.' **Lack Confidence on inference**: **R**: 'Did you feel like you understood how Pip was feeling during that text?' **P3**: 'Was he nervous?'			**Reduced ambiguity**: **P3**: 'You know where you stand with it, social communication is like in real life you haven't got a clue.' **Real world utility**: (After being asked if it helps in reality) **P3**: 'Yeah maybe? No, not with the kind of books I read.'

5. Escapism: sub-themes include 'Escaping reality', 'Immersion', 'Transportation'.
6. Concentration issues: sub-themes include 'reading attention barriers', 're-reading behaviour', 'stress influence'.

A further study, also using Framework Analysis and involving a larger sample size, is currently underway.

* * *

Here is an excerpt from the passage of 'social dialogue' (taken from Charles Dickens' *Great Expectations*) which participants were asked to read at the interview.

> Pip, a young orphan, has gone to meet Miss Havisham, a rich older lady who has invited Pip to her house. At Miss Havisham's house Pip meets a young girl, Estella. The passage begins with Pip and Estella playing cards together.
>
> 'He calls the knaves, Jacks, this boy!' said Estella with disdain, before our first game was out. 'And what coarse hands he has! And what thick boots!'
>
> I had never thought of being ashamed of my hands before, but I began to consider them a very indifferent pair. Her contempt for me was so strong, that it became infectious, and I caught it.
>
> She won the game, and I dealt. I misdealt, as was only natural, when I knew she was lying in wait for me to do wrong; and she denounced me for a stupid, clumsy labouring-boy. …
>
> 'Estella, take him down. Let him have something to eat, and let him roam and look about him while he eats. Go, Pip.'
>
> I followed the candle down, as I had followed the candle up, and she stood it in the place where we had found it. Until she opened the side entrance, I had fancied, without thinking about it, that it must necessarily be night-time. The rush of the daylight quite confounded me, and made me feel as if I had been in the candlelight of the strange room many hours.
>
> 'You are to wait here, you boy,' said Estella; and disappeared and closed the door.
>
> I took the opportunity of being alone in the courtyard, to look at my coarse hands and my common boots. My opinion of those accessories was not favourable. They had never troubled me before, but they troubled me now, as vulgar appendages. I determined to ask Joe why he had ever taught me to call those picture-cards, Jacks, which ought to be called knaves. I wish Joe had been rather more genteelly brought up, and then I should have been so too.
>
> She came back, with some bread and meat and a little mug of beer. She put the mug down on the stones of the yard, and gave me the bread and meat

without looking at me, as insolently as if I were a dog in disgrace. I was so humiliated, hurt, spurned, offended, angry, sorry—I cannot hit upon the right name for the smart—God knows what its name was—that tears started to my eyes. The moment they sprang there, the girl looked at me with a quick delight in having been the cause of them. This gave me the power to keep them back and to look at her: so, she gave a contemptuous toss—but with a sense, I thought, of having made too sure that I was so wounded—and left me.[46]

Jude Robinson, Ellie Gray, Melissa Chapple, 'Methodological Strengths and Limitations'

The demonstration of three different qualitative approaches offered by this chapter helps to mutually illuminate the relative strengths and limitations of each method for capturing the value of literary reading in relation to mental health.

Certain limitations are contextual. For example, in respect of the ethnographically informed study of prison reading groups, constraints were imposed on the research process by the custodial setting. The researcher was not permitted to talk to the women in their rooms, and depending on the participant and setting, some encounters had to be arranged in view of a member of the security staff, which may have inhibited disclosure. As part of disciplinary procedures, some women's free time was restricted or withdrawn, and, as the women were only able to attend approved activities, they were not available to talk to the researcher outside these times and sometimes were even unable to attend the groups. Conflicting (legal or health) appointments could also limit women's availability. The researcher needed to be escorted by custodial staff which further limited interview time depending on their availability. Some of the sessions were also interrupted by early 'movement', in which women were required to immediately return to their rooms, and the researcher was unable to speak with them. Although it was made clear that participants could refuse permission to have the groups observed, or decline consent for interviews, some women may have preferred not to join the groups during the study. Given the brief and sporadic nature of the research visits, there may also have been women attending the groups that the researcher never met and/or never spoke to individually.

Ethnography's commitment to close observation of individual and group behaviour and acceptance of the value of brief exchanges and informal conversations made it possible to work productively within these constraints where a more systematic experimental approach (using a control group, for example, engaged in a comparison activity) might have been unworkable in practice, however desirable in theory. Similarly, while the findings from the study would have been enhanced by quantitative analyses derived from standardised assessment instruments such as measures of anxiety, depression or quality of life (see Chapter 12), the availability of participants at critical points (baseline/pre-intervention and post-intervention) might have proved an obstacle. In addition, the introduction of such measures, reminiscent of the many other assessments women entering the criminal justice system undergo, may have affected the women's willingness to engage with the researchers in the more participatory, open conversations inherent in an ethnographic approach and to accept their presence when observing the reading groups.

IPA is one of several qualitative approaches united by their emphasis on meaning and experience, but distinguished by their goals, methodologies and epistemologies.[47] IPA differs from grounded theory in that the latter, rather than creating an interpretative account of lived experience, seeks to generate a high-level conceptual account (or theory) of social processes occurring in a particular context.[48] Discourse analysis (DA), rooted in linguistics, is concerned with the role of shared language systems in creating meaning, and in enacting identities and relationships (Starks & Trinidad, 2007). While IPA endorses DA's social constructionist viewpoint that language is a fundamental aspect of reality construction, it argues for moving beyond linguistic interaction in order to fully understand experience, because language alone 'does not speak to the empirical realities of people's lived experiences' (Eatough & Smith, 2008, p. 184). In contrast to DA, IPA researchers, drawing on the social-cognitive paradigm, are nonetheless concerned, in addition, with inner mental states. This focus seemed especially pertinent to a study of reading where subjective processes are likely to dominate even within a Shared Reading setting. IPA has similarities with narrative analyses in its commitment to interpretative meaning- making and experiential emphasis (Eatough & Smith, 2008). However, narrative researchers focus more on the structure and organisation of stories (e.g. beginning-middle-end, plots) and relate this to meaning-making within a context of temporal continuity.[49] The emphasis implies a sense of 'journeying', more suited perhaps to the exploration of experience where a journey is prominent (e.g. the experience of illness from diagnosis to recovery), and less appropriate to the study of the presentness and in-the-moment experience of the reading group. Indeed, one of the potential limitations of IPA—principally chosen for its capacity to facilitate an understanding of how participants in a reading group with mental health issues derive meaning from the experience—was the reliance on retrospective recall. Recent reading studies have used video-recorded footage as a stimulus to recall within the interview (see Chapter 10) and use of this method might enhance future IPA studies of reading. It should also be pointed out that, while the idiographic nature of IPA makes it inappropriate to generalise the findings of the current study to a wider population (Pringle et al., 2011), researchers can aim for theoretical transferability rather than empirical generalisability, such that theoretical concepts may be applied more broadly to help make sense of the findings.

As the final section of the chapter makes clear, Framework Analysis permits researchers to *develop* and *test* a pre-conceived framework, which can be from theory, relevant research findings, pilot findings, or other justifiable resources that lead to specific assumptions about how the results might look (Parkinson et al., 2016). The advantage of Framework Analysis is its incorporation of all relevant findings for the development of a more informed analytical approach, and its encouragement to use as much data as possible, thus reducing data loss that may impact resulting findings. Framework Analysis was selected in preference to Thematic Analysis, where analysis takes place without any assumptions having been made about the data. This is more advantageous in areas where there are no theories or research that relate to the data, or no examples that would depict it well. (For this reason, thematic analysis remains a strong contender as the qualitative method of choice for exploratory studies in relation to reading and health.[50]) Although it is true that theories in the area of autism research, such as the E-S theory, do not maximally explain the link between autism and reading habits, individual findings such as those from Barnes (2012) provided useful insight. Thematic Analysis would thus have been limiting compared to Framework Analysis, as relevant findings helped organisation and interpretation of the data in such a way that it could be critically compared to autism theory.

The point of these concluding reflections is not to endorse certain qualitative approaches in respect of reading and mental health but to offer a demonstration of how the selection of method will be determined by the reading model and the population which experiences it, as well as by the specific aims of the study.

Notes

1. The study was supported by funding from the National Personality Disorder Team/Ministry of Justice, UK, and received ethical approval from the Northern and Yorkshire Research Ethics Committee (UK) and the National Offender Management Service (NOMS, UK).
2. See, for example, Billington et al. (2011), Dowrick et al. (2012, Chapter Five, Notes 2 and 3).
3. In all, 35 women were recruited to the study, the age range was 18–62. For full details of participants and recruitment procedure, see J. Billington, E. Longden, and J. Robinson, 'A Literature-Based Intervention for Women Prisoners: Preliminary Findings', *International Journal of Prisoner Health*, 12.4 (2016), 230–43 (p. 233); J. Billington and J. Robinson, *An Evaluation of a Pilot Study of a Literature-Based Intervention with Women in Prison* (University of Liverpool, Centre for Research into Reading, Literature and Society, 2013), pp. 18–20.
4. P. Atkinson, *Ethnography: Principles in Practice* (London: Routledge, 1995).
5. K. O'Reilly, *Ethnographic Methods* (Abingdon: Routledge, 2005).
6. R. Sanjek, *Fieldnotes: The Making of Anthropology* (London: Cornell University Press, 1990).
7. R. Emerson, R. Fretz, and L. Shaw, 'Participant Observation and Fieldnotes', in *Handbook of Ethnography*, ed. by P. Atkinson, A. Coffey, S. Delamont, J. Lofland, and L. Lofland (London: Sage, 2007), pp. 352–68. All initial 'jottings' were later written up into more complete fieldnotes, or field records, in the days following the visit. P. Atkinson, *The Ethnographic Imagination: Textual Constructions of Reality* (London: Routledge, 1990).
8. C. Geertz, *The Interpretation of Cultures* (London: Fontana Press, 1993).
9. C. Riessman, *Narrative Methods for the Human Sciences* (London: Sage, 2008).
10. A. Coffey and P. Atkinson, *Making Sense of Qualitative Data: Complementary Research Strategies* (London: Sage, 1996); D. Silverman, *Interpreting Qualitative Data* (London: Sage, 2012).
11. J. Robinson, 'Focus Groups', in *Handbook of Qualitative Research in Education*, ed. by S. Delamont (Cheltenham: Edward Elgar, 2012), pp. 391–404.
12. See E. Gray, G. Kiemle, P. Davis, and J. Billington, 'Making Sense of Mental Health Difficulties Through Live Reading: An Interpretative Phenomenological Analysis of the Experience of Being in a Reader Group', *Arts & Health*, 8.3 (2016), 248–61.
13. M. Larkin, S. Watts, and E. Clifton, 'Giving Voice and Making Sense in Interpretative Phenomenological Analysis', *Qualitative Research in Psychology*, 3.2 (2006), 102–20. See also, Edmund Husserl, *General Introduction to Pure Phenomenology* (1931), trans. by W. R. Boyce Gibson (London: Routledge, 2012).

14. V. Eatough and J. A. Smith, 'Interpretative Phenomenological Analysis', in *Sage Handbook of Qualitative Research in Psychology*, ed. by C. Willig and W. Stainton-Rogers (London: Sage, 2008), pp. 179–94 (p. 180).
15. J. A. Smith, P. Flowers, and M. Larkin, *Interpretative Phenomenological Analysis: Theory, Method and Research* (London: Sage, 2009).
16. K. Reid, P. Flowers, and M. Larkin, 'Exploring Lived Experience', *The Psychologist*, 18.1 (2005), 20–23.
17. J. A. Smith, 'Evaluating the Contribution of Interpretative Phenomenological Analysis', *Health Psychology Review*, 5.1 (2011), 9–27.
18. B. Giorgi and A. Giorgi (2008), 'Phenomenology', in *Qualitative Psychology: A Practical Guide to Research Methods*, ed. by J. A. Smith (London: Sage, 2008), pp. 26–52; J. Pringle, J. Drummond, E. McLafferty, and C. Hendry, 'Interpretative Phenomenological Analysis: A Discussion and Critique', *Nurse Researcher*, 18.3 (2011), 20–24. See also Martin Heidegger, *Being and Time* (1927), trans. by Joan Stambaugh (New York: New York State University Press, 2010) and Chapter 10.
19. J. A. Smith and M. Osborn, 'Interpretative Phenomenological Analysis', ed. by Smith (2008), pp. 51–80.
20. J. A. Smith, 'Semi-Structured Interviewing and Qualitative Analysis', in *Rethinking Methods in Psychology*, ed. by J. A. Smith, R. Harré, and L. Van Langenhove (London: Sage, 1995), pp. 11–26.
21. P. Fonagy and M. Target, *Psychoanalytic Theories: Perspectives from Developmental Psychopathology* (London: Whurr, 2006). See also Chapters 13 and 15.
22. J. Bowlby, *A Secure Base: Clinical Applications of Attachment Theory* (London: Tavistock, 1988).
23. S. Baron-Cohen, 'Editorial Perspective: Neurodiversity—A Revolutionary Concept for Autism and Psychiatry', *Journal of Child Psychology and Psychiatry*, 58.6 (2017), 744–47.
24. L. Kanner, 'Early Infantile Autism', *Journal of Pediatrics*, 25.3 (1944), 211–17.
25. E. Müller, A. Schuler, and G. B. Yates, 'Social Challenges and Supports from the Perspective of Individuals with Asperger Syndrome and Other Autism Spectrum Disabilities', *Autism*, 12.2 (2008), 173–90.
26. N. Bauminger and C. Kasari, 'Loneliness and Friendship in High-Functioning Children with Autism', *Child Development*, 71.2 (2000), 447–56.
27. S. W. White and R. Roberson-Nay, 'Anxiety, Social Deficits, and Loneliness in Youth with Autism Spectrum Disorders', *Journal of Autism and Developmental Disorders*, 39.7 (2009), 1006–13.
28. M. O. Mazurek, 'Loneliness, Friendship, and Well-Being in Adults with Autism Spectrum Disorders', *Autism*, 18.3 (2014), 223–32.
29. S. Baron-Cohen, T. Jolliffe, C. Mortimore, and M. Robertson, 'Another Advanced Test of Theory of Mind: Evidence from Very High Functioning

Adults with Autism or Asperger Syndrome', *Journal of Child Psychology and Psychiatry*, 38.7 (1997), 813–22.
30. M. V. Lombardo and S. Baron-Cohen, 'The Role of the Self in Mindblindness in Autism', *Consciousness and Cognition*, 20.1 (2011), 130–40.
31. S. Baron-Cohen, 'Autism: The Emphathizing-Systemizing (E-S) Theory,' *Annals of the New York Academy of Sciences*, 1156.1 (2009), 68–80.
32. R. A. Mar and K. Oatley, 'The Function of Fiction Is the Abstraction and Simulation of Social Experience', *Perspectives on Psychological Sciences*, 3.3 (2008), 173–92. (See also Chapter 15.)
33. D. C. Kidd and E. Castano, 'Reading Literary Fiction Improves Theory of Mind', *Science*, 342.6156 (2013), 377–80. (See also Chapter 13.)
34. M. J. Tirado and D. Saldaña, 'Readers with Autism Can Produce Inferences, but They Cannot Answer Inferential Questions', *Journal of Autism and Developmental Disorders*, 46.3 (2016), 1025–37.
35. E. Koopman and F. Hakemulder, 'Effects of Literature on Empathy and Self-Reflection: A Theoretical-Empirical Framework', *Journal of Literary Theory*, 9.1 (2015), 79–111.
36. S. Baron-Cohen, S. Wheelwright, R. Skinner, J. Martin, and E. Clubley, 'The Autism-Spectrum Quotient (AQ): Evidence from Asperger Syndrome/High-Functioning Autism, Males and Females, Scientists and Mathematicians', *Journal of Autism and Developmental Disorders*, 31.1 (2001), 5–17.
37. S. Baron-Cohen and S. Wheelwright, 'The Empathy Quotient: An Investigation of Adults with Asperger Syndrome or High Functioning Autism, and Normal Sex Differences', *Journal of Autism and Developmental Disorders*, 34.2 (2004), 163–75.
38. K. E. Bodner, C. E. Engelhardt, N. J. Minshew, and D. L. Williams, 'Making Inferences: Comprehension of Physical Causality, Intentionality, and Emotions in Discourse by High-Functioning Older Children, Adolescents, and Adults with Autism', *Journal of Autism and Developmental Disorders*, 45.9 (2015), 2721–33.
39. K. D. Ten Eycke and U. Muller, 'Brief Report: New Evidence for a Social-Specific Imagination Deficit in Children with Autism Spectrum Disorder', *Journal of Autism and Developmental Disorder*, 45.1 (2015), 213–20; J. Craig and S. Baron-Cohen, 'Creativity and Imagination in Autism and Asperger Syndrome', *Journal of Autism and Developmental Disorders*, 29.4 (1999), 319–26.
40. I. E. Boerma, S. E. Mol, and J. Jolles, 'Reading Pictures for Story Comprehension Requires Mental Imagery Skills', *Frontiers in Psychology*, 24.7 (2016), 1630.
41. J. Barnes, 'Fiction, Imagination, and Social Cognition: Insights from Autism', *Poetics*, 40.4 (2012), 299–316.
42. N. K. Gale, G. Heath, E. Cameron, S. Rashid, and S. Redwood, 'Using the Framework Method for the Analysis of Qualitative Data in

Multi-Disciplinary Health Research', *BMC Medical Research Methodology*, 13.1 (2013), 117.

43. S. Parkinson, V. Eatough, J. Holmes, E. Stapley, and N. Midgley, 'Framework Analysis: A Worked Example of a Study Exploring Young People's Experiences of Depression', *Qualitative Research in Psychology*, 13.2 (2016), 109–29.
44. NVivo was helpful at this stage, as it reduced the chances of data loss and allowed viewing and editing of the organisational framework until it worked best.
45. Using NVivo for stage 3 and 4 allowed the framework from stage 2 to be manipulated into the final codes, sub-themes and themes, and again reduced data loss.
46. Charles Dickens, *Great Expectations* (1861), ed. by Charlotte Mitchell (Harmondsworth: Penguin Books Ltd., 2003), pp. 60–62; this extract also appears in Angela Macmillan, *A Little Aloud: An Anthology of Prose and Poetry for Reading Aloud to Someone You Care For* (London: Chatto & Windus, 2010), pp. 39–46.
47. H. Starks and S. B. Trinidad, 'Choose Your Method: A Comparison of Phenomenology, Discourse Analysis and Grounded Theory', *Qualitative Health Research*, 17.10 (2007), 1372–80.
48. K. Charmaz and K. Henwood, 'Grounded Theory', in *Sage Handbook of Qualitative Research in Psychology*, ed. by C. Willig and W. Stainton-Rogers (London: Sage, 2008), pp. 240–59.
49. M. Murray, 'Narrative Psychology', in *Qualitative Psychology: A Practical Guide to Research Methods*, ed. by J. A. Smith (London: Sage, 2003), pp. 111–31; M. Murray and S. Sergeant, 'Narrative Psychology', in *Qualitative Research Methods in Mental Health*, ed. by D. Harper and A. R. Thompson (Chichester: Wiley-Blackwell, 2012), pp. 163–75.
50. V. Braun and V. Clarke, 'Using Thematic Analysis in Psychology', *Qualitative Research in Psychology*, 3.2. (2006), 77–101.

10

Qualitative Methods II: Developing Innovative Qualitative Approaches in Research on Reading and Health

Josie Billington, Philip Davis, Grace Farrington, Kelda Green, Fiona Magee, Mette Steenberg and Thor Magnus Tangeraas

Josie Billington and Philip Davis, 'Reading Live: A Qualitative Method for Analyzing Reading in Real Time'

In this section, we describe the evolution of what began as an experimental qualitative approach to the analysis of group literary reading which has crystallised into an indispensable methodology. While we offer it as a standalone method here, it can also be powerfully combined with the methods outlined in the sections and chapters which follow.

The first step in the development of this method came with the decision to audio-record all reading groups in the first mixed methods study of reading and mental health undertaken by the Centre for Research into Reading, Literature and Society (CRILS), which investigated the value of

J. Billington (✉) · P. Davis · K. Green · F. Magee
Centre for Research into Reading, Literature and Society,
University of Liverpool, Liverpool, UK
e-mail: jbilling@liverpool.ac.uk

P. Davis
e-mail: phildav@liverpool.ac.uk

G. Farrington
The Reader, Liverpool, UK
e-mail: graceframe@thereader.org.uk

J. Billington (ed.), *Reading and Mental Health*,
https://doi.org/10.1007/978-3-030-21762-4_10

Shared Reading for people experiencing depression (see Chapters 2 and 5). The audio-recording itself was at this stage mostly a functional means to an end. In addition to the standard measures of depression taken before and after the twelve-month reading group, we wanted to understand how the dynamic of the group—the relative contributions of (often socially isolated) individuals and the interaction between them—changed over time. The most powerful standard qualitative methods for capturing these components were linguistic ones—conversation analysis in particular—and the recordings were initially intended simply to collect the primary data for transcription and linguistic analysis.

The transcripts proved rich material indeed. We found very quickly that many features *required* the combined literary-critical and linguistic expertise of the team. When interpreting a pause or silence, or when weighing the significance of a sentence begun and not completed, we found ourselves applying to the transcripts, the kind of literary close reading skills which the participants were applying to the literature they were reading.[1] These interpretative issues often compelled us to return to the recordings during the course of analysis, in order to understand a precise second or two of hiatus in dialogue, or a particular instance of broken syntax in their live, dynamic context. Indeed, even at this early stage, we were keen to analyse micro-happenings and to use the available technology to substantiate objectively our more subjective interpretations. Computerised analysis of the sound recordings, millisecond by millisecond, showed the subtle and intricate 'intonation signals' given off both by group members *and* by the poem on its being read aloud.[2] This offered powerful corroboration of our intuition that Shared Reading aloud produces a kind of interpersonality[3] both with the book, its author and characters, and with other group members. But in the course of these findings, it also became abundantly clear that the audio-recordings alone were missing a potentially huge amount of valuable data in relation to what constituted this phenomenon.

M. Steenberg
Aarhus University, Aarhus, Denmark
e-mail: mette.steenberg@cas.au.dk

T. M. Tangeraas
Department of Communication and Design,
Kristiania University College, Oslo, Norway
e-mail: ThorMagnus.Tangeras@kristiania.no

In our second study of reading in relation to community mental health,[4] therefore, we filmed and sound recorded reading groups. Our experience had taught us that the recordings would need to be 'read', using the interpretive tools of open-minded literary criticism.[5] But to maximise the quality and range of understanding in relation to a real-life mental health context, that 'reading' needed to be undertaken by literary and linguistic specialists in collaboration with psychologists also. We met as a group, therefore, over a number of weeks to witness together the reading as a live phenomenon. We were not at this stage seeking consensus or reliability. This was classic data immersion as practised in qualitative research (see Chapter 9) combined for the first time, as far as we know, with the expertise of literary-critical close reading. We waited to see what (at the level of theme, category, concept) emerged. In what follows, we re-create what happened on our first viewing of the footage.

The reading group is made up of three men and three women between the ages of 25 and 60 who are attending a community reading group for those experiencing mental health issues.[6] In the third weekly session of the group, they are reading George Eliot's nineteenth-century novella, *Silas Marner*—specifically, here, the reaction of the protagonist, a miser and hermit, to the loss of his horde of gold. As demonstrated in Part II, the literature is read aloud, live, with the help of a group leader:

> Group Leader (reading):
> Since he had lost his money, Silas had contracted the habit of opening his door and looking out from time to time, as if he thought that his money might be somehow coming back to him, or that some trace, some news of it, might be mysteriously on the road and be caught by the listening ear or the straining eye. It was chiefly at night, when he was not occupied in his loom, that he fell into this repetition of an act for which he could have assigned no definite purpose, and which can hardly be understood, except by those who have undergone a bewildering separation from a supremely loved object.[7]

Most group members continued to look down, thoughtfully, at the book. It was Fred who took our attention, as he immediately looked up, eyes keenly alert, saying, a little self-consciously:

> I knew a case of that myself. My grandfather, when he retired from work, actually used to go out on the road, the same time every morning, stand at

> the bus stop and let the bus go. He'd never get on the bus. He'd just wait for it to come, religiously every morning, 7.15, go down, get his paper and then come home, make my breakfast and get me ready for school. Just why—I could never work it out. I'd say 'why?' and he'd say, 'broken hearted that's why, because my work was everything and a whole lot'. Made an awful long day for him. That pattern of behaviour went on for a year or more.

'It's the habit?' (the group leader gently prompts), 'the loss of the job is really painful, but the habit is a comfort?'. Now Linda, another group member, says:

> It's the anchor isn't it. It'd give him something to hold onto. It's as though he needed to see the bus coming and going just to make sure that - to reassure him the world was still carrying on.
> Fred: That's right (turning to Linda and nodding). I think he ached for normal service to be resumed. That was it.

What struck us about this moment was the felt presentness of this memory in Fred's recounting of it. (Fred, now in his fifties, was speaking of forty years ago.) Significantly (as the linguists noted), the story is mostly told *not* in the simple past tense of narrative ('I knew', 'when he retired') but in the continuous past of 'he used to', 'He'd never get on the bus. He'd just wait for it to come'. Of course, this is the grammatical index of the 'pattern of behaviour' which Fred's grandfather puts in place of what is no longer there—his working life. But, in the moment, it is strongly suggestive of what remains deeply unresolved in Fred himself. 'Just why I could never work it out.' Here, he softly shakes his head, looking down, his hands open. It is as if Fred is again the child asking 'why?'

The quick involuntariness of Fred's response was one crucial feature which the research team found repeated across the recordings, and to which participants gave ample testimony at interview (see Chapter 10, 'Josie Billington, Philip Davis, Grace Farrington, Fiona Magee, "Qualitative Interviews 2: Video-Assisted"').

> I went in there, not knowing; I didn't know I was going to come across that. I was totally taken aback and it felt so important. I felt it mattered and should be pursued.
> I felt quite … quite emotional there – and wasn't expecting to. The reading just touched something in me…I had no idea where that was going to go.

Critical here is 'having no idea', 'not knowing' in advance. The literary text, is experienced—these accounts suggest—*pre*-cognitively, creating the ground for affective responses which happen live and in the moment, as a kind of surprise or awakening. Reading, at such moments is a form of immediate *doing*, actively and dynamically in the moment. The starting-point for thus '*doing* reading', was a felt inner experience, implicitly registered in response to the text.

Here, as was quite common, the awakening took the form of personal anecdote. Indeed, one finding was that personal story was often an enabler to individual *and* group response so long as it was intrinsically triggered by the text and did not break the emotional atmosphere created by it. Autobiographical material had the power to deepen the field of *resonance* radiating from the literary story—in this case the moved bafflement in the face of the 'repetition of an act [with] no definite purpose, which can hardly be understood, *except by those who have undergone a bewildering separation from a supremely loved object*'. When Frank instinctively inhabits, via personal memory, the final move of this sentence (as though 'except' were not a mere prosaic conjunction, but a cue and catalyst for a human-imaginative shift), the circle of feeling within which the work remains live is expanded (Linda: 'He needed to see the bus ... to reassure him that the world was still carrying on').[8]

Compare Heather's response, later in the same session, to Robert Frost's famous poem 'The Road Not Taken', which brought with it the memory of her experience of hospitalisation over seven years with anorexia, while her twin sister was taking the more conventional path of university. Usually very quiet, this was the first time Heather spoke at length.

> I think from childhood, people have expected us to do the same. I think even I expected we would do the same at least up until the age that we are now-21. We kind of assumed our lives would follow similar paths, and – they haven't. Over the last seven years I think she's taken the more conventional path that I always thought I would travel – but I haven't – for various reasons. So it's almost like I can *see* what I *could* have done in this other person.

This is not a routine anorexia story told with the facility of familiarity, but a moment of surprised admission—'*Even I* expected we would do the same'—and of energetic recognition: 'I can *see* what I *could* have done'. The conventional path not taken is not simply a matter for regret but a subject-matter to be engaged with from a different place or perspective. Significantly, this shift of place or position happens at precisely the point in the poem where the autobiographical 'I' is most thrown out of linear story in the final stanza. The two paths diverge:

and I –
I took the one less travelled by[9]

For a fraction of a second, the poem occupies the otherwise uninhabitable space between a self in potentia, which has already long been left behind, and a self yet to be, that has already been realized. When Heather explores the two roads of Frost's poem in relation to her own twin life, she embodies the poem's mental terrain, holds its existential meaning, as if on behalf of the group, almost *becoming* a version of the poem.

When the depressed person's past life story cannot be changed, says Christopher Dowrick, it is the possibility of changed 'understanding' that matters: 'Meaning does not simply exist: it emerges'; 'It is possible to turn memory into a source of energy either by drawing new implications from old memories or else by expansions, incorporating the memories of others'. What is key is that a person's life 'makes sense emotionally, that at least some of the problems posed by living are worthy of commitment and engagement'.[10] Fred's and Heather's responses offer small instances of how life matter that might have stayed a static and inert part of the past, is given, even momentarily, the expansion and space, via literary reading, to find a vital and meaningful place within a person's story.

Even at this first stage of analysis, then, we were beginning to speculate on the mental health outcomes of these awakenings. But what we found, across the recordings, was that, without this initial emotional resonance in the first place—arousal, surprise, aliveness—nothing to meaningful purpose followed in the second. Awakening was not necessarily characterised by a single nameable emotion (as in 'the poem is *about sadness*') but more a felt and often adjectival sense (signalled initially by shorthand deictic phrases such as 'It's sad', 'This is tender') out of which more complex explicit thoughts would later emerge and open.

Thus, as a research team, we concentrated above all on what we took to be individual 'breakthrough' moments when, in a two-way interaction, the literature seemed both to get through to participants and itself to come alive through them, via the resonance it triggered. In order more reliably and consistently to pinpoint these instances of live 'happening'—moments of change, or breakthrough—we developed a rating system (refined over successive studies to ensure inter-rater reliability) in relation to William James's description of 'emotional excitement':

> There are dead feelings, dead ideas, and cold beliefs, and there are hot and live ones; and when one grows hot and alive within us, everything has to re-crystallize about it. These hot parts are the centres of our dynamic energy, whereas the cold parts leave us indifferent and passive in proportion to their coldness.[11]

It is the 'hot' and 'alive' feeling and thinking we are looking for, both for their own sake in disclosing the power of literary reading, and because—as James (founder of modern psychology) insists—these are the centres of healthy shift and growth in the individual. Our rating system thus consisted of a 5-point scale, where 0 = cold/dead, 5 = hot/live. In a two-stage process, we initially used the system to identify blocks of time—ranging from 2 to 10 minutes—within each recording. Then we rated 30-second intervals in order to isolate salient happenings more specifically.

We have continued to use this rating system to identify instances for analysis at multi-dimensional levels (see Chapters 11 and 13). But during the course of successive studies, thematic categories or characteristics of breakthrough have emerged, outlined below and briefly exemplified,[12] which now help to frame our qualitative analysis.

Creativity
The effect of aroused emotion and not knowing in advance produces emergent feeling and thought and a shift away from default responses or automatic language. Often the new language is visibly inflected by the language of the poem or story. So it is when a group of people living with chronic pain and associated depression were reading Laurie Sheck's 'Mysteriously Standing', which describes 'intervals of withdrawal where I am a burned field... little Stonehenge of the heart'[13]:

> Tim: 'little Stonehenge' – Is that someone describing how something that you don't think has feelings might feel?

The poem's effort to make 'something' that is not there, *there*, substantial, summons a vocabulary other than labelling, which here has an impact upon syntax. Such formulations occur in contrast to the norms of pre-programming—the speech patterns associated with the untroubled register of information and opinion—as a rediscovery of language in place of familiarised automaticity. A related use of creatively intelligent negative syntax occurred when Hannah read Rainer Maria Rilke's poem 'Evening':

> the lands grow distant in your sight,
> One journeying to heaven, one that falls;
> and leave you, not at home in either one,[14]

> Hannah: It's about everything that isn't. There's everything you can be and there's everything that you're not, and they're both there at the same time. That's why it's called 'Evening', not 'Night'.

The responsive creativity which generates a language for itself rather than finding one ready-made, brings readers close to the heuristic processes of the writers by whom they are moved. It is related to the 'creative inarticulacy' identified by linguistic analysis (see Chapter 11) when a word, a line, a sentence becomes an achievement.

Articulate Contemplation

The literature helped to provide a language for verbalized recognition, in place of passive suffering (see Chapter 4), in areas of (painful) experience otherwise difficult to locate or speak of without reduction of meaning. The example below comes from a group for older adults reading Edward Thomas's poem 'Adelstrop'. Joan, on a second or third reading and after a long silence, began to speak but only in the words of the poem. '"No one left and no one came"',[15] she read, as if musing at the possible meaning. Then she looked up and directly round at the group. 'That's how it is for me,' she said in a different tone of voice, more certain, deliberate.

> Joan: I don't know if there is anyone there. I put words out but I don't know if there is anyone really there to pick them up. There's no evidence. One can't be sure. One hopes. 'No one left and no one came.' No, it seems I am quite alone, but I trust there is someone there to receive it.

After a silence, Jean read the poem's final stanza: '"And for that minute a blackbird sang/Close by"' (Thomas, p. 36). 'I hear birds outside sometimes early in the morning. That's a good sound.' In this instance, lyric's special power (as we saw with Heather) is to offer a vocalised place where something immaterial existing inside oneself—something not fully known or named or not even had ('It seems ... I trust')—is momentarily held and realised.

Enlivened Thinking
Some of the keenest thinking happened where uncertainties or under-used dimensions of self and so-called negative experiences were actively used rather than denied or regretted. In relation to the Laurie Sheck poem, for example, Kim said:

> Kim: 'a burned field' – that's a really really *really* good way of describing yourself sometimes isn't it?

'Really really *really* good'—in its energy of tone and thought, and emphatic use of repetition—is notably separate from the suffering Kim recognizes and feels at another level. She can speak of her past and ongoing distress with a manifestly excited vivacity that belongs to a released capacity to think the thoughts of one's life whatever their content. Reading Joanne Harris's short story, 'Faith and Hope Go Shopping', in which two elderly women escape from a care home and travel up to London to visit the shoe department of Fortnum and Mason's, Ellie (who is herself beset by neurological difficulties which affect her sight) spoke of how the disability of one of the old women in the Joanne Harris excursion was actually a benefit:

> Ellie: I was going to say I wonder whether Hope's blindness is actually working in their favour because she can't see how posh it is when Faith can ...

At this level the binary distinction between so-called 'negative' and 'positive' experiences also becomes transformed. Experiences that were painful, denied, seen as useless or suffered as shameful are usefully triggered in relation to the text, in the way that a writer might use his own her own experience to create the poem or story.

This enlivened thinking, moreover, was not separable from the precise and close imaginative *attention* to the language and syntax of the poem. Reading the Sheck poem, Tim pointed out the 'strange placing' of the words when he read the poem out loud.

> Mysteriously standing, its distinct construction odd and uninjured in this yellow
>
> Light. (Sheck, p. 41)

> Tim: I thought that was strange how 'Light' kind of went across the line, the yellow light. It's like the light's separate from the withdrawal isn't it? It does really separate the two – it comes after.

In relation to Robert Herrick's seventeenth-century lyric 'To Anthea, Who May Command Him Anything', Ellie (with no formal experience of studying literature since school) saw how important sonically was the poem's repeated use of the comma ('Bid me to live, and I will live', 'Bid me to weep, and I will weep'[16]) in making the lover's pledge more freely rather than automatically given. 'Each "I will" is a definite promise – only one step away from "I do".'

The challenge of poetry offers an alternative discourse to (sometimes clichéd or stereotypical) modern forms of expression, enabling a move away from safe, habitual or default models for personal thinking. The 'difficulty' and linguistic depth of the literary text works as a profitable obstacle to simple facility, literal explanation or automatic opinion—accessing areas of experience for which the reader has no ready language yet which they need to work at and express or 'get out'.

Enhancement of Mental Processes

One key characteristic of Shared Reading, as Fred and Heather's responses showed, are frequent instances of reappraisal of past experience. When we showed Heather the breakthrough moment in relation to 'The Road Not Taken' at interview, she explained the process like this:

> With the poems and the readings, when it touches on something personal in your life or your experience, it doesn't necessarily make you think about it in a way - it doesn't make you form a new opinion of it but maybe it … makes you realize what your opinions are on it. That you hadn't necessarily consciously thought about before.

This is language of 'realization', in an amalgam of old, long-felt content and sudden new perspective, which the poem tacitly calls for.

> It makes you think about things on a level you can actually see, you know in your head. You can see what you're thinking rather than it just being part of your general feeling on life, you know, you kind of pinpoint things more. It made me realize what … what I already knew, even though I hadn't articulated it necessarily.

Think and feel. This is a special, unique kind of meta-thinking in which the language in which to examine a feeling exists simultaneously *with* the feeling which that same language recreates or recalls. Literature's loyalty to life offers a place for thinking *about* it without ceasing to be *in* it. To be in it without being able to think about it is our usual state—what T. S. Eliot called having the experience but missing the meaning. To think about it without being in it is what education all too often offers—abstract consciousness cut off from its subject-matter, as in text-books or self-help books, offering remedies wholly separate from the feel of the griefs they purport to cure.[17]

Community

Across all of these characteristics, and perhaps enabling them, there emerged the sense and feel of a close community from a gathering of individuals. The imaginative power of shared literature catalysed, we found, the formation of a small-group community by creating a space for shared emotional meditation (rather than conventional or vulnerably exposing confession). The relation between private and public was closer than conventionally allowed, creating a small alternative human society out of the interaction of individual, group and text.[18]

What was particularly remarkable was that the group did not really exist save as a static or notional unit *until*, through the text and the group leader serving it, live connections were made between one individual and another. Then the movements, connections and reconfigurations, between different individuals at different moments in relation to different texts, were unpredictable. Thus, sudden shifts from one participant to another made for a dynamic process of grouping and re-grouping in the course of any session. The video-recordings allow a strong visual sense of these shifts, centres and relations. It was not simply that the groups were notionally democratic and respectful: there was a genuine and unpredictable mobility across age and class whereby at a key moment of realisation one group-member or another changed role—became a version of the Group Leader or the novelist, or the temporary spokesperson for the poem, or the sudden realizer of the personal meaning. This un-fixedness of roles within the group, the experience of never knowing on whom the experience will 'land', is part of the phenomenon of emergence, and of democracy, intrinsic to the nature of the sessions.

The linguistic and physiological indices of this community are explored in Chapters 11 and 13. Currently, we are working on developing a research study exploring the deep structures of interaction using our archive of filmed recordings. The aim is to perform the kind of micro-analysis of Shared Reading which Colin Trevarthen and Daniel Stern applied to the dynamics of intersubjectivity in parent–child interaction.[19]

* * *

We conclude with an instance from the close of the group reading of *Silas Marner* which represented, for this session, a definitive breakthrough. Here, Silas has just awoken from a trance-like state to discover what he at first believes is his lost gold returned.

> He felt his heart begin to beat violently, and for a few moments he was unable to stretch out his hand and grasp the restored treasure. The heap of gold seemed to glow and get larger beneath his agitated gaze. He leaned forward at last and stretched forth his hand; but instead of the hard coin with the familiar resisting outline, his fingers encountered soft warm curls. In utter amazement Silas fell on his knees and bent his head low to examine the marvel; it was a sleeping child, a round fair thing with soft yellow rings all over its head. Could this be his little sister come back to him in a dream—his little sister whom he had carried about in his arms for a year before she died, when he was a small boy without shoes or stockings. That was the first thought that darted across Silas's blank wonderment. *Was* it a dream? (*Silas Marner*, p. 99)

Linda: His preoccupation of thinking about his money, has completely - it has not even come to the forefront of his mind. He doesn't think about the gold *at all*. It had been central to his being until then.

Group-leader (re-reading): 'and bent his head low to examine the marvel: it was a sleeping child - a round, fair thing, with soft yellow rings all over its head.'

Linda: What he thinks is his gold, what he touches is something warm, and real …

Group-leader: Yes …

Linda: Real gold.

Group Leader: Straightaway he says, 'Could this be his little sister come back to him in a dream?' It's funny about the dream.

Linda: Well [shaking head] he just cannot … imagine … this is reality.

Group-leader: Yes -

Linda: It's too wonderful.

Group-leader: Yes, yes

Linda: And the joy. It's … he just [again gently shaking head] cannot comprehend.

'Cannot' is stressed twice here (accompanied by a shaking of the head) in a reversal of the conventional negative. Rather than being cynically dismissed as 'too good to be true', the real in Linda's formulation—'too wonderful', too new and wholly unexpected—has become almost paradoxically what defies imagination. This example of the breaking down of expected norms and barriers as to what reality is and can be, is a culmination of the reawakening and reappraisal process involved in this reading-group experience. It is the result of the process of unpredictability or not knowing in advance which ends here in a transcendence of reductive, habitual or depressed frameworks of understanding. Such awakenings are vital, never merely negligible, says Dowrick, for people who might be passively in the thrall of a depression. 'In imaginatively aiding the emergence of meaning, the doctor must use every detail however small, in the reality of the patient's life, to locate hope through the glimpse of an alternative' (Dowrick, 2009, p. 198). Literature offers the best model of this implicit 'reality', where its meaning is never readily offered in terms of cases or cures and is invariably *more* than any paraphrase or categorisation can hold. Our research helps to show that the meaning hidden inside people who feel small or diminished needs literature's 'holding ground'[20] in order not to be wasted, lost or forgotten.

Mette Steenberg (Qualitative Interviews 1), 'The Micro-Phenomenological Interview as a Methodology for Analysing and Enhancing Reading Engagement'

Mette Steenberg is a researcher at Aarhus University, Interacting Minds Center and Director of The Danish Reading Society (Laeseforeningen), a sister organization to The Reader, UK, which has been promoting Shared Reading in Denmark. (See also Chapters 4, 12 and 18.)

In this section, I give a brief introduction to the micro-phenomenological interview as developed by Claire Petitmengin[21] and demonstrate briefly how the technique can be used to both study and enhance reading engagement. At the close, I discuss how the methodology can be used to formulate hypotheses on the reading process to be tested in subsequent hypothesis-driven mixed method designs.

Starting from the hypothesis that reading engagement is a mediating factor in transformative reading experiences, it is important for research into the therapeutic effects of Shared Reading, and literary reading more generally, to understand when and how reading engagement happens, and in response to which factors in the Shared Reading process; quality of voice, textual features, group dynamic and physical setting. Moreover, the micro-phenomenological interview mirrors the mode of reading that facilitators aim for in Shared Reading groups: thick descriptive explorations into what something 'feels like'. It is thus not only a method for studying the kinds of reading engagement that may afford therapeutic processes; it is also a method for enhancing reading engagement in itself, and thus facilitating therapeutic processes in reading.

Within phenomenologically grounded empirical studies, engagement is the term used to analyze the ways in which readers' transactions with literary texts engage the self. Previous research indicates that certain modes of engagement may lead to 'self-modifying feelings'[22] or 'emergent thinking' (Longden et al., 2015; Davis et al., 2016) both hypothesised to be vital for 'change' or 'transformative' reading experiences.[23]

The micro-phenomenological interview (earlier referred to as 'elicitation interview technique' in Petitmengin, 2006) is a method developed for becoming aware of, and being able to describe, pre-reflexive dimensions of subjective experience. Originally developed by Vermersch[24] to help professionals within the field of education gain awareness of the implicit part of their teaching practices, it has been adapted by Petitmengin (2006, 2018) as a second person methodology within cognitive science to provide detailed and minute accounts of subjective experience. The need for such accounts grew out of the limitations of a neuroscientific account of consciousness based on 'neural correlates', and laid the foundations of what has been termed neurophenomenology.[25] The micro-phenomenological interview is a reiterative process in which the aim is to enhance insight into the 'felt sense'[26] and the cognitive processes of an experience. The method consists of a questioning technique in which the interviewer brings the interviewee back to 're-live' an experience.

The brief example described here was the first of several I conducted with readers who had reported experiences they themselves identified as 'significant reading moments'. I conducted the interview with the aim of developing a research protocol for subsequent studies into reading engagement. The micro-phenomenological interview is often used as a two-phase research methodology; first it works inductively to establish categories and on this basis, secondly, it develops a research protocol and formulates a hypothesis to be tested deductively on a larger sample. In this sense, the approach is akin to grounded theory framework (see Chapter 9), with concern for cognitive and affective processes.

- The micro-phenomenological interview consists of two parts: (1) Establishing the temporal unfolding of the experience in order to define the boundaries of the experience and (2) Broadening of the synchronic dimension.

This particular interview took place several months after the interviewee had read in a Shared Reading group 'Romanesque Arches' by the Swedish Nobel laurate poet Thomas Tranströmer. The interviewee (X) reported having had a very strong experience as we read the poem and agreed to be interviewed about it. The interview took 30 minutes. First, I identified what kind of experience the interview was going to focus on. It was in X's own words an experience of 'getting on some form of a roller-coaster, it's like…I feel I come to, come to some other place emotionally in my mind', of becoming 'confused' and entering 'another state of mind' and eventually experiencing a blackout' and a feeling of being 'no longer myself'.

In the next step I identified the temporal unfolding of the experience. As I established the temporality, I became aware that X had experienced the 'being no longer myself' as a sequential experience following the temporal sequences described in the poem:

1. the arches (standing inside the church)
2. meeting the angel (experiencing the 'roller-coaster' and entering a state of 'blackout')
3. being pushed out on the plaza (and emerging back into consciousness).

Having established the temporal order, I went on to explore and broaden the experiential dimensions within each of these sequences:

> The arches. I guided the interviewee back to the moment of standing within the Romanesque church experiencing the arches by asking questions such as whether the experience was seen from inside or outside of the scene and subsequently went on to explore sensations (of light, sounds, smells, spatial and kinesthetic sensation) and feelings as X stood in the room (atmosphere, mood).
> Meeting the angel. This is how the interviewee describes the scene in his own words: 'it's relatively well-known, you experience it for instance when you are in love or experience great art, very, very moved; a movement… and I don't know any longer if I'm the same, in a way I'm no longer the same, and that you could call another state of mind, I'm not the same as I was before…'
> Emerging into the plaza and into consciousness. X described the 'change' of consciousness or perception as a 'spiritual experience' or a feeling of 'being in love'.

In order to relive the experience, the interviewer might at any moment during the interview bring the interviewee back by saying: What we're going to do together, now, is to go back in time, as though we had a video recorder. To do this, I want you to go back to the moment when I asked you: 'when you were standing under the arches, what did you see?'. From this point you can as an interviewer broaden the synchronic dimensions using what Petitmengin calls 'Ericksonian language': 'And when you do nothing, what do you do? And when you don't know, what do you know? How do you know that you don't know?' (Petitmengin, 2016, p. 250), or as I did in this case: 'When you experience a roller-coaster, what do you experience?', and 'how do you know that you have come to a different place of your mind?' and further 'can you describe this place for me (going into sensations and feelings)?'

As we were broadening the dimensions, I became aware that the strong 'spiritual' experience was mediated by X's embodied identification with the narrator: 'there is a shift here (upon meeting the angel), he is able to make me part of his, or he writes me into, into a….or what shall I say…that confusion the author describes after having met this angel, I also feel I have that feeling, I feel a kind of …I don't experience it from the outside, I am part of the experience after I have met this angel and received the message from the angel, me or him, and then I am simply confused in the same way as he describes in the poem'. The same embodied identification happens in the last sequence: 'then he is pushed out…he shares with me, Tranströmer shares with me, the experience of having, you know of having had a very spiritual experience in this church…and when he has that… he is pushed out of the church out on the plaza'. When I asked X to describe the blackout and the re-emerging back into consciousness on the plaza, X responded: 'there I'm actually glad that I've got the author with me and that I can lean myself on the lines, if not I may not have gotten out of that church, then I would have stayed in there…it's a kind of blackout, I have a kind of blackout…' I repeatedly tried to come back to the dimension of the blackout by asking: 'and when you experience a blackout, what do you experience'. The reply was 'I think in a sense I'm inside of the author/narrator' and X went on to explain that, as he had lost consciousness, so had she. In other words, X had embodied the perception of the narrator and had no knowledge outside of the consciousness of the narrator.

Through the interview a relation was established between deeply immersed and absorbed engagement in literary reading and experiencing an embodied identification with the viewpoint of the narrator and feelings of no longer 'being the same'.

This is interesting, in so far as bibliotherapy as it was first theorised by Caroline Schrodes[27] is based on identification, a hypothesis constantly repeated in the literature[28] and founded on the assumption that the therapeutic outcome is driven by a thematic-oriented cognitive insight into a previously defined 'problem'.[29] This interview, however, demonstrates that identification can happen without being 'theme', or 'problem'-driven by 'theme'; rather, it seems to be driven by a more fundamental mechanism of embodied identification created by means of narrative stance and descriptive details of kinesthetic experiences.

On the basis of this first interview I have subsequently explored identification in various different texts that differ both in terms of narrative stance and theme, in order to be able to establish a research protocol and a hypothesis on the role of identification in Shared Reading. The aim is to develop yet better-mixed method studies (see Chapter 12) which relate reading process and outcome measures.

Josie Billington, Philip Davis, Grace Farrington, Fiona Magee (Qualitative Interviews 2), 'Video-assisted'

In a further methodological innovation developed by CRILS, in tandem with its multi-disciplinary analysis of video-recorded reading groups, selections from the video-recordings were shown to group participants at individual interview. The short clips (of no more than several minutes) were chosen from those instances which were regarded as salient by the multi-disciplinary team (see Chapter 10, 'Josie Billington and Philip Davis, "Reading Live: A Qualitative Method for Analyzing Reading in Real Time"'). The primary purpose of this approach initially was further to 'check' the research team's findings. This was to be the experience-near qualitative data which would complement the formal linguistic analysis to which the transcripts of the video-recordings were subject (see Chapter 11). We looked to the interviews, as we looked to the linguistic analysis, to test, correct and fine-tune some of the hypotheses already suggested by the research team as well as to elicit free-ranging responses. But this method offered a richness we had neither anticipated nor consciously sought.

'Live' recall (a variation on second-person elicitation technique/the micro-phenomenological interview?)
Participants abundantly attested at interview that an involuntary emotional and neo-physical connection to the literary work, anterior to the level of considered response, was often the first point of entry: 'When you're reading a well-written, powerful poem, it sort of hits you in the face even though it physically can't'; 'The reading can get to feelings very quickly: it's almost condensed'; 'You can feel it deep inside'; 'The poem really zeroed in on my feelings, laid them bare'; 'It has really - hit me; right there [points to heart], the whole poem'.[30] Such testimony verified our finding that the literary material was putting the readers in touch and in place with resonant areas of deep and real human experience otherwise difficult to locate or recover. As Claire Petitmengin says, in seeking to access inner processes, a person usually begins with explanation or judgement or with what he or she believes or imagines he or she is doing. 'A particular effort is necessary for the person to gain access to his or her experience itself, which lies underneath his or her representations, beliefs, judgements and comments. To carry out this task, guidance is useful' (Petitmengin, 2006, p. 235). The video recordings help us to see how literary reading can trigger access to subterranean or 'underneath' experience in place of effort or guidance. Without the readers' trying, quite involuntarily ('The poem kind of shortcut into a feeling when I was least expecting it. It just happened quite – suddenly'), the reader's attention is 'stabilised' and instantly re-directed 'from outside to inside', focussed on an inner dimension and interior sensation.

What was palpable at the video-assisted interviews was that feelings first experienced by participants in the group were often powerfully re-experienced when they viewed the video clips. So, when Angela witnessed her response to John Clare's poem 'I am':

> Group Leader (reading final stanza):
> I long for scenes where man has never trod,
> A place where woman never smiled or wept,
> There to abide, with my creator, God,
> And sleep as I in childhood sweetly slept:
> Untroubling and untroubled where I lie,
> The grass below – above the vaulted sky.[31]

> Angela: It feels, there's something about peace isn't there, because it's not even talking about being happy. 'Never smiled or wept': it's about peacefulness and to be untroubled.

Seeing this clip at interview, Angela said immediately (without further prompt):

Angela: I do remember that. I mean I clearly felt quite ... quite emotional there – and wasn't expecting to. It just touched something in me about how I was feeling at the time. There was lots of talk there about the Creator and God. It wasn't about any kind of religious touching in me – it was about the sense of turmoil and not feeling at peace [pause]. It's particular words I remember, something about turmoil and being tossed on the sea of [looking back at the poem, reads silently for a few seconds, then, from stanza 2, reads aloud]

> I am, and live—like vapours tossed
> Into the nothingness of scorn and noise,
> Into the living sea of waking dreams,
> Where there is neither sense of life or joys,
> But the vast shipwreck of my life's esteems;

I feel it now actually, watching it again. For me it wasn't even in the past, it was current. It was something that kind of, was sort of was going on at the time—you know, still is, really.

'Now', 'past', 'current', 'at the time', 'still'. This involuntary blurring of past and present, where the reader is returned via the video-clip to the moment of reading in its embodied immediacy, is a common feature of the interviews. Ellie, watching her response to Robert Herrick's seventeenth-century lyric 'To Anthea, Who May Command Him Anything', said 'That almost made me feel a little bit tearful just then! It's quite moving isn't it. I remembered again when you showed me it, my first thought was oh it's only ... it's from ages ago'. Linda, on viewing her response to *Silas Marner* (see above, 'Josie Billington and Philip Davis, "Reading live: A Qualitative Method for Analyzing Reading in Real Time"'): 'It's just like a portal, like a portal into another person's consciousness... You know exactly what George Eliot's describing in Silas... [quoting] "The thoughts were strange to him now, like old friendships impossible to revive". Although it's described in words, it makes a kind of wordless knowledge inside your mind'. Keith, watching a recording of his response to Shakespeare's Sonnet 29 ('When in disgrace with fortune and men's eyes', see Chapter 5) spoke of the expression of his own sense of self-disgust in relation to the line 'Yet in these thoughts myself almost despising': 'Once you become aware of something, you cannot turn back, you can't unknow. So, right now [i.e. at interview] when I see these things in print, they strike home'. Print strikes home, as though the reader is almost unavoidably caught by the immediate translation of something previously elusive into something definitive.

These instances demonstrate how the video-assisted interview helps overcome another of the principal barriers Petitmengin has identified to getting in touch with subjective experience: namely, that 'real-time access is impossible' (Petitmengin, 2006, p. 237). An inner process cannot be reflected upon or verbalised while it is happening, and is often too fleeting to capture anyway. Subsequent reflection upon it always risks distortion of it. To become conscious of the process, the participant 'must re-enact it several times, play it out again in an inner way' (Petitmengin, 2006, p. 238). This replay—which is the basis of Petitmengin's micro-phenomenological approach (Petitmengin, 2006, 2007, 2011, 2018) as demonstrated above ('Mette Steenberg, "The micro-phenomenological interview as a methodology for analysing and enhancing reading engagement"')—happens in a literal sense when reading participants, reviewing the video-recorded highlights, are able to re-inhabit the feel of significant but small passing moments rather than recalling them post hoc.[32]

Above all, the evidence from our study of live reading (from observation of the group experience through to individual interview) is that literature per se helps overcome what Petitmengin regards as an essential obstacle to establishing a relationship of 'contact' with our own inward experience—the difficulty of putting our inner experience into words:

> The vocabulary at our disposal to describe the various dimensions of our subjective experience is very poor, and this poverty can probably be put down to the fact that in our culture it has been little explored. For example, we have no precise words to describe synesthetic sensations, or the subtle internal processes. (Petitmengin, 2006, pp. 238–39)

Literature, in fact, is the one area of our inherited culture which does seriously explore the inner life. Our customarily impoverished language for first-person data—the fact that the underlying rawness is hard to get down to—is why we need poetry's and fiction's dedication to articulate recognition of subjective experience. When Angela picks out and re-reads from John Clare's poem, 'the vast shipwreck of my life's esteems', she is not so much quoting from the text, as inhabiting the emotional reality of the poem which itself is coming to life again through her. It is an important example of how poetry has potential at once to 'hit' inner trouble *and* help unfold it into articulate expression. The challenging depth of the emotion, together with the relative difficulty and unfamiliarity of the literary language, blocks simple facility and literalistic opinion, galvanising a new kind of probing, exploratory language ('not about being happy', 'something about not being at peace') which is often spontaneously creative ('You can't unknow'; 'It makes a kind of wordless knowledge in your mind'). It is as if, at such times, the literary text replaces the micro-phenomenological interviewer. In this way, literature and literary reading is a potentially vital tool in phenomenological science's endeavour to 'develop rigorous methods' and a 'create a language' for 'the very precise study of subjective experience' (Petitmengin, pp. 230, 261).[33]

Certainly the video-assisted interviews have helped to create a more 'precise', nuanced or finer language for the study of shared literary reading. Susan, for example, spoke thus of how the literary text was at the centre of the group, a vocally embodied presence and 'power' when read aloud:

> I'm interested in our body language. At the time I did feel engaged in it, but I hadn't realised how much, till I saw us leaning into it if you like. It was as though there was a power in the middle of the table, or around the Group Leader as she was reading, and it was pulling us in.

Ann spoke in interview of how, at its best, 'each moment became totally a world in itself for appreciation'. This meant, she said, that the group were not talking together 'about' something—an issue or feeling—but talking together 'within' it. As Arthur put it (describing the experience of getting to grips with complex writings not difficult for their own sake but because sited in important emotional areas): 'It means that your mind is in action at the same time as your feelings are in action. You're not just talking about feelings but actually *doing* feelings'. Heather said: 'It makes you think about things on a level you can actually see, in your head. You can see what you're thinking and feeling rather than it just being part of your general feeling on life. You pinpoint things more' (see above, 'Josie Billington and Philip Davis, "Reading Live: A Qualitative Method for Analyzing Reading in Real Time"'). Such terms—thinking *within* not about, the mind in action, *doing* reading/*doing* feelings, *seeing* mental and emotional processes—have become staples of our research vocabulary in identifying a special form of 'metacognition' involved in literary reading, in which one can have the thought about the feeling while still *feeling* the feeling, via the literary text.

Not Therapy, Not Cases

One feature of the interviews was that, re-immersed in the recorded reality of particular reading moments, participants repeatedly drew a contrast between the almost involuntary, unfiltered emotions which Shared Reading demanded and their experience of formal therapy groups. Keith, a member of a reading group in an addiction rehabilitation centre, spoke of no longer 'having to remember' to maintain defensive pretence.

> Books and poems make you look at things honestly. And it's harder to tell lies around them. This, it's about feelings, so you're talking about feelings. That [therapy groups] you're talking about actions, behaviours.

Feelings here mean a deep level of serious personal involvement, entered into all the more honestly because accompanied by some reluctance and resistance. In an addiction therapy group:

> What I thought they wanted to hear was - 'Yeah I had a really bad day the other day, I really fancied a drink but I sat down and I thought No, it won't be just one, it's never just one, so I got through it,' and they'll go, 'Oh well done'. If I was getting only comfortable thoughts, I would not change my behaviour.

Shared Reading was (beneficially) not 'comfortable' because the abrupt and unexpected emotional involvement freed the reader from the set vocabulary of cases in therapy or conditions in recovery. As Heather said (whose anorexia meant that, unusually for someone of her age, she had experienced many therapeutic groups):

> This is less … *miserable*, I suppose. You're not sitting around talking about how you feel terrible, everything's going wrong; you're talking about [long pause] not always good things but things [pause] in a better context.

Literary reading, this suggests, enables profitable ('better') contemplation of the apparently negative or the ostensibly *un*comfortable in human experience, through stimulating a wider and more spontaneously human discourse.

Indeed, of deep importance to many participants at interview was how sharing human situations offered by literature enabled them not to think of themselves as 'cases'. Peter: 'Oh I'm not going mad, someone else has had this experience. Somebody else is feeling that way'. For these readers, literature broadens and enriches the human norm, accepting and allowing for troubles, traumas, inadequacies and other experiences usually classed as negative or even pathological. Poetry and fiction creates a special kind of emotionally contemplative time-out, a healthy environment not least because it allows—within its safety, informality and good fellowship—material that is painful and risky and in need of expression. One participant in a chronic pain reading group, Alistair, gave his own compelling analogy for the kind of democracy created by Shared Reading:[34]

> No one is dominating. It's a bit like an opera. The parts will all be singing at the same time, and you have a baritone solo over there and the tenor will come in and they are all singing their own part, like in counterpoint harmony. It's incredible really; it is quite unique.

'No one is dominating' includes, says Helen (a member of the same group), the group-leader:

"There's no return to the therapist: You are not asked to relate personally: you just *do*' (see Chapter 8). Personal relation to the literature is discovered entirely voluntarily, at the participants' own pace and in their own time, rather than programmatically. Shared Reading, as one participant put it, is 'therapy by stealth'.

Therapeutic Value of Interviews?

Jane exclaimed, when seeing her response to *Great Expectations*: 'Oh goodness, I am starting to feel'; 'I was coming across quite well there. Quite confident'. Donald was amazed how, since he was 'not an assertive person', he had 'sort of spilled over'; 'It's a kind of reminder that there is a self in there.' 'You suddenly think, God! I have got an imagination,' reported Peter, 'whereas your world was very small often, on your own and lonely':

> It makes you feel like a fully-functioning person again. You know, like a member of society. I like what I'm seeing more than probably I ever have ... I think he's all right that guy.

In the context of these often difficult lives, sometimes the greatest surprise is that of suddenly valuing oneself and one's experience. The participants, we felt, deserved the close attention they themselves often paid to the works they read; in their readings, there are moments of extraordinary achievement, which, though transient and intricate, merited greater recognition, not least by the participants themselves. One of the central uses of video-assisted interviews was this further opportunity for participants to develop the capacity for self-reflection, consolidating some of the insights momentarily arising in the reading-group sessions, keeping the literature present and also deepening the person's relation to it. Here are two brief examples.

Example 1.
Donald, a member of a local community group, has suffered depression through loss of work and purpose in the world. At interview, he sees the moment where he found himself responding to a seventeenth-century love lyric by Robert Herrick:

> Bid me to live, and I will live
>   Thy protestant to be:
> Or bid me love, and I will give
>   A loving heart to thee.
>
> A heart as soft, a heart as kind,
>   A heart as sound and free,
> As in the whole world thou canst find,
>   That heart I'll give to thee.[35]

Donald's usual way of speaking is peppered with 'nots'—'I'm not a confident person'—marking all his deficiencies, and what he won't or can't do. But here he said this:

> Certain words touch nerves with me [pointing to poem on the page and reading]- 'Heart as soft, heart as kind'. See it's that commitment thing. I just find loyalty, commitment, really good things, which I've not had. Softness, kindness, I like those traits.

Admitting to 'softness', taken from the words of the poem, was not something he would usually do, Donald said. Most striking amid Donald's nots is 'things which I have *not* had': in an imaginative transformation of the negatives of lack, 'not having' is not simply a cause for depression, here, but a basis for still generously valuing.

Example 2:
Anita, is a middle-aged woman, whose care for her own aging mother, as well as her own physical disablement, has left her isolated and depressed for many years. At interview, she watched her response to Joanne Harris's short story 'Faith and Hope Go Shopping' in which two elderly women escape from a care home and travel up to London to visit the shoe department of Fortnum and Mason's. Where other group members talked of the 'kindness' of the young shop assistant in bringing shoes for the women to try when they were never going to buy them, Anita had said:

I don't think it was just kindly. This was deeper. I felt this man was at his ordinary day job and suddenly – what he did [kneeling to put on the shoe for Faith and to see if it fits], was absolutely unfaltering. He realized - it was an experience for *him as well.*

The interview:

Anita: I suppose I've been brought up to ensure - that the other person is physically comfortable, to notice their needs. And therefore I felt he in a way had the same feeling I was putting on him; that he was taking into account that it wasn't bodily comfort but the emotional comfort, to ensure the absolute care for that person. I am not talking about old people care or children care, but just – human care. For many years, I couldn't go into a shop and for them to have that experience ...

Interviewer: There is lot of your experience coming through – the daughter, the person who has not gone out of the house.

Anita: Yes, I am both at that moment – the trapped old woman and the carer. Probably because it is **not me**, it is coming from the page, it isn't me, I am almost taking a backseat and the text is speaking. It wasn't something that was being narrated, it was unfolding at that moment, and you had to just watch it and see. It wasn't me thinking 'I have this sorted', it was something that was happening, an actual moment happening.

At its most insightful, the use of the reader's own experience in relation to the text is dual in being both a giving to it and a learning from it, in imagination as well as memory. Part of the 'happening' here is that Anita, in identifying with both characters at the same time, is released from both her habitual life roles, and is occupying the space between them. This is a big internal move, closer to a creatively literary (or writerly) than a 'depressed' one.

One function of the elicitation of subjective experience, says Petitmengin, is therapeutic. When a person becomes conscious of the operations and processes of the inner life, it opens up 'the possibility of transforming it' (Petitmengin, 2006, p. 260). This chapter has illustrated how the combination of two qualitative interview methods might further that possibility.

It should be noted in conclusion that the video-assisted method also enabled an unusual degree of 'triangulation' of qualitative data. For example, the author Joanne Harris herself viewed the moment described above, saying: 'What she feels is quite true. Everywhere these two old ladies went, they touched another person, something unusual happened there and he too was part of the experience and he felt changed which was why he behaved in the way he did. It is quite understated in the story; I really appreciated the way she brings that out'. The video clips were also shown (with the participants' consent) to carers and health professionals. A pain consultant viewing the reading group for chronic pain held his clinic, said: 'Some of the things we spend hours trying to "teach" [in CBT for example] come out here on their own. They're more convincing learnt this way because the patients get there on their own. They find what they need to know in their own way, as if it is coming from themselves individually not from outside'.

Thor Magnus Tangeraas (Qualitative Interviews 3), 'Intimate Reading'

Thor Magnus Tangeraas is Associate Professor of Communication at Westerdals Department of Communication and Design, Kristiania University College, Oslo. He recently completed his PhD thesis, '"How Literature Changed my Life": A Hermeneutically Oriented Narrative Inquiry into Transformative Experiences of Reading Imaginative Literature' at Oslo-Met University.

This chapter explicates the method of 'Intimate Reading', a hermeneutically oriented narrative inquiry, which I developed to investigate life-changing reading experiences.

A central premise in hermeneutics is that 'the work of art has its true being in the fact that it becomes *an experience that changes the person* who experiences it'[36] and that 'self-understanding is mediated by the conjoint reception – particularly through reading - of historical and fictional narratives'.[37] Previous qualitative research has shown that many readers have found a particular work of fiction to be of significant help to them in dealing with personal issues, and experimental studies have revealed that readers experience self-modifying feelings during the act of reading. How transformative reading experiences may produce lasting change and become integrated into the person's life-story had not been studied empirically. How would I go about producing such knowledge?

I initially opted for a narrative inquiry. According to Polkinghorne, 'Narrative is the form of hermeneutic expression in which human action is understood and made meaningful.'[38] Furthermore, narrative is fundamentally about processes of change. However, I encountered certain methodological problems with narrative inquiries. To address these problems, four critical procedures were developed: (i) *subservation*, the mode of attending to the readers' communication of their experience; (ii) *text production,* from a manuscript matrix of transcripts and memos a narrative is presented; (iii) *critical selection of the narratives,* through a preliminary comparative analysis those narratives that correspond most closely to the construct of Life Changing Experience of Reading Fiction are selected; (iv) *idiographic* interpretations based on the hermeneutic logic of anteroduction. In this chapter I have decided to mainly concentrate on one of these procedures, that of text production, which I will exemplify by reference to the story of Sue's encounter with Matthew Arnold's poem 'The Buried Life'. But I shall also briefly explicate the other three.

i. *Interview as subservation*

What approach to data collection does using a narrative method entail? There is no consensus on this, although most narrativists assume an interactionist position, where 'the researcher does not *find* narratives, but instead participates in their creation'.[39] I call this method *subservation.* Whereas 'observation' comes from 'ob' + 'servare', meaning 'attending to' by being placed 'in front of' or 'before', there is a fundamentally different way of attending to something. When we subject ourselves to something, we are not gathering information, but are rather undergoing the contemplation of that something: it acts upon us. Thus, when talking to people about their experience, I can either gather information about something, or I can listen attentively to fathom the depth of their subjective experience, which is to *subserve* that experience in order to understand the meaning of it. Unlike in observation, where the researcher's presence is seen as a problem as it can influence objectivity and create bias, in subservation the researcher's presence is vital, aiming to have a *positive* influence on the intimant's communication.

This means that data production is envisaged as *subservation:* empathically listening to the other's intimation of their experience. But how does one combine this with paying attention to the literary work that occasioned the life-changing experience? Inspired by Wengraff's biographical narrative interview method[40] and the dialogic reading method of Shared Reading, I have developed an approach to data collection that tries to resolve this issue. The procedure is one of Single Question Induced Narrative (SQUIN): 'Please tell me about your experience'. This is supplemented by an invitation to read out loud significant passages from the work in question.

The aim is to facilitate *intimation.* In intimation, the interviewee speaks from an embodied utterance position. Intimation involves more than the interviewee's conscious expression and the interviewer's conscious understanding. By intimation is meant the interviewee's communication of their lived experience, encompassing both telling and reflecting; there may be an *implicit* level of communication not directly expressed in words and perhaps not even fully in the person's awareness, and the response of the interviewer to this expression can only be an approximation to the full meaning of the communication. The interviewee does not have a ready-made story to convey, nor is one 'co-constructed' in the dialogue. The interviewer's main task is *active listening*. The aim is to enable the intimant to speak *from* and *within* the felt emotional reality, expressing it as their emotional truth.[41] The facilitation of intimation and the authentic responding to its expressions is to *subserve* the intimant; this necessitates that I as interviewer *subject* myself to their experience as it is lived in the interview. I must *respond* to the person's intimation. The 'instrument' of subservation is the interviewer's empathy. What I attempted to bracket was the notion that I was going to *elicit stories* of life-changing reading experiences. I would endeavour not to be evaluating their experience as we spoke. Thoughts like 'is this really a life-changing experience?' and 'Is it detailed enough?', although these might appear in consciousness at certain junctions, were to be suspended.

ii. *Selection of prototypical narratives based on comparative analysis*

According to Hiles and Chernak narrative analysis can range from the 'straightforward collection of stories to be categorized and classified (into genres, etc.), through a more in-depth analysis of stories [...] to a more closely focused micro-analysis of the narrative sense-making process and the psychosocial context'; they emphasise that narrative data analysis is still an area 'in need of considerable, radical development'.[42] I have chosen to regard narrative analysis as a preliminary analysis with the view to *critically selecting* narratives for interpretation. The ensuing interpretation of a narrative is a *hermeneutic* concern to address the question of validity.

The preliminary analysis of the 16 narratives produced revealed that there was variation with respect to the following seven factors:

Proximity: how close to the work of fiction does the dialogue take us? Does the intimant point to specific passages and discuss the work in depth in the interview, or does she speak of her story without much reference to the work?

Ascription: When reading the narrative, is it reasonable to attribute the life-change to the reading of the book rather than to contextual factors?

Concentration: If the dialogue diverts too much away from the life-changing reading experience, then the narrative is not sufficiently concentrated.

Coherence: The narrative must have sufficient coherence. If I during the interview or in reading the transcript afterwards find it difficult to gain a sense of coherence as to what the life-change is all about, or to understand what the person means, the narrative must be excluded.

Integrated memory: The reader must have represented the reading experience as life-changing prior to the interview. For example, one of the intimants reported that it was only upon seeing the question posed by my poster, 'has a book changed your life?', that he began to think of his reading experience as life-changing.

Resolution: The reader must be judged to have achieved a stage of resolution of crisis, so that the experience is 'complete'. For instance, if the person says the reading experience helped her through her depression, and yet at the time of the interview she is still receiving psychiatric treatment, then the crisis may not be fully resolved.

Love of the book: The reader must still harbour strong positive feelings associated with the book. If the intimant has largely forgotten about the book, merely regarding it as instrumental in bringing about change, then the work itself may not have made a lasting, deep impression.

In view of these factors I developed the following construct of a Life-changing Experience of Reading Fiction (LCERF):

> A narrative is of an LCERF if the work of imaginative literature is proximal in the dialogue; the change can unequivocally be ascribed to that work; the dialogue is highly concentrated on the experience; the narrative is coherent and intelligible; the experience was already integrated in memory as life-changing; the crisis has been resolved; there is a lasting love of the book; and the person has shared the affective experience of reading significant passages from the work in our dialogue.

Based on this definition I then selected the six narratives that I understood to be prototypical of LCERF, one of which was Sue's encounter with Arnold's *The Buried Life*.

iii. *Transcription, editing and narrative representation*

In discussing the 'difficult interpretive decisions' involved in transcribing interviews, Riessman raises the following question: '[...] How to represent narratives from these conversations?'[43] It is precisely this question I will discuss in the following. I regard the narrative representation of an interview as a matter of turning transcript into manuscript, into text. This interpretive process involves choices related to the transcription of interviews, the editing of these transcripts, and the adding of elements from pre- and post-interview memos to the edited transcripts. This three-stage process is ultimately a philological procedure of transforming the witnessing and recording of an oral narrative into an authoritative textual edition presented for interpretation.

Oliver et al. argue that despite being a central and pivotal element in qualitative data collection, transcription practices remain superficially examined.[44] They suggest that the constraints and opportunities of transcription choices be reflected upon, and reflected into, the research design. They place transcription practices on a continuum of two dominant modes: *naturalism*, which attempts to represent every detail, verbal and extra-verbal, of the communication; and *denaturalism*, which removes all non-verbal signs and involuntary vocalisations. A main problem related to the continuum is that 'choosing a naturalised approach could provide detail that might obfuscate the substance of the interview [...]. A denaturalised approach could result in *white-washed* data' (Oliver et al., p. 1281). With the former approach, participants may be represented in an insensitive way, whereas with the latter data may be lost or distorted. Oliver et al. recommend that in order to solve this dilemma two versions of the transcript can be retained. The first would be a naturalised version for the purpose of in-depth analysis, the second would be a denaturalised version used for member-checking and content analysis. I have appropriated this form of thinking, but conceptualise it as a two-stage process of (i) transcription, and (ii) editing from a manuscript matrix consisting of transcript, recording and memos—rather than as two versions of the transcript.

In my view, a major weakness in methodological discussions about transcription is the unquestioned assumption that transcription is a *final* stage, the text on which interpretation is based—and that one presents excerpts from the transcript to the reader. I regard the transcript as a necessary intermediate stage on the way to the full presentation of the data. The transcript is a suspended communication, halfway between recorded oral communication and a written document, a text. A text is, according to Ricoeur, 'any discourse fixed by writing'.[45] Thus data production consists of interview, recording, transcription, editing of transcript and memos and presentation of textual narrative. I suggest that instead of two versions of the *transcript*, one operates with two distinct stages: the semi-naturalised transcript is turned into a 'denaturalised' script, or text which contains the whole narrative. The first stage is one of accurate transcription, using an appropriately fine-grained level of naturalism. This is also an act of interpretation, as all information recorded cannot possibly be represented in a transcript. The second stage is an editing of the transcript, in the process of which the transcript is made into a written document that is denaturalised. Why is this necessary? If the transcriber opts for a highly denaturalised transcription straight away, too many interpretive choices are left unreflected upon. The critical reader will have no means of checking how one went from recording to a text. To attempt faithfully to represent as much of the interaction as possible makes the researcher aware of interpretative choices. Presenting a naturalised transcription rather than a written text is problematic for reasons of ethos: the speaker comes across as a less-articulate and reflective person than how she was perceived in the oral dialogue context. By 'cleaning up' the transcript and editing it, the intimant is represented not in an idealised way but corresponding to my impression of the person in the interaction. In actual terms, this means that I take up a position at the denaturalism end of the continuum when it comes to the end data product. It is by showing how the data were transformed at each stage, that *reliability* is ensured.

A naturalised transcript in fact distorts the speaker's 'voice': if a person comes across as less articulate than what she really is, she will be perceived as less knowledgeable. Editing the transcript is thus an exercise in *rhetoric*, in so far as the speaker's *ethos* must be protected, *logos* must be rendered faithfully, and the figures of *pathos* must not be smoothed out. Importantly, the speaker's ethos in the interview situation must be reflected in the text. The principal challenge in transforming the transcripts into texts is to distinguish between redundant utterances and significant expressions. I will here present a short excerpt from the transcript of the interview with Sue, juxtaposed with the corresponding text passage, before discussing the major alterations and their implications.

<u>Excerpt from transcript of interview with Sue</u>

Interviewer: Thank you (short pause) what, what was it like to read it here and now?

Interviewee: it's quite a long time since I've read it in its entirety actually hmmm erm good (pause) yeah it's, I mean, there's lots lots more in it really you know, that, bits that I didn't remember or erm it kind of feels erm, you know it still, it still has the same kind of power really, for me, you know? (long pause)

Interviewer: Yeah.

Excerpt from corresponding passage of Narrative of Sue

Thor: Thank you. What was it like to read it here and now?

Sue: It's quite a long time since I've read it in its entirety, actually. Hmm, I mean, there's lots more in it really, bits that I didn't remember. But it still, it still has the same kind of power for me, you know? (*Tears in her eyes. She pauses*)

The psychologist Russell T. Hurlburt, in reflecting on his interviews with people describing moments of inner experience, discusses the effects of 'undermining expressions' that take attention away from the experience. Among such 'undermining expressions' he lists e.g. 'like', 'I guess', 'you know'. He argues that such expressions generally 'undermine confidence in descriptions'.[46] As is evident in the transcript excerpt, there is a high frequency of 'I mean', 'you know', 'I think', 'like', 'kind of'. These expressions can undermine the speaker's ethos. However, I did not really notice them much as we spoke together *during the interview*. They become significantly more *obtrusive* when transcribed. Why does Sue use them? Hurlburt argues that they may be understood either as 'subjunctifiers', signs that the speaker does not really believe in what she says, or as 'ornaments', habitual expressions that may reflect socio-linguistic factors in the language environment to which the speaker belongs. As Sue displayed the same expressions in another context in which I met her, I think it is safe to assume that in Sue's case, these are 'ornaments', habitual expressions. Hence, I chose to remove most of them. If presented with this semi-naturalist transcript, Sue might have been negatively surprised and perhaps objected to being represented in such a way. However, the problematic aspect is that sometimes she will use these expressions as signals that she is thinking, actively searching for the right word or phrase. In these instances, such expressions are not merely ornaments, but 'tools' or 'handle-bars' to help her get a grip on her thought. Therefore, it was an interpretative issue when to include such markers. In these instances, they are not *undermining* but *mining* expressions, mining for the right expression of thought that resides on the periphery of the field of awareness.

A second interpretative issue is representation of syntax. A naturalised transcription would not contain any commas or full stops; instead each pause would be measured in milliseconds. Unless these transcripts are read *out loud,* one cannot realise them as communication. As such, a transcript reads much like a *scriptura continua*[47] or unseparated text. In turning the first statement of Sue into three full sentences, I have had to approach the transcript syllable by syllable while re-listening to the recording, in order to interpret the *scriptura continua* and turn it into written text. I kept the 'hmm' to signify that Sue is pondering at this point. The decision to render the third sentence as 'But it still, it still has the same kind of power' is neither straightforward nor obvious. Sue does not in fact use the word 'but'—it is an interpretation on my part to use this disjunction. In the transcript, the repetition of 'still' looks like a sign of hesitancy, whereas it may also be taken as a marker of pathos. The latter alternative is brought into the foreground more clearly in the written text, although both alternatives are viable.

The general concern regarding the ethos of Sue was to represent her as a person who has to *feel* her way into her thoughts, who takes the time to look for the right metaphor or phrase. Moreover, she does not come across as a person prone to exaggeration. Therefore I decided to include a certain number of the 'mining expressions', such as 'I guess' or 'kind of'. These expressions are not simply habitual, nor do they betray lack of confidence in one's assertions. The overall impression of Sue was of someone who was almost physically *moulding* her expressions; groping, kneading, extracting words to clothe her lived experience. I have in this excerpt deleted my introjections of 'yeah'. They add nothing to the unfolding meaning of the narrative. However, they were important in the unfolding of the dialogue in the actual interview.

The amendments from transcript to written text are not restricted to deletions and contractions, however. Moreover, in parentheses I have included a reference to a non-verbal sign: *tears in her eyes.* This of course does not appear in the transcript, but was interposed afterwards. It is taken from the post-interview memo where such emotional reactions and the points at which they occurred were noted. It is significant because it illustrates that she is being moved by the re-reading. Furthermore, I have amended the neutral designations 'interviewer' and 'respondent'. At the time of transcription, I had not yet decided upon which pseudonyms to use, nor had I decided to conceptualise the interviewee as 'intimant'.

What does not transpire from these excerpts are two fundamental decisions: I have not edited the order of segments in the unfolding dialogue. The discourse corresponds to the order in which events were related in the interview. Also, the entire dialogue is included except for initial chit-chat and practical stuff relating to the completed informed consent form that the intimant would give back to me before the start of the interview proper. This is the same for all the interviews. In some interviews, there was a break midway through. What should be apparent to any reader from this comparison of transcript and text, is that there is a whole variety of interpretive choices being made in every passage. However, if I had presented a naturalised transcript, the reader would then be confronted as if with a *scriptura continua*, and would have had to realise it as text. What is important is that the reader should be given an informed insight into how the transformation has been carried out.

According to Polkinghorne, there are two ways of using narrative data and including them in the research report. Either one uses 'paradigmatic' analytic procedures to produce categories out of the common elements (coding-based approaches), or the researcher produces a narrative, as in a case study report.[48] I find this dichotomy far too simple. What both these approaches have in common, is that *excerpts* or *segments* of a participant's story is included into the researcher's discourse—either to exemplify a category or as direct quotes in the reporter's scientific report. My approach belongs to neither of these types. I present the *entire* dialogue as a narrative, and subsequently interpret this as a whole text. I find it to be a general problem in qualitative studies that the reader is presented with quotes from participants, as if they could unproblematically be taken out of context. Moreover, such quotes are used to *illustrate* a point, and presented as if the utterance was transparent and not in need of interpretation. Thus presenting the intimant's whole narrative is an integral part of subservation.

The transformation of the interview into a textual narrative is an example of what Stephen Nichols calls a 'new philology'.[49] The transcript along with the recording and memos constitute the manuscript matrix to be interpreted, and from which the edited text is created. The text supplants the transcript, the recording, and my memos, to produce a narrative. Several different texts could be created from this matrix, just as a variety of different transcripts can be created from the same recording. What is important is not arriving at the single correct and transparent text, but arriving at *one* justified version, which I authorise through explicating my decisions. This version then becomes the authoritative text which any interpretation must refer to.

iv. *The anteroductive logic of interpretation*

A narrative of an LCERF implies a series of transformations from the original reading experience: remembering this reading experience as life-changing; telling the researcher about this in a dialogic exchange; recording the oral aspects of the dialogue and writing memos afterwards; transcribing the record of the dialogue and producing a text; critical selection of texts for interpretation; and interpreting the texts ideographically. From one stage to the next, there is a transformation of meaning. I am not concerned with what is lost at each point, or with what *really* happened during the reading. With each step, something essential is distilled and carried forward to be *realised,* or appropriated. Meaning is carried forward towards a telos: this is literally a process of *anteroduction.* What each step involves, in itself and in relation to the others, has not been adequately addressed in narrative approaches or in qualitative approaches in general. In other words, anteroduction has not been fully elaborated as a logic of inquiry in its own right. As Ricoeur states: 'The text must be unfolded, no longer towards its author, but towards its immanent sense and towards the world which it opens up and discloses'.[50]

My interpretations are organised in accordance with the tripartite narrative structure of beginning–middle–end identified through the preliminary comparative analysis of transcripts: *life-crisis, transaction with the literary work,* and *resolution* or subjective change. Each interpretation thus follows a similar trajectory. First, I explicate and amplify the nature of the crisis, objectifying it in terms of psychological research but also intermediating between participants' expressions on the one hand and literary and affective terms on the other. For instance, Sue's crisis is objectified as a depression, and metaphorically viewed as a loss of soul. Next, the transaction is studied in terms of two main categories: *affective realisation,* the qualities of being moved, and *mode of engagement.* All participants speak of realising something important, and that this realisation was deeply felt. Furthermore, they describe and indicate the way they have engaged with the structural, thematic and stylistic components of the work. To bring out the emerging properties of these intimations, I have 'carried forward' classical terms that have either become lay-terms and thus lost or altered their precise meaning, or are restored from obscurity. There is no one discourse, theory or conceptual field that 'covers' these readers' experiences. If a fusion of horizon is to occur, my pre-understanding must be modified and expanded, and the intimant's expression must be clarified, amplified and enriched. I offer in summary here my interpretation of Sue's experience of reading Matthew Arnold's 'The Buried Life'.

Of the six reading experiences I studied, only Sue's originally have unfolded in a group setting. Her experience of 'The Buried Life' being a moment of shared feeling, I understood Sue to be concerned lest she no longer may speak from *within* the experience, but be restricted to talking *about* it. Not only did she feel that her experience was difficult to convey in words; I took her to imply that successfully relating her experience to me would depend on a moment of meeting occurring between *us,* in our dialogue. So I invited her to read the poem for me again, in its entirety. Here is one passage that was key for Sue:

Only—but this is rare—
When a belovèd hand is laid in ours,
When, jaded with the rush and glare
Of the interminable hours,
Our eyes can in another's eyes read clear,
When our world-deafen'd ear
Is by the tones of a loved voice caress'd—
A bolt is shot back somewhere in our breast,
And a lost pulse of feeling stirs again.
The eye sinks inward, and the heart lies plain,
And what we mean, we say, and what we would, we know.
A man becomes aware of his life's flow,
And hears its winding murmur; and he sees
The meadows where it glides, the sun, the breeze.[51]

I do believe that Sue's own fullness of feeling was revived in our meeting. In his phenomenological investigation of subjective experience that leads to change, Daniel Stern suggests that conscious present moments be divided into three different kinds. The first kind is the regular, ordinary present moment. Secondly, there is the *now moment*. This is a present moment that 'suddenly pops up and is highly charged with immediately impending consequences'.[52] Thirdly, there is a *moment of meeting:* 'This is a present moment in which the two parties achieve an intersubjective meeting' and each becomes aware of the other's experiencing. 'They share a sufficiently similar mental landscape so that a sense of "specific fittedness" is achieved'.[53] These moments of meeting usually follow immediately upon now moments, and, argues Stern, constitute 'the key moments of change in psychotherapy' (Stern, p. xi). Stern gives two pertinent examples of potential moments of meeting that resemble those in 'The Buried Life': 'looking at someone in the eyes who is looking at you, and taking a deep breath while talking to someone' (Stern, p. xv).

My interpretation revolves around several such moments of meeting: Sue and 'The Buried Life'; Sue and I in dialogue; my own reading of the poem; and my understanding of her story. In my view, her affective realisation is a form of *eparetic ekstasis:* she is *lifted up* in the encounter with the poem. Sue's mode of engagement with the poem can be termed a *synesis*, an interaffective attunement that opens up contact with a deep source of vitality. Because this experience transforms Sue's entire understanding of what poetry is and how it has changed the course of her life, I think her story can be called an Epiphany.

Essentially, such *intimate reading* is a dialogic process where different understandings, vocabularies and traditions interpenetrate, and serve to intermediate between the horizon of the researcher and the participants' voices. Not only do the classical and psychological terms throw light on the readers' experiential accounts, but importantly, the readers' accounts also enable a deeper, concrete and specific understanding of the classical tradition's affective language. This hermeneutic approach may thus lead to a renewed engagement with the classical literary tradition's language of affection.

Kelda Green (Qualitative Interviews 4), 'Diary-Assisted'

Kelda Green recently completed a PhD study at the University of Liverpool, entitled 'When literature comes to our aid: investigations into psychological understanding in the writing of Seneca and Montaigne, Wordsworth and George Eliot'.

This study combined literary study with experimental psychology with the aim of exploring the therapeutic potential of private reading. The challenge was to design an experimental methodology which would:

1. Create a space for readers to engage carefully with a complex and unfamiliar work of literature, on their own personal terms and in extended, reflective privacy, rather than as an academic or explicitly therapeutic exercise.
2. Offer a means through which first hand acts of private reading could be captured and analysed, helping to reveal the implicit, hidden effects of reading while avoiding reductive oversimplification or narrowing categorisation.

The work of the Romantic poet William Wordsworth was chosen as the basis of the experimental study. He is the archetypal 'healing poet'[54] and his writing has had a well-documented therapeutic effect on readers, fellow poets, and importantly here, on some of the earliest pioneers of the discipline of Psychology.[55] It was hoped that the distinctly slow pace of his long poem 'The Ruined Cottage' would encourage participants to engage in daily, careful contemplation and to build a relationship with the text over time. The poem's central character, The Wanderer, is a Wordsworthian reimagining of an ancient Stoic sage, a representative of the philosophy in which many modern-day therapeutic interventions are rooted.[56]

After securing ethical approval from The University of Liverpool, a group of eighteen adults were recruited via advertisements displayed across the campus and in public libraries in Liverpool and London. Participants were aged between 19 and 71 and consisted of 11 females and 7 males. The only inclusion criterion was fluency in English. Participants were divided into two groups. Age, gender, profession, education and reading habits were taken into account during the allocation process.

The nine participants allocated to group one were given a blank notebook and asked to spend thirty minutes per day for fourteen consecutive days writing about anything that they felt to be important to them. This group were not asked to read any poetry. A further nine participants in group two were given a 'poetry diary' containing a copy of Wordsworth's 'The Ruined Cottage'. The 1009 line poem had been split into fourteen sections of approximately seventy lines each. Participants were asked to spend thirty minutes per day for fourteen consecutive days reading a section of the poem and writing about anything that seemed important to them within it in their reading diary.

Two weeks after the completion of their diaries, each participant was invited to attend a semi-structured interview that lasted between one and two hours. During interviews, extracts of the diaries that participants had written, and/or passages of the poetry that they had studied, were read back to them, triggering further discussion. Thematic analysis was selected as an analytical methodology in both experiments due to its flexibility and capacity to 'potentially provide a rich, detailed, yet complex account of data'.[57] Themes identified during the analysis of the diaries and interview transcripts were verified by a cross-checking group consisting of post-graduate researchers qualified in qualitative analysis.

A sample of the diaries produced by participants in the two groups, alongside corresponding interview transcripts, are presented here in order to demonstrate some of the range, variety and nuance of individual responses to the reading and writing tasks and to indicate the value of the diary-assisted reading methodology as a means of generating data for study of the complex subtleties of private reading.

Group One

One distinctive characteristic of each of the diaries written by those in group one was their overwhelming focus on the present. Participants wrote about their daily routines, everyday interactions and concerns. The tone of these diaries was casual and chatty and there was little or no change in focus, depth or language across each person's fourteen diary entries. One participant, for example (here designated P1), wrote on day seven:

> Had a fantastic day! Not done anything like bike mechanics before but I really enjoyed it. It was something my hubby wanted to do but because I'm scared to go out on my own on the bike in case I get a puncture, he enrolled me on it.

Independent cross-checkers noted that the set of ten diaries written by participants in group one were 'not emotionally deep', commenting that, 'Participants struggle to think about what is important to them. Diaries are less contemplative and cover a less diverse set of topics. They are event driven and the main themes are: work/life balance, exercise, family, daily routine, anticipation/anxiety'.

While it may have been easy to characterise these diaries as prosaic, during the interviews, a number of those in group one—including participant P1 quoted above—explained that the process of daily writing had been somewhat beneficial to them:

> I don't know if it's just the modern world where you just rush from place to place and you never just sit down with a blank page in front of you and just think. It was nice just to sit down and write. Yeah, I think it was just that putting things down on paper.

Regardless of the content of the diary, the task appeared to force this participant to fit a short period of quiet contemplation into her daily routine, giving her what was perhaps a rare opportunity to 'just think'.

One participant (here designated P2) was of particular interest in this regard. He wrote a highly confessional diary in which he described at great length his struggles with depression. He focussed exclusively on the present in each diary entry, making no reference at all to either his past or future:

> This week, a friend told me not to admit to anyone about my depression and treatment as it could make me a scapegoat or a psycho in the group. Perhaps I was too eager to tell everybody.

The tone of each diary entry is self-critical and hopeless. However, during his interview, this participant spoke about how writing the diary had helped him:

> This actually reminds me of the method of psychodynamic psychotherapy that I took in the past. At first I got annoyed when I was saying a lot about my problems but finding the therapist was silent. Later I realised that just

> expressing my problem made me think about it in a different way, I was trying to guess what the other person might be thinking. I often find new ideas about my problems after a period of silence. Even if I'm writing for myself, I am thinking what a reader might think, so I am thinking in a different way.

P2 connects the act of writing on the blank pages of the diary with speaking into the silence of the therapy room. In both cases there is somebody listening to and observing him from behind the silence, either the therapist or a real or imagined reader. It is the silence—or in the case of the diary, the blank page—which allows P2 to get outside of his own mind.

The interview stage was particularly significant for this participant because he was no longer simply imagining 'what a reader might think'; he was faced with his actual reader and had to listen to them reading his own words back to him:

> **Does hearing me read the diary back to you help to process the experience in any way?**
>
> Yes, actually I am quite surprised about how much we have really processed it. I'm really glad, I'm really happy that this has happened. I didn't expect it to look like this.
>
> **Imagine if you had a son and your son had written this diary. If you read it, what advice would you give him?**
>
> I'm thinking of my own father and I think a lot of what I am doing is trying to make myself different … well, it's not like he was horrible, but he was very structured. I'm uncomfortable about my own father. Well, maybe it's hard to … it is a challenge. The challenge to be different, in some meaningful way, to your parents.

P2 is beginning to separate the version of his self that is inside the diary from the self that is on the outside reading the diary, and to find some room for manoeuvre in the space between these two selves. Writing can perhaps lead to the development of more objective and less punishing attitudes by creating a way for somebody to look in at themselves from an external perspective, particularly when combined—as here—with a secondary process of being read.

Group Two

While participants in group one focused on their daily activities and concerns within their diaries, those in group two (who were reading 'The Ruined Cottage') tended to write about the wider span of their lives, almost entirely avoiding the present in order to focus—often with great specificity—on memories of the past. The group of independent cross-checkers noted that 'the poem acts as a trigger for memories and the diaries contained very detailed and emotive memories as participants reflect on the poetry in relation to their own lives'. The following two examples give some evidence of the broader scope and corresponding depth of thought which was characteristic of this set of diaries.

Participant 3 (P3) is the head teacher of a secondary school. She teaches English and has studied English literature to post-graduate level. She is familiar with the poetry of Wordsworth and in her initial diary entries she frequently referred to what she had formerly learnt about Wordsworth at university. However, over the course of the task she appeared to move away from her default 'academic' mode, shifting to a more personal way of reading and writing. The independent cross-checkers noticed this shift from academic to personal, commenting that, 'The writing has changed from earlier entries, it sounds almost poetic. The poem seems to be influencing the reader in a reflective way, which is influencing how they see the world'. At the very start of her interview, P3 acknowledged how her attitude and approach to the task had changed over the course of the two weeks:

> Well I'm an English teacher for a start, so before you know you start going into the tried and tested ways of reading and analysing that you have learned to do for a really long time. Initially I was very much trying to find the answer to what stuff meant in that kind of English student kind of way. That's where I defaulted to. Whereas as it went through, you probably can tell in the writing, I was much more personally connected to the poem and finding space to think. It's a combination not just of the task but of the subject matter as well. It's the poem that takes you there actually.

It was on day seven of the task that this participant read a passage of the poem in which The Wanderer describes the overgrown remains of the garden he is standing in. It is a garden that once belonged to Margaret—a woman who died following a long period of emotional decline—after being abandoned by her husband:

> It was a plot
> Of garden ground run wild, its matted weeds
> marked with the steps of those, whom, as they passed,
> The gooseberry trees that shot in long lank slips,
> Or currants, hanging from their leafless stems,
> In scanty strings, had tempted to o'erleap

The broken wall.
[…]
'I see around me here
Things which you cannot see: we die, my Friend,
Nor we alone, but that which each man loved
And prized in his peculiar nook of earth
Dies with him, or is changed; and very soon
Even of the good is no memorial left.[58]

In response to this passage, P3 wrote:

> I had quite a shock then, reading a description of the overgrown garden, with words like 'matted', 'leafless', 'long lank', 'scanty strings' leading then into the man saying what he says about death, and all that we 'prize' changing and going with us as we die. I wasn't wanting to think about that, as mum prepares for her op. I'm thinking about gentle pauses, her lovely garden staying just fine at home for her while dad waits for her to recover and all proceeding forward as it should.

She finds the passage uncomfortable to read but it is the shock of being faced by this image of decay that forces her to drop her previous detached, academic default mode. The poem leads her to consider what—in the aftermath of a period of illness for her mother—her mind had been working hard to avoid. In this case, her re-quoting of words from the text is a good thing to come out of her student/teacher experience as it creates a more focused, live reading of the poem.

Two weeks later at her interview, I read aloud this same passage of poetry about Margaret's overgrown garden and P3 spoke again about the fear that it had initially triggered in her:

> Not wanting anything to alter or adjust at all and how the processes of nature happen anyway no matter what you do and that is quite scary. I like that, I really love that passage and I really connected with it but at the same time it showed a really powerful advancing of time and nature that is a little bit scary, especially if you are faced with illness. The garden itself reminded me of where we lived as kids, they or we had a big garden and I imagine it now, I imagine it like that, even though they don't live there now. Mum's getting better, but if she wasn't, there would be that sense of that happening there, and how sad that is. I think that that is a really overwhelmingly sad passage, really powerfully, really powerfully. I don't like going and revisiting places particularly because I often find that the experience you had is altered and not always in a good way. I think that's why that spoke to me as well really strongly in terms

of mum's illness, because I don't like going back to where we lived as children in case it's all gone wrong. You know that sort of idyllic quality is gone.

The default academic mode has been abandoned here and is replaced with a strong sense of emotional connection. The poetry appears to be triggering a certain quality of memory that is not simply reminiscence but rather a form of reimagining. Reading can perhaps be one way of imaginatively restoring a place that cannot be returned to in reality.

The capacity of the poetry to take participants into more unconscious or unexpected areas of thinking as they wrote, and to trigger particular qualities of thought, is also demonstrated in the responses of Participant 4 (P4), who left school aged sixteen, enjoys reading for pleasure but has no formal qualifications in English Literature. He approached the task with some trepidation and for the first two days wrote long descriptive summaries of the poetry that he had been reading. However on day three of the task he abruptly changed his approach. He stopped paraphrasing the poetry and instead began to write much briefer notes about how the task was making him feel and what he was learning from it. He subsequently went on to write about deeply personal topics. In particular, he wrote about the different experiences of grief that he and his mother had gone through after the death of his father.

On day twelve, he read a passage of the poem in which The Wanderer recalls the effect that Margaret's grief over the loss of her husband had had on her baby child:

> Her infant babe
> Had from his Mother caught the trick of grief,
> And sighed among its playthings. (l.868-870)

In response he wrote:

Grief is Contagious.

- It seems strange to me that she would seem so affected by her husband's grief yet so unaffected by the death of her child. Or I suppose her husband's death had so affected her that the remainder of him (her child) was a burden.
- Makes me jealous of that kind of love.
- You want to scream at her 'pull yourself together' which makes me feel as though I'm unsympathetic and dead inside myself. This poem has made me think about myself as someone who may have been affected by grief unknowingly.

He is writing simultaneously about both Margaret and his own mother, about Margaret's husband and his own father and about Margaret's child and his own self (as the 'remainder' rather than 'reminder' of the father). The poem is allowing him to get close to his own parallel experiences and to think and say what would be difficult—if not impossible—for him to say to his mother: 'Pull yourself together' or 'I'm jealous of that kind of love'.

During his interview P4 spoke about his conscious decision on the third day to shift away from his default tactic of superficial description and towards a more emotional approach:

> I thought I'm just describing the poem rather than doing anything of any difference. I'm basically rewriting it in a really stupid way. I think that from the look of it, the more I absorbed the less actually I wrote down. I read back the first one and I thought, this is just a complete waste of time. I'm gonna have to start bullet-pointing it. I'm getting as much down doing bullet points as I am sentences. You know, in terms of emotional delivery.

As his responses became increasingly personal the diary entries became significantly shorter and more fragmented. All the unnecessary paraphrase was stripped away and instead he appeared to focus on the task of getting closer to the emotional core of the poem.

During his interview P4 spoke again about how reading the poem had led him to think about his own grief in a way that he might otherwise have avoided:

> **You wrote in a few places about being 'unknowingly' affected by grief, what did you mean by that?**
>
> Yes. Because I have only become a little more tolerant of talking about my own father in the last year or so. Because I never really liked talking about it and I can't say I was consciously affected by it at the time. In the poem it talks about this old woman, and I very much saw my own mum in it. Because she is not the same woman … even now. She is nowhere near what she was. I was quite happy go lucky really before that … you know … because I don't like saying it was … you know because I can't say I ever got on with him, I can't say I ever really liked him, I can't say it was a big loss personally. It was just that thing of how it affected my mother and subsequently how that affected me. Because that was in the poem, I think I just couldn't not write what I wrote.

This participant's feelings hang unspoken in his pauses and behind his negative sentences, for he finds it easier to say what it is that he can't say—'I can't say I ever got on with him, I can't say I ever really liked him, I can't say it was a big loss personally'—than explicitly to say what it was that he did feel towards his father. The final double negative, 'I just couldn't not write what I wrote', suggests the struggle taking place between wanting to articulate his feelings, being pushed into certain thinking areas by the poem, and his habitual instinct to avoid the topic.

* * *

While each of these brief examples offer only a snapshot of the rich and varied case studies compiled over the course of this research study,[59] they are used here to illustrate how the methodology of diary assisted reading alongside interviews can offer a means of collecting nuanced data which both illuminates and respects the process of private reading. Through compiling these individual accounts of private reading, we can begin to understand the implicit therapeutic properties of literature and the ways in which literature offers readers a space outside of the everyday, enabling them to cast off default patterns of thought and to quickly get into the thick of their inner, emotional lives.

Notes

1. J. Billington, C. Dowrick, J. Robinson, A. Hamer, and C. Williams, 'An Investigation into the Therapeutic Benefits of Reading in Relation to Depression and Well-Being' (University of Liverpool: Centre for Research into Reading, Literature and Society [CRILS], 2011), pp. 25–54.
2. See Billington et al., pp. 46–51, and C. Dowrick, J. Billington, J. Robinson, A. Hamer, and C. Williams, 'Get into Reading as an Intervention for Common Mental Health Problems: Exploring Catalysts for Change', *Journal of Medical Humanities,* 38.1 (2012), 15–20 (p. 18).
3. J. Davis, 'The Art of Medicine: Enjoying and Enduring: Groups Reading Aloud for Wellbeing', *The Lancet*, 373.9665 (2009), 714–16 (p. 716).
4. P. Davis, J. Billington, R. Corcoran, V. Gonzalez-Diaz, S. Lampropoulou, G. Farrington, F. Magee, and E. Walsh, 'Cultural Value: Assessing the Intrinsic Value of The Reader Organization's Shared Reading Scheme' (University of Liverpool: CRILS, 2015): see also, E. Longden, P. Davis, J. Billington, S. Lampropoulou, G. Farrington, F. Magee, E. Walsh, and R. Corcoran, 'Shared Reading: Assessing the Intrinsic Value of a Literature-Based Health Intervention', *Journal of Medical Humanities*, 41.2 (2015), 113–20.
5. I. A. Richards, *Practical Criticism* (London: Kegan Paul, 1929).

6. The research (see note 4) was funded by the Arts and Humanities Research Council UK, approved by University of Liverpool Research Ethics Committee.
7. From George Eliot, *Silas Marner* (1861), ed. Juliet Atkinson (Oxford: Oxford University Press, 1998), p. 98.
8. At interview, participants said that the private stories and often vulnerable identifications offered by an individual other than themselves in the group usually had a genuine and educative place in the discussion, rather than being gratuitously indulgent (Davis et al., p. 35).
9. E. C. Lathem, *The Poetry of Robert Frost* (New York: Henry Holt, 1988), p. 105.
10. Christopher Dowrick, *Beyond Depression,* 2nd edn (Oxford: Oxford University Press, 2009), pp. 169–70, 172, 185.
11. W. James, *Varieties of Religious Experience,* ed. by Martin E. Marty (Harmondsworth: Penguin Books Ltd., 1985), p. 197.
12. These examples, and those in iii (below) are taken from Davis et al. (see note 4) and from two later studies (both approved by UK NHS Research Ethics Committees): J. Billington, G. Farrington, S. Lampropoulou, K. McDonnell, J. Lingwood, A. Jones, J. Ledson, A.-L. Humphreys, and N. Duirs, 'A Comparative Study of Cognitive Behavioural Therapy and Shared Reading for Chronic Pain' (University of Liverpool: CRILS, 2016); P. Davis, F. Magee, K. Koleva, and T. M. Tangeras, 'What Literature Can Do' (University of Liverpool: CRILS, 2016).
13. L. Sheck, *Captivity* (New York: Alfred A. Knopf, 2007), p. 41.
14. Quoted in *Poems to Take Home*, trans. by David Constantine (Liverpool: The Reader, 2010).
15. R. S. Thomas, *Selected Poems* (London: Faber & Faber, 1964), p. 36.
16. C. Ricks (ed.), *The Oxford Book of English Verse* (Oxford: Oxford University Press, 1999), p. 144.
17. P. Davis and J. Billington, 'The Very Grief a Cure of the Disease', *Changing English Special Issue: Uses of Poetry,* 23.4 (2016), 396–408 (p. 399).
18. Participants across CRILS's studies have reported: an active sense of belonging, within a 'place', psychological as much as physical, from which further development (flexibly and at their own pace) can ensue (J. Billington, A. Jones, A. L. Humphreys, and K. McDonnell, 'A Literature-Based Intervention for People with Chronic Pain', *Arts and Health: An International Journal for Research, Policy and Practice,* 8.1 (2014) 13–31); a sense of acceptance, within an environment that is at once practically structured and emotionally 'warm' through the creation of a personalised ethos (Davis et al., 2014); a renewed belief in the value of their own contribution, welcomed by those who have hitherto felt themselves to be in various ways redundant (Gray, 2016, see Chapter 8 [A]); humane recognition of their worth as individuals (Davis et al., 2014); a sense of the social as more than

contact with others or the overcoming of isolation, but as an inherent value (Longden et al., 2015).

19. See, for example, S. Malloch and C. Trevarthen, *Communicative Musicality* (Oxford: Oxford University Press, 2009); Daniel Stern, *The Interpersonal World of the Infant* (London: Karnac, 1998).
20. P. Davis, *Reading and the Reader* (Oxford: Oxford University Press, 2013), Chapter 1, pp. 1–48.
21. C. Petitmengin, 'Describing One's Subjective Experience in the Second Person: An Interview Method for the Science of Consciousness', *Phenomenology and the Cognitive Sciences,* 5.3–4 (2006), 229–69; C. Petitmengin, 'Towards the Source of Thoughts; The Gestural and Transmodal Dimension of Lived Experience', *Journal of Consciousness Studies*, 14.3 (2007), 54–82; C. Petitmengin, 'Describing the Experience of Describing? The Blind Spot of Introspection', *Journal of Consciousness Studies,* 18.1 (2011), 44–62; and C. Petitmengin, A. Remillieux, and C. Valenzuela-Moguillansky, 'Discovering the Structures of Lived Experience: Towards a Micro-Phenomenological Analysis Method, *Phenomenology and the Cognitive Sciences* (2018). https://doi.org/10.1007/s11097-018-9597-4
22. D. Kuiken, D. S. Miall, and S. Sikora, 'Forms of Self-Implication in Literary Reading', *Poetics Today*, 25.2 (2004), 171–203 (see also Chapters 12 and 16.)
23. S. Sikora, D. Kuiken, and D. S. Miall, 'Expressive Reading: A Phenomenological Study of Readers' Experience of Coleridge's The Rime of the Ancient Mariner', *Psychology of Aesthetics, Creativity, and the Arts*, 5.3 (2011), 258–68. See also Davis et al. (2016).
24. P. Vermersch, *L'Entretien d'Explicitation en Formation Initiale et Continue* (Paris: ESF, 1994/2014).
25. F. J. Verela, 'Neurophenomenology: A Methodological Remedy for the Hard Problem', *Journal of Consciousness Studies*, 3:4 (1996), 330–49.
26. E. T. Gendlin, *The Practising Professional. Focusing-Oriented Psychotherapy: A Manual of the Experiential Method* (New York: Guilford Press, 1996).
27. Caroline Schrodes, 'Reading and the Emotions', *The Reading Teacher*, 9.1 (1955), 24–29.
28. G. Katz and J. Watt, 'Bibliotherapy: The Use of Books in Psychiatric Treatment', *Canadian Journal of Psychiatry*, 37.3 (1992), 173–78; R. S. Lenkowsky, 'Bibliotherapy: A Review and Analysis of the Literature', *Journal of Special Education*, 2.2 (1987), 123–32; and L. I. Silverberg, 'Bibliotherapy: The Therapeutic Use of Didactic and Literary Text in Treatment, Diagnosis, Prevention and Training', *Journal of the American Osteopathic Association*, 103.3 (2003), 131–35.
29. J. T. Pardeck and J. A. Pardeck, *Bibliotherapy: A Clinical Approach for Helping Children*, vol. 16 (Langhorne, PA: Gordon and Breach Science Publishers, 1993).
30. See note 12 for the source of these quotations.

31. J. Clare, 'I am' (1848), in Jane Davis (ed.), *Poems to Take Home* (Liverpool: The Reader, 2011), p. 10.
32. Petitmengin holds that some degree of retrospective access is always necessary because it is impossible for us to direct our attention at one and the same time onto the 'what' and the 'how', onto the object of the process and the way in which we carry it out'. She quotes John Stuart Mill, '"A fact may be studied through the medium of memory, not at the very moment of our perceiving it, but the moment after: and this is really the mode in which our best knowledge of our intellectual acts is generally acquired. We reflect on what we have been doing when the act is past, but when its impression in the memory is still fresh." (Auguste Comte and Positivism [Ann Arbor: University of Michigan, 1882/1961], p. 64)'. 'In any case,' Petitmengin continues, this retrospective access is not trivial. Even when an experience has just finished, its 're-enactment' or 'presentification' is a complex cognitive process' (Petitmengin, 2006, p. 238).
33. Literature operates to produce, we are suggesting, the kind of enrichment, freshness and refinement of language (see also Chapter 10, section 'Josie Billington and Philip Davis, "Reading Live: A Qualitative Method for Analyzing Reading in Real Time"') that Petitmengin is seeking when she says: 'If he perseveres, the interviewee then discovers that he can use words differently, to make them say something new, and that it is possible for him to describe his experience in a fresh way, with an unexpected level of precision. The use of words that enable him to precisely describe new facets of his subjective experience has the effect of refining the perceptions of the interviewee: in a subsequent interview for example, drawing on this vocabulary that is shared with the interviewer, he will provide a description that is even more precise. It would seem therefore that we can gradually enrich our language with words and with more precise descriptive categories enabling us to refer to our own experience' (Petitmengin, 2006, 253–54).
34. A phenomenon which the video-recorded evidence particularly impressed upon the research team (see Chapter 10, section 'Josie Billington and Philip Davis, "Reading Live: A Qualitative Method for Analyzing Reading in Real Time"').
35. R. Herrick, 'To the Virgins, to Make Much of Time', in *The Oxford Book of English Verse*, ed. by Christopher Ricks (Oxford: Oxford University Press, 1999), p. 143.
36. H.-G. Gadamer, *Truth and Method*, 2nd ed., trans. by Joel Weinsheimer and Donald G. Marshall (New York: Continuum, 2003), p. 103.
37. P. Ricoeur, *Philosophical Anthropology*, trans. by David Pellauer (Malden: Polity Press, 2016), p. 229.
38. D. E. Polkinghorne, *Narrative Knowing and the Human Sciences* (New York: State University of New York Press, 1988), p. 145.

39. K. Neander and C. Skott, 'Important Meetings with Important Persons: Narratives from Families Facing Adversity and Their Key-Figures', *Qualitative Social Work: Research and Practice,* 5.3 (2006), p. 297.
40. T. Wengraff, *Qualitative Research Interviewing: Biographic Narrative and Semi-Structured Methods* (London, Thousand Oaks, and New Delhi: Sage, 2001).
41. C. Petitmengin, 2006.
42. D. Hiles and I. Cermak, 'Narrative Psychology', in *The Sage Handbook of Qualitative Research in Psychology,* ed. by C. Willig and W. Stainton-Rogers (London: Sage Publications, 2008), pp. 147–64.
43. C. K. Riessman, *Narrative Methods for the Human Sciences* (Los Angeles and London: Sage Publications, 2008), p. 42.
44. D. G. Oliver, J. M. Serovich, and T. L. Mason, 'Constraints and Opportunities with Interview Transcription: Towards Reflection in Qualitative Research', *Social Forces,* 84.2 (2005), 1273.
45. P. Ricoeur, 'What Is a Text? Explanation and Understanding', in *Hermeneutics and the Human Sciences,* trans. by John B. Thompson (Cambridge: Cambridge University Press, 1995), p. 145.
46. R. T. Hurlburt, *Investigating Pristine Inner Experience: Moments of Truth* (New York and Cambridge: Cambridge University Press, 2011), p. 117.
47. P. Saenger, *Space Between Words: The Origins of Silent Reading,* 2nd ed. (Stanford, CA: Stanford University Press, 1997).
48. D. E. Polkinghorne, 'Narrative Configuration in Qualitative Analysis', *Qualitative Studies in Education,* 8.1 (1995), 5–23.
49. S. G. Nichols, 'Introduction: Philology in a Manuscript Culture', *Speculum,* 65.1 (1990), 1–10 (p. 2).
50. Ricoeur, *Hermeneutics and the Human Sciences,* p. 53.
51. M. Arnold, 'The Buried Life' in *The Poems of Matthew Arnold,* ed. by Kenneth Allott (London: Longmans, Green & Co. Ltd., 1965), pp. 271–76 (p. 275).
52. D. N. Stern, *The Present Moment in Psychotherapy and Everyday Life* (New York: W. W. Norton, 2004), p. 151. I assume that this understanding of the present moment closely resembles the common conception of the epiphanic. Stern himself refers to it, somewhat misleadingly, as kairos.
53. *The Present Moment in Psychotherapy and Everyday Life,* p. 151. Stern's basic assumption is that 'change is based on lived experience. In and of itself, verbally understanding, explaining or narrating something is not sufficient to bring about change. There must also be an actual experience, a subjectively lived happening' (p. xiii). I concur with his view.
54. M. Arnold, 'Memorial Verses' (1850), in *Matthew Arnold Selected Poems,* ed. by M. Allott (Oxford: Oxford University Press, 1995), l.63, p. 96.

55. Including J. S. Mill, Matthew Arnold, John Ruskin and William James see: Ralph Bardon Perry, *The Thought and Character of William James*, 2 vols. (London: Humphrey Milford, 1935), i, p. 322
56. J. Evans, *Philosophy for Life and Other Dangerous Situations* (London: Rider Books, 2012), pp. 3–4
57. V. Braun and V. Clarke, 'Using Thematic Analysis in Psychology', *Qualitative Research in Psychology*, 3.2 (2006), 77–101 (p. 78).
58. W. Wordsworth, *The Excursion*, ed. by S. Bushell, J. A. Butler, and M. C. Jaye (Ithaca: Cornell University Press, 2007), Book I, Line 452–74.
59. K. Green, '*When Literature Comes to Our Aid: Investigations into Psychological Understanding in the Writing of Seneca and Montaigne, Wordsworth and George Eliot*', PhD thesis, The University of Liverpool, 2018.

11

Linguistic Approaches

Sofia Lampropoulou, Kremena Koleva, Kevin Harvey, Gavin Brookes, with Josie Billington and Philip Davis

Sofia Lampropoulou, Kremena Koleva, Josie Billington and Philip Davis, 'Linguistic Analysis of Transcribed Video-Recorded Reading Groups'

This section focuses on the contribution of linguistic analysis to the study of video-recorded Shared Reading groups considered in Chapter 10, ('Josie Billington and Philip Davis, "Reading Live: A Qualitative Method for Analyzing Reading in Real Time"'). The methods of qualitative linguistic analysis applied to the transcripts of the video-recordings are outlined, together with salient findings. (Across these studies, the linguistic evidence proved essential in helping to corroborate the qualitative findings from the multidisciplinary team.)

S. Lampropoulou (✉)
Department of English, University of Liverpool, Liverpool, UK
e-mail: S.Lampropoulou@liverpool.ac.uk

K. Koleva
University of York, York, UK
e-mail: kremena.koleva@york.ac.uk

K. Harvey
University of Nottingham, Nottingham, UK
e-mail: Kevin.Harvey@nottingham.ac.uk

J. Billington (ed.), *Reading and Mental Health*,
https://doi.org/10.1007/978-3-030-21762-4_11

Approaches

Qualitative analysis of selected transcripts related expressions to their context, to the functions they served, and how these functions related to the relationship between participants and text (involvement, for example). Discourse analysis identified how the texts being read helped to shape conversational contributions.[1]

(Abbreviated) Findings

Deixis

Two key linguistic findings were that (i) shared group reading elicits personal autobiographical memories and narratives of self-disclosure—often vulnerably painful for the teller—of the kind usually fostered among intimates, and that (ii) this phenomenon occurs in live relation to the text. The linguistic clue here is deixis (cues and phrases, that require contextual information to convey any meaning: personal pronouns for example). In discussing the text, readers characteristically maintained the text's original deixis for identification of person, time and space, rather than shifting it to signal the perspective of the reading group, indicating a strong degree of involvement between participants in the group and the protagonists in the text. As a result, the text was not detached but transferred to the here and now of the reading group interaction. This related also to the characteristic use of the present tense in discussion, so that even past life was not distant. Deixis can also signify an initial pointing activity, an act of instinctive location ahead of the ability for further articulation. For example: 'I've been *there*'

G. Brookes
Department of Linguistics and English Language,
Lancaster University, Lancaster, UK
e-mail: g.j.brookes@lancaster.ac.uk

P. Davis · J. Billington
Centre for Research into Reading, Literature and Society,
University of Liverpool, Liverpool, UK
e-mail: jbilling@liverpool.ac.uk

P. Davis
e-mail: phildav@liverpool.ac.uk

was one participant's shorthand way of explaining, amid pain, her need to leave the room during a reading of John Clare's 'I am' on mental breakdown. (Compare 'That bit there'—Lorraine's way of designating the lines 'From sullen earth sings hymns at heaven's gate; For thy sweet love remembered …' in Chapter 5.) This linguistic evidence strengthens the emergent finding that 'live thinking' as witnessed on the video-recordings is the outcome of the translation of personal experience or material into and out of the literature (see Chapter 10, 'Josie Billington and Philip Davis, "Reading Live: A Qualitative Method for Analyzing Reading in Real Time"' and 'Josie Billington, Philip Davis, Grace Farrington, Fiona Magee, "Qualitative Interviews 2: Video-Assisted"').

Creative Inarticulacy

There were pronounced linguistic traces in respect of the creativity identified in the video-recordings. A much-repeated locution, unconsciously adopted by participants of different social background and educational experience, is the phrase 'it is as though' or 'it's almost as if' or 'it is almost like' or 'I feel as though'. It is commonly the prelude or bridge to a bold and interesting breakthrough in thought (as opposed to the tonal opinionatedness of, say, 'I just/still think'). Here is one example, again in relation to John Clare's 'I am':

> *Alice*: It feels, there's something about peace isn't there, because it's not even talking about being happy.
> *Heather*: Yes, it's almost like he wants like freedom from mental turmoil or something like that, you know just to not kind of cause anyone any trouble.
> *Kate*: It's almost as if the everyday life, almost as if he's thinking that is what he may interpret as paradise. You know the people everyday, or it's almost as if people are untouched by illness, grief, happiness.

Arising out of an uncertainty or hesitation that is nonetheless far from disabling, 'almost as if', 'something like' are tools that allow time, space and permission for what is tentative or provisional, on the borderline between language and thought, in the form of imaginative interpretation and inference close to the intrinsic spirit of literary thinking itself.

Of key importance, too, were the instances where a person pauses or even stops without quite finishing a sentence. Take this example in relation to George Eliot's novella, *Silas Marner* (see Chapter 10 'Josie Billington and Philip Davis, "Reading Live: A Qualitative Method for Analyzing Reading in Real Time"'):

Linda: I think sometimes if you've lost something, be it for example this character losing his money, or even like it might be a drastic change, for example you're retiring and suddenly your life's different, it's wondering what—it's a future that you don't know. In the past the future's always been—there.

'Wondering what …': Linda's uncompleted, non-naming locution is a characteristic of the recorded sessions which was particularly connected with the uncertainty and unpredictability of not-knowing-in-advance or not being clear about where a thought is going. The effect at such times is more of a full silence than an empty one. An emergent live thought seems not so much blocked as continuing to exist suggestively and unspoken in the resonant atmosphere of the group without a ready-made category or framework. As one group facilitator put it: 'You can see it, you can feel it as a facilitator, so, you know, you can see the *birth* of it as you're reading'. These are the shoots or seedlings of reconceptualisation.

Sometimes these 'stops' or 'hangings', situations in which speakers abandon a thought or leave it uncompleted, are less like the linguistic probing described above and closer to a 'processing halt', at which gestures often take over. Jane, responding to a passage relating to the protagonist's early childhood in Charlotte Bronte's *Jane Eyre,* said 'And I think the expression on her face and her physical disposition or, or certain … It's not physical violence, it's psychological violence, it's more damaging … it remains for the rest of your life … if you hurt your arm or whatever, it might heal up but [points to head]'. 'Hangings' sometimes appear symptomatic of the realisation or recreation of what has powerfully stopped lives in the past or hesitancy and uncertainty in relation to the future. Jud, from a group in a setting for people suffering from psychosis, reading Arnold's 'The Buried Life', was asked directly by the group leader whether he himself had any buried original plan as the poet suggested: 'Um, yes, possibly, but it seems to be far removed from the reality I am in now'. Smiling ruefully, Jud leaned forward to hear again the final words of the poem:

> And then he thinks he knows
> The hills where his life rose,
> And the sea where it goes.[2]

'Yes, it seems to be quite a distance between the person you once were – hoping to be, and the person you have become, so … ur …'. The stop here is to do with the difficulty experienced by a person who in the present looks back to the past, but a past which seems now to have lost the future it once had—hence the lack of an immediately articulatable future now. These complicated time loops, affecting the imagined understanding of time itself (compare Linda's 'In the past, the future's always been – there') are experienced in the linguistic hesitations: it is not only the distance between the person you have become and 'the person you were' but also 'the person you were – hoping to be'.

At other times, these are instances of group members sensing of an 'intangible reality' or higher plane of reality in the face of which conventional language appeared powerless or floundering. Group members' hesitancy or groping—'something … it …. what … kind of … sort of … like'—is an effort to grasp this new reality, sometimes reaching for metaphor or conceit in a process of sought-tangibility equivalent to the creation of poetry itself. 'It splits up the darkness' (of Robert Hayden's poem, 'Those Winter Sundays', in which a father's unthanked love is lovingly remembered); 'This Wordsworth poem raises an enormous sky over all we fear or we hold dear'; 'It's quite a quandary: you're a prisoner who is thinking you are free to do whatever you want'; 'Something you can't actual explain but it is an invitation, a light inside the house, to come in by'.

Speech stalls or struggles or has to reinvent itself because of the sudden experience of something *more than* any paraphrase or categorisation can express. Those moments are full of what the philosopher-psychologist Eugene Gendlin calls the 'implicit' meaning involved in the coming of words. 'You want to go on. In an implicit way you feel what should be next, but you do not know what to say. The phrases that come do not precisely say it. Something implicit is functioning in your rejection of them'.[3]

Mobility of Mind

One of the main impediments to well-being is a feeling of what one participant at interview called 'stuckness'—the sense of inescapable predicament, a felt inability to change, repetitive thinking. Linguistic analysis found two linguistic traces for mobility: a flexible movement of mind between pronouns, and in respect of negatives.

Pronouns:

The flexibility of thinking which crosses from the self to the text and back again, and also extends imaginatively to a range of perspectives within the text or in the group, is reflected in a series of linguistic habits, particularly the barely conscious use of pronouns. In *The Secret Life of Pronouns*, James

W. Pennebaker suggests that an implicit indicator of mental health is an increasing shift from I-centred discourse to discourse more concerned with others.[4] The transcripts of Shared Reading groups show a subtler mobility—from 'I' to 'he' or 'she', or 'we'—where the shifts are achieved with seamless rapidity in live thought. Most significantly, they feature a particular usage of 'you' not in the second person but as a third-person informal version of 'one'. One striking finding in comparing Shared Reading with a conventional therapeutic intervention (Cognitive Behavioural Therapy) for people living with chronic pain, was the widespread and consistent replacement of repetitively negative first-person singular formulations characteristic of CBT—'I am not who I was before my pain', 'I don't do anything … anymore. I can't even speak … about it anymore'—with a more thoughtfully speculative 'you' syntax. Struck by Scrooge's ability in Dickens's *A Christmas Carol* not to be stuck but to alter his future, one participant, Hannah, said:

> I suppose it's the change in perception that's important. 'I am not the man I was.'[5] For the future you've got to learn from your past, even the smallest things can teach you. He's learned not just who he was but who he needs to be.

This mobile use of 'you'—moving causally between he, I, and we— is an instinctive instrument of thought, offering an imaginative middle ground for thoughtful exploration of the relation between 'the text' and 'me', as well as between 'me' and 'others' (be they 'we' or 'he, she, they', in the text or in the group).

The uses of the negative:
As Scrooge's 'I am not the man I was' was not a merely negative utterance, so one characteristic of group-readers most involved contributions was the use of the double-negative. We have seen instances of this in Chapter 10, ('Josie Billington and Philip Davis, "Reading Live: A Qualitative Method for Analyzing Reading in Real Time"' and 'Josie Billington, Philip Davis, Grace Farrington, Fiona Magee, "Qualitative Interviews 2: Video-Assisted"'): 'Cannot imagine, cannot comprehend'; You can't unknow'. Hannah (quoted above) said of Scrooge. 'He can't unsee what is shown to him'. Very often this usage, like the hesitation and 'stumbling' witnessed above, appears to have threshold-crossing significance.

When Ona, for example, read Dorianne Laux's poem 'For the Sake of Strangers' in a group for older people, she said: 'That feeling there … disengaged to the world – I … I … I remember that feeling. I was aware of things but not aware of things. I wasn't part of it. The words in the poem

"No matter what the grief, its weight, we are obliged to carry it".[6] I'm afraid I know that. I can't say I don't know that because I do'. Ona had previously found it difficult to speak of the death of her husband. Here, amidst the hesitation ('I ... I ...'), 'I can't say I don't' comes like a sudden blurting, triggered by emotion and memory, which momentarily and spontaneously obliterates previous barriers between past and present, self and others. As with Donald saying in relation to the Herrick poem, 'These are things I haven't had' (Chapter 10), the negative syntax here is actually a signal of the release into active use of uncertainties, under-used dimensions of self and so-called negative experiences hitherto denied, regretted or neglected as redundant.

At other times, the double negative mark the turns of syntax that participants often instinctively use in sensitively feeling out the space they are having now to occupy and explore. When Jud says on Tessimond's poem, 'Day Dream': 'I think he's saying there... that it's do-able, I guess... there's nothing that couldn't be done... I guess', it is the signature double negative ('nothing that couldn't') that lets in the chink of possibility. Hannah, reading Rainer Maria Rilke's poem 'Evening' ('The lands grow distant in your sight,/One journeying to heaven, one that falls;/ and leaves you, not at home in either one'), noted 'It's about everything that isn't. There's everything you can be and there's everything that you're not, and they're both there at the same time. It's a space between dark and light' (see Chapter 10, 'Josie Billington and Philip Davis, "Reading Live: A Qualitative Method for Analyzing Reading in Real Time"'). Such language locates a dimension of thought *between* ordinary or 'stuck' fixities. Arguably, this is mental health forming itself at micro-level.

Kevin Harvey and Gavin Brookes, 'The Corpus Approach'

The transcripts analysed in the practical demonstration below derive from a multi-disciplinary mixed-methods study comparing the benefits of Shared Reading with Cognitive Behavioural Therapy for people living with chronic pain[7] (see Chapter 12 for fuller details of the study). The authors of the analysis in this section were not involved in the original study in which, in terms of linguistic analysis, qualitative (conversation) analysis only was applied. All CBT and reading sessions were audio-recorded and transcribed. One transcript from each data set—both recorded early in the 'intervention'—is analysed here using techniques from ***corpus linguistics****. These independent findings are then cross-referenced with qualitative and quantitative findings from the original study to exhibit the* *potential value and need for dynamic interplay* ***across*** *disciplinary approaches in the study of reading.*

In this section of the chapter, we analyse the transcripts of the Shared Reading group and CBT session using techniques from corpus linguistics. Corpus linguistics is a collection of methods that use specialist computer programs to study linguistic patterns in large collections of naturally occurring language data. Such a collection of language is known as a corpus (pl. *corpora*). To make them amenable to computational analysis, it is essential that the text(s) contained in a corpus are stored in an electronic, machine-readable format. Corpora are not, strictly speaking, randomly compiled collections of language, but are designed in a careful and considered way so as to ensure that they represent a particular language or linguistic variety of interest. Corpora come in two main types: general and specialised. Where general corpora are designed to represent entire languages or varieties (usually at a particular point in time), specialised corpora are designed to represent language use in more specific contexts. Because they are designed to represent language on a broad scale, general corpora tend to be very large in size, typically comprising thousands of texts and millions (sometimes billions) of words. Specialised corpora, on the other hand, tend to be smaller, comprising fewer genres, texts and words.[8] The transcripts analysed in this chapter constitute specialised corpora; they represent language used in very specific contexts and as such are relatively small and genre-constrained. The Shared Reading group corpus contains 20,193 words, while the CBT corpus is just over half the size and contains 11,820 words.[9]

One advantage of studying corpora is that their (usually) large size allows analysts to account for a wider range of variation in the type of language or texts being studied, and therefore produce more generalisable findings based on more substantial and representative textual evidence than would be possible using manual, qualitative approaches alone. Yet, the advantages afforded by corpus data are not restricted to large corpora alone, for even smaller corpora—such as our corpora of Shared Reading and CBT transcripts—offer a series of benefits to analysts. The specialist computer programs that are used to study corpora—such as *WordSmith Tools* (Scott, 2016), *AntConc* (Anthony, 2019) and *CQPweb* (Hardie, 2012)—afford analytical perspectives on the language in the corpus that would be impractical (if not impossible) to adopt without the help of a computer. This includes: searching for every occurrence of a word or combination of words in the data, generating frequency information about linguistic phenomena of interest (e.g. words, chains of words, grammatical types), performing statistical tests to measure the significance or strength of relationships between phenomena, as well as presenting the data in ways that render it more amenable to qualitative analysis.[10] These procedures can reveal patterns in the data that might run counter to human intuition or, in the case of larger corpora containing many texts, which feature sparingly in one or two texts but become significant when considered as part of a larger whole.[11] Computer programs also offer the practical advantage that they can perform frequency counts and complex statistical calculations with greater speed and reliability than the human mind.

Because their analyses are guided by more objective criteria, such as frequency information and statistical significance, corpus methods can also help to reduce the influence of human bias on the research (Baker, 2006). This increased objectivity is also supported by corpus linguistics' commitment to methodological transparency, underpinned by two guiding principles: (i) no systematic bias in the selection of texts included in the corpus (i.e. do not exclude a text because it does not fit a pre-existing argument or theory) and (ii) total accountability (all data gathered must be accounted for) (McEnery and Hardie, 2012). Combined, these principles of methodological transparency can help analysts to overcome the accusation that their analyses are based on convenient texts or examples, cherry-picked to support the researcher's argument or theory.[12]

At this point, it is also important to acknowledge that it is not possible for the influence of human bias to be removed from the corpus linguistic research process completely. The human researcher is required to make a number of important methodological decisions over the course of a corpus linguistic analysis, including those involved in constructing or selecting a corpus and choosing which analytical techniques to use and deciding on their parameters. These are all decisions which will have some bearing on the findings. Furthermore, it is important to bear in mind that the frequency and statistical output that corpus methods provide are not ends in themselves. Computers alone cannot provide explanations for the linguistic patterns in a corpus; it is up to the researcher to interpret the significance of such patterns and explain why they occur. At this point in the analysis, it can be useful to supplement the aforementioned quantitative approaches with more qualitative analysis of linguistic features of interest in their original contexts of use (see Part I).

In this section of the chapter, we will analyse the Shared Reading group and CBT transcripts using three well-established corpus techniques: frequency, keywords and concordance, which we accessed using the *WordSmith Tools* computer program.[13] Rather than introducing these techniques in detail here, we will instead introduce them over the course of our analysis, thereby providing worked demonstrations of their use. Our analysis will not address any specific research question but will have a broadly comparative agenda—to explore some of the most frequent or statistically salient similarities and differences between the language used in our Shared Reading group and CBT transcripts.

Frequency

The frequency technique does what it says on the tin—it provides a list of all the words that are present in our corpus and tells us how often each one occurs. Frequency can provide a good starting point for corpus analysis, as it affords rapid insight into the types of words that tend to be used most often in the language we are analysing—in this case, in the Shared Reading group and CBT interactions. Tables 11.1 and 11.2 provide a list of the ten most frequent words used in the Shared Reading group and CBT corpora,

Table 11.1 Top ten words in the Shared Reading group

Rank	Word	Freq.	Frequency per 1000 words
1	*the*	846	42.08
2	*it*	574	28.55
3	*and*	502	24.97
4	*i*	480	23.88
5	*to*	445	22.14
6	*you*	433	21.54
7	*yeah*	411	20.44
8	*that*	391	19.45
9	*a*	343	17.06
10	*she*	342	17.01

Table 11.2 Top ten words in the CBT transcript

Rank	Word	Freq.	Frequency per 1000 words
1	*i*	453	38.38
2	*the*	366	31.01
3	*it*	343	29.06
4	*and*	324	27.45
5	*you*	291	24.66
6	*that*	249	21.10
7	*to*	240	20.33
8	*a*	225	19.06
9	*of*	182	15.42
10	*yeah*	158	13.39

respectively.[14] For ease of interpretation, and to facilitate comparison between the datasets, we have also normalised the figures in these tables to express the frequency of each word per thousand words in its dataset.

The top ten words in both datasets, or corpora, are dominated by grammatical or 'function' words, such as 'the', 'it' and 'and'. This is not particularly surprising, since the most frequent words in most varieties of English are function words, and so these types of items regularly dominate the top word frequency lists. However, even grammatical words can be revealing of interesting similarities and differences between corpora. In this case, we note the higher frequency of the first-person pronoun 'I' in the CBT data compared to the Shared Reading group. As well as being the most frequent word in the CBT transcript, this word is also relatively more frequent in this dataset compared to the Shared Reading group. Where 'I' is used approximately 38 times for every thousand words in the CBT data, it is found only 23.88 times per thousand words in the Shared Reading group. This might suggest that the CBT context is more likely than the context of a Shared Reading group to elicit disclosure of opinions and experiences from a first-person perspective, with participants more likely to talk from their own subjective experiences (e.g. '**I**'m now defined by my pain rather than me defining who **I** am through my actions **I** don't do anything **I** don't see anybody **I** don't go anywhere you know prior to this **I** ran my own business **I** worked full time…').

On the other hand, the third-person pronoun 'she', which is ranked tenth in the Shared Reading group but does not appear among the ten most frequent words in the CBT data, indicates that the participants in the Shared Reading group are perhaps likely to talk about the experiences and perspectives of the character in the book they are talking about (Mrs Manstey)[15] (e.g. 'Because of it and this is the way **she**'s going to feel (.) it's going to close her in'), as well as their own. At the same time, although these differences in pronouns point to some differences in the language used in the corpus, these are not absolute differences (i.e. presence vs. absence) and they are not likely to be statistically significant, so we need to be careful not to over-interpret these frequency differences.

Other pronouns in the frequency list point to similarities between the two datasets, specifically the second-person singular you, which features in both wordlists and gestures towards the interactional nature of both contexts, whereby the speaker is addressing another fellow interlocutor (e.g. 'Do **you** mean that she could have social life but she chooses not to (Shared Reading group), um do **you** think that's an important part of it or not really' [CBT]).

However, in both datasets, the word 'you' functions most often as a form of general reference, whereby the speaker expresses their own perspective or experience as being generalisable and so shared with others involved in the interaction.

Aside from these pronouns, the remainder of the words populating both of these word lists are grammatical words, including the word 'yeah', which tends to function as an affirmative in spoken language[16] and so indicates the tendency for the participants in both contexts to agree with one another and construct discussions around topics to do with pain in a collaborative way. Although looking at frequent grammatical words can therefore prove revealing of the linguistic characteristics of the text(s) under study, to explore similarities and differences between the thematic content of our datasets, it is more productive to focus on lexical or 'content' words. To focus on such words, we usually have to filter out high-frequency grammatical words. However, this is not ideal, as corpus linguists are generally reticent to prima facie disregard any word in the data, particularly if that word occurs with a high frequency. Moreover, even grammatical words, which often fail to excite on initial impressions, can sometimes turn out to be significant for analyses.[17] Our analysis therefore makes use of a more statistically robust method of accessing content words—the keywords technique.

Keywords

Keywords are words that are unusually frequent in one corpus when it is compared against another corpus (a reference corpus). The reference corpus typically represents a norm or 'benchmark' for the type of language under investigation. For this analysis, we investigate the differences between the two datasets by comparing them against each other. The resulting keywords are then taken to be characteristic of the language used in each context—Shared Reading group or CBT—when it is compared against the other. Another decision we have to make relates to the statistical measure we use to determine and rank the keywords in our data. In this analysis, we used log ratio—a measure which ranks keywords according to the strength of the difference in frequency between the two corpora that have been compared to generate keywords.[18] Starting with the transcript of the Shared Reading group, Table 11.3 shows the keywords for this dataset when we compared it against the CBT transcript.

As this table shows, the keywords procedure produced five keywords for the Shared Reading group interaction. Before commenting on these keywords, it is useful to first clarify how they have become keywords. Although frequency is a driving factor in identifying keywords, high frequency alone is not sufficient for a word to be flagged as 'key' by the computer. What is most important in determining whether a word is a keyword is the relative frequencies of the word between the two corpora being compared. For example, although the word 'window' is less frequent than the word 'her', it has been assigned a higher keyness value (log ratio) score because, where 'her' features 4 times in the CBT data, 'window' does not appear at all. Thus, the difference between the two frequencies has been judged by the computer to be stronger in the case of window, which means that it has a much higher log ratio score.

The most striking thing about the keywords in Table 11.3 is that most of them ostensibly refer to the main character in the story being discussed by the group—Mrs Manstey ('mrs', 'manstey', 'her' and 'she'). The remaining keyword, 'window', reflects the fact that the majority of Mrs Manstey's activities take place by the window in the place where she lives. These keywords therefore reflect the fact that, when it is compared against the CBT

Table 11.3 Shared Reading group keywords, ranked by log ratio

Rank	Keyword	Freq. in Shared Reading	Freq. in CBT	Log ratio
1	*Mrs*	117	0	141.57
2	*Manstey*	64	0	140.70
3	*Window*	51	0	140.37
4	*Her*	227	4	5.05
5	*She*	342	12	4.06

Table 11.4 CBT keywords, ranked by log ratio

Rank	Keyword	Freq. in CBT	Freq. in Shared Reading	Log ratio
1	*Tablets*	17	0	139.56
2	*Hurt*	15	0	139.38
3	*Brain*	15	0	139.38
4	*Chronic*	14	0	139.28
5	*Damage*	13	0	139.17
6	*Ten*	29	2	4.63
7	*Pain*	100	8	4.42
8	*Part*	26	5	3.15
9	*Um*	92	25	2.65
10	*Uh*	36	10	2.62

transcript, the Shared Reading group can by characterised by discussion about Mrs Manstey and her surroundings and activities. Now, turning our attention to the other dataset under study, Table 11.4 displays the keywords for the CBT transcript when compared against the Shared Reading group data.

The first thing to note about Table 11.4 is that the computer produced twice as many keywords for the CBT transcript (10) as the Shared Reading group (five). On first impressions, this suggests that CBT interactions are linguistically more varied than the Shared Reading group discussion and there are more words that are, computationally speaking, characteristic of it. Most of the keywords relate to the concept of chronic pain, its causes and cures, including words which denote chronic pain ('hurt', 'chronic', 'pain'), the brain ('brain'), brain damage ('damage'—which tends to relate to tissue damage) and medication ('tablets'). The word 'ten' refers to discussion around a pain score, while 'part' tends to be used in discussions about the factors that contribute towards pain (i.e. parts which contribute towards a whole). In addition to this, we have particles that are characteristic of spoken communication ('um', 'uh').

The frequency and keywords measures provide useful analytical entry points, as both offer effective means for identifying prominent and statistically salient linguistic themes in our corpora. However, to explain why such words (and the themes they denote) are frequent or statistically salient, it is necessary for us to follow them up in more fine-grained, qualitative fashion. We can do this using the corpus procedure of concordance.

Concordance

The concordance technique provides a way of viewing the data that allows us to examine every occurrence of a word or phrase in its original linguistic context, with the search word or phrase highlighted in bold, and several surrounding words displayed to the left and right. Concordance analysis is right at the heart of any close reading of a corpus, providing a useful means for spotting patterns that might be less obvious during more linear, left-to-right readings of the data. In Examples 11.1 and 11.2, we produce two sets of randomly chosen concordances which feature the word 'pain'. *Pain* is a keyword in the CBT data but also occurs, albeit only 8 times, in the Shared Reading data. These concordances offer some intriguing textual insights into the uses of this word across both datasets.

1. features of the other (.) you can be at one end of the spectrum of nerve type **pain** and and the nociceptive type pain but the vast majority of people
2. those people who say (.) because there's a nerver block it must be a neuropathic **pain** and I'll say yes what's happened is all the cartilage has been
3. the central nervous system and the peripheral nervous system nerves spinal cord brain um are transmitting **pain** impulses in the same way as they transmit hot and cold uh um vibrations another one
4. generally come to the conclusion that everyone we've seen their pain their **pain** is totally different to] everybody else
5. The **pain** like the throbbing pain I was getting is going away but everywhere you touch is aching
6. Yeah (.) well if you notice we don't say what's you're **pain** score over ten because we [know that it varies]

Example 11.1 Sample concordances for occurrences of *pain* in the CBT transcript

In the above examples, the CBT group users discuss pain not so much in personal, lay terms, but in a pseudo-technical language, adopting therewith standpoints of knowledge and authority associated with the use of such discourse. The participants adopt a scientific and clinical register, a variety of language which is reflective perhaps of the group members' familiarity with medical and therapeutic discourse, and their socialisation in a counselling-based community of practice.[19] We might see this bent for technical description as an instance of proto-professionalisation, the process whereby lay persons adopt a psychologising approach to their disclosures, framing their knowledge and personal experiences of chronic pain in what de Swaan (1990) describes as 'proto-professional' terms,[20] where the emphasis on clinical symptoms and a medical, technical understanding of psychological distress mixes lay and professional beliefs. Note, for example, how the participants refer to the anatomical nature of pain, presenting themselves as experts in its physiological provenance: 'you can be at one end of the spectrum of nerve type pain and and the nociceptive type pain' (1) and 'the central nervous system and the peripheral nervous system nerves spinal cord brain um are transmitting pain impulses in the same way as they transmit hot and cold uh um vibrations' (3). Pain is qualified in precise, expert terms 'neuropathic pain' (2), and is spoken about in relation to diagnostic charts and assessment criteria 'well if you notice we don't say what's you're pain score over ten because we [know that it varies]' (6).

Yet at the same time, though less frequently, there is also recourse to a more demotic register to articulate and pinpoint the inescapably personal and idiosyncratic nature of pain: 'The pain like the throbbing pain I was getting is going away but everywhere you touch is aching' (5). The use of the metaphor 'throbbing pain' illustrates how, despite the possibility of framing one's personal pain in a more technical, clinical manner (as often appears to be the case with this group of proto-expert participants), figurative discourse might step in when pain escapes such professional encoding, when pain resists straightforward objectification through off-the-shelf literal language. As this instance reveals, metaphor isn't simply a rhetorical flourish that colours and embellishes, but is rather an essential and 'powerful resource of the imagination that literally extends the boundaries of our shared world'.[21] The

7. **pain** Yeah Yeah and how it kind of it keeps you in one place (.) and you kind of think about well if I move It how you become cocooned in pain And it hold it holds you in one place

8. Yeah It pins you in one place as well cos it's that thought of well I'm in **pain** now (.) so if I move It'll be worse I've got this and that (.) and it kind of / it does pin you

9. dressed this time (.) not just now getting ready to go out but earlier in the day it was harder for her wasn't it Yeah it was It's like when you're down over something everything seem / **pain** or not matter what it is it always seems much larger doesn't it

10. then other days you feel like you're scraping yourself off the floor to do it Or even moments isn't it [Yeah] [Yeah] It feels like just a moment Well this is like when you're I **pain** this little bit here isn't it

11. It pins you in one place as well cos it's that thought of well I'2m in **pain** now (.) so if I move It'll be worse I've got this and that

12. That's what it feels like Cos it's (.) sorry] [I also felt] that um (.) the looping string twined around my chest and holds me (.) I can I can link that to **pain**

Example 11.2 Sample concordances for occurrences of *pain* in the Shared Reading transcript

'throbbing pain' metaphor might be conventional but it still allows the participant to reify what is otherwise an 'interior and unsharable experience'.[22] Indeed, without recourse to metaphor, it would be all but impossible to faithfully articulate the personally felt experience of pain.

Interestingly, in Example 11.2—concordance lines taken from the Shared Reading group—an arguably less conventional use of metaphor is in evidence.

In examples 7–12, there is a relative absence of technical language to express pain. Rather, the felt experience of pain is externalised through the recurring use of the container metaphor, where pain takes on a spatial dimension, is vividly described as something with its own agency that 'cocoons' the person and holds them in place (7), or 'pins you in one place' (8), or is a 'looping string' (12) wrapped around the body that 'holds' the sufferer. Such agentive tropes, as Biro (2010, p. 16) observes, serve a dual function: first they enable the sufferer to validate their pain, and second, help them better understand it. In example 8, for example, the speaker confirms (validates) what one of their fellow interlocutors has communicated and the exchanges between the participants collaboratively move forward, forging new shared perspectives and alignments, as though pivoting around or taking inspiration from the trope.

But of course it also needs to be pointed out that these novel tropes are not produced in a social or linguistic vacuum. Their expression derives, to a significant extent, from the subject of their talk—namely, the literary text which the group members are presently discussing after having shared it live together. As is often the case with literary works, the text under discussion is a linguistic resource that offers an external outlet for interior events (Scarry, 1985, p. 8). For example, the participants use the story as a vehicle for articulating the uniqueness of their own pain, while at the same time appreciating that their own suffering is not entirely unique, that others have experienced similar physical and emotional travails. The literary text, and the participants' live engagement with it, therefore offers a way round the intrinsic problems of communicating pain to others (Biro, 2010, p. 17). The literary text, as is evident here, enables the participants to see the issue of pain from another perspective, and then to reflect on it and to appreciate that, though pain separates us from others, it might have a common underlying structure (Biro, 2010, p. 18).

One could of course say more of these two sets of concordance lines, and what they reveal, among other topics and issues, about the problem of pain formulation. One important issue that both sets of concordance lines help illustrate is that, whether spoken about in a group therapy or Shared

Reading setting, pain is an unignorably personal phenomenon. But when communicating pain there is always the prospect that others might potentially fail to appreciate how the speaker actually, individually, uniquely experiences it. As Scarry argues, 'To have pain is to have certainty; to hear about pain is to have doubt' (Scarry, 1985, p. 13). In other words, one's own felt experience is incontrovertible and undeniable but others hearing about it might not necessarily confirm it. It is therefore not surprising that the participants in the two datasets adopt a range of strategies to render 'the sentient fact' of their pain knowable to others, harnessing discursive strategies which are, to a large extent, determined by the specific context of the two groups, with their unique sets of attributes, shared values and purposes.

In short, this brief corpus analysis, though of course by no means comprehensive, provides some discursive insights into the two sets of transcripts, linguistic insights which might otherwise be overlooked (or not so readily apprehended) by an exclusively manual, qualitative analysis. That said, any corpus analysis is only as good as the analyst who conducts it: even if a computer sorts the data into formats that throw up numerously promising patterns of language use, the analysts themselves still have to interpret and tease out the significance of such patterns, and decide which to pursue and which to abandon.

* * *

What follow are reflections: first from Josie Billington (JB) on the relation of this independent corpus analysis to quantitative and qualitative findings from the original chronic pain study; second from Kevin Harvey and Gavin Brookes (KH/GB), responding to JB; finally, Kremena Koleva (KK) brings her own qualitative-linguistic interest in 'intangibles' to the same transcripts studied quantitatively above.

JB

Corroborations

The 'higher frequency of the first-person pronoun "I" in the CBT data compared to the Shared Reading group' resonates with the finding from the conversation analysis of 'consecutive self-disclosure' among CBT group members. Likewise, the prevalence in the reading group of the third-person pronoun 'she', and the direct relation of the transcript's keywords to the protagonist of the story—both indicating participants' engaging with the experiences and perspectives of the character in the book—are corroborated by the qualitative evidence that discussion is 'triggered' by fictional story in Shared Reading. The finding that 'in CBT, most of the keywords relate to the concept of chronic pain, its causes and cures' correlates exactly with the finding from conversational analysis that 'in the CBT session the chronic pain theme is consistently maintained and there is no deviation' (see also Chapter 12). There is also strong synergy between the demonstration in conversation analysis that 'the facilitator is constructed as expert' by participants, and the finding in the corpus analysis that participants tend (deferentially) to 'frame their personal pain in a technical, clinical manner'. Yet, where conversation analysis finds 'a clear distance between coordinator/expert and participants/sufferers', corpus analysis suggests, rather differently, that participants seek to align themselves with a standpoint of expert knowledge by adopting a proto-professional discourse and technical understanding of their suffering. (One query: can corpus linguistics distinguish between the technical language used by the facilitator of CBT and that used by the participants? Is this where qualitative analysis is essential?)

Dynamic cross-references

The finding that there were 'twice as many keywords for the CBT transcript (10) as the Shared Reading group (five)' and the (first) impression therewith that 'CBT interactions are linguistically more varied than the Shared Reading group discussion' might be usefully combined with some of the original study's statistical results. As Chapter 12 will show more fully, the study asked participants in both interventions to keep 12-hour mood/emotion diaries alongside pain diaries given the close correlation of the two in chronic pain. One unexpected finding was that the *number* and *range* of words used following SR sessions was significantly expanded, and more intense in terms of emotion expressed, good and bad (e.g. energised, vibrant, refreshed; frustrated, restless) as compared with words used following CBT which were considerably fewer and more bland and/or factual in content (e.g. happy; tired). This relates, of course, to your final discussion of language and expression taking its cue from the literary text in Shared Reading. I'm wondering whether it's possible that the phenomenon of fewer keywords might actually denote a concentration and intensity (cognitive, imaginative, emotional) which in turn fosters an expanded expressive repertoire—one partly borrowed from the text itself but also engendered by deepened engagement, awareness and openness in relation to it?

A surprising area of apparent contradiction in the original study occurred between the qualitative evidence derived from conversation analysis, on the one hand, and from the video-assisted qualitative interviews on the other hand. The former found 'more collaboration and construction of "in-groupness" between participants (through agreement, repetitions and collaborative overlaps) compared to Shared Reading'; where in the latter, participants uniformly emphasised the intimacy of the Shared Reading group as compared to the CBT group: 'we're a little team you know'; 'a bit like brothers and sisters'; 'part of a family', 'a little serious community'; 'it's quite telepathic really'. We surmised that community in Shared Reading developed more implicitly beneath explicit linguistic markers and capturing this process might require the kind of physiological measures described in Chapter 13. In this context, it is especially compelling that corpus analysis finds the 'recurring use of the [non-conventional] container metaphor, where pain takes on a spatial dimension' is a catalyst for 'participants collaboratively [to] move forward, forging new shared perspectives and alignments, as though pivoting around or taking inspiration from the trope'. Across the transcripts, the use of metaphor might be a pattern to pursue. (See also Chapters 15 and 16, on metaphor.)

KH/GB
Although corpus linguistics can offer powerful insights into discourse, revealing patterns about empirical language use that human intuition is likely to fail to apprehend and/or appreciate, the utility of the corpus approach is dependent on the design and structure of the corpus in question, along with the nature of the research questions asked of the corpus. In relation to the kind of questions posed above—which are moot and difficult to answer—the corpus linguistic approach in itself offers little by way of solution to these intriguing conundrums. For example, in relation to the query respecting whether corpus linguistics can distinguish between the technical language used by the facilitator of CBT and that used by the participants, it really depends on how the corpus is structured in the first place. The corpus is not composed in such a way to see this separation of distinct voices (though it could be if the corpus were resolved into separate corpora for the different participants) so in this case the easiest way is just to search for some of these terms in the original transcripts to see who tends to use them, although undertaking this process might be relatively time-consuming. Accordingly, this is where more qualitative-based techniques come in—a fine-grained analysis which can pay attention to the moment-by-moment unfolding of discourse and thereby pinpoint any minute instances of interest and revelation. But even here the corpus approach still has a potential place, since the qualitative researcher can use the corpus search facility to identify terms of interest and then, once located, use them to drill further down into the discourse to flush out more intricate and context-bound instances of linguistic use, even if the process is somewhat laborious.

There could well be something in the observation that the phenomenon of fewer keywords might suggest a concentration and intensity which engenders an expanded expressive repertoire. There is surely a prima facie claim for this. That said, the generation of keywords in this case pivots around a statistical algorithm which takes into account a range of factors between the target and reference corpora (the two corpora compared against one another in order to generate keywords), and it's difficult to pinpoint one particular factor that accounts for the smaller amount of keywords. Again, further qualitative investigation would be necessary to answer this intriguing question.

KK
Language fails us when we most need it—to avoid feeling lonely and isolated—because loneliness is avoided only if one has been understood and being understood goes beyond understanding the words we say.

It hurts.

This is the first thing a participant utters after the coordinator invites the group to help them define chronic pain. You, a listener, can hear a fusion of the speaker's angry defiance, paralysing helplessness, desperate hopelessness. This is not in the syntax or semantics of the utterance, it's in its **brevity** which creates a heart-stabbing experience. The list of similarly short utterances after this one creates the illusion of a prolonged stabbing experience, each utterance a new stab.

I dare say it is heart-stabbing only for people who have felt a pain similar in its intensity to the one the speaker is talking about. I am not convinced whether the same utterance will have the same force, and therefore the same expressiveness, to an alien who is not acquainted with the human condition. This difference in listeners is vital because very often you try to talk about your pain to someone who has not gone through any particularly painful experiences in their lives (i.e. an alien to pain) and if you tell them *It hurts.* they would not know exactly what you mean. They just don't have the necessary reference point, a painful experience of their own of similar intensity. So, I think some of the message of *It hurts.* is over and above its syntax and semantics; I will call it a *communication potential.* I say potential because it relies on the ability of a listener to retrieve it; it's a potential that vibrates on different wavelengths waiting to be picked up on, so to speak; it may be picked up on, but it may not be. It's a potential.

All of this is illustrated in the transcript by the proliferation of phrases such as 'if you know what I mean', 'if you see what I mean' and also tag questions such as 'isn't it' that invite some sort of confirmation from the listeners. All of this suggests that without this confirmation, without the listener's ability to *see* what the speaker means there is no real communication and speakers are forced to remain lonely and isolated in their pain.

Previously, when I spoke of 'intangibles' (see above, 'Sofia Lampropoulou, Kremena Koleva, Josie Billington and Philip Davis, "Linguistic Analysis of Transcribed Video-Recorded Reading Groups"') I had in mind speakers who are groping for words to express something of which they have some awareness, but it seems not enough to capture its enormity in mere words. There is a bit of it here too. Look at the following utterance *I it's **a life ch/** to me it's been **a life change** uh (0.5) for me it was **a life changing event** in 2008 so //...* To me it is a good example of 'live thought'—the highlighted bits suggest the gradual access to thought, cognition, a reality outside language. Again, part of the meaning is not in the syntax and semantics, it's in the gradual nature of accessing this reality. In other words, it's communication potential.

In many ways, I am groping for words to express something that struck me a while back, in my youth, when I read Kundera's *The Unbearable Lightness of Being*. I am adding the passage here by a way of conclusion:

> Now, perhaps, we are in a better position to understand the abyss separating Sabina and Franz: he listened eagerly to the story of her life and she was equally eager to hear the story of his, but although they had a clear understanding of the logical meaning of the words they exchanged, they failed to hear *the semantic susurrus of the river flowing through them.* (my italics)[23]

Notes

1. J. P. Gee, *An Introduction to Discourse Analysis: Theory and Method* (Abingdon: Taylor & Francis, 2014); B. Jonhstone, *Discourse Analysis*, 3rd edn (Oxford: Wiley-Blackwell, 2017).
2. M. Arnold, 'The Buried Life', in *The Poems of Matthew Arnold*, ed. by Kenneth Allott (London: Longman, 1965), pp. 271–76 (p. 275).
3. E. Gendlin, 'The New Phenomenology of Carrying Forward', *Continental Philosophy Review*, 37.1 (2004), 131.
4. J. W. Pennebaker, *The Secret Life of Pronouns* (New York and London: Bloomsbury, 2011), p. 108.
5. C. Dickens, *A Christmas Carol*, ed. by Michael Slater (Harmondsworth: Penguin Books Ltd., 1965), p. 126.
6. D. Laux, *What We Carry* (Brockport, NY: BOA Editions, 1994), p. 23.

7. J. Billington, G. Farrington, S. Lampropoulou, J. Lingwood, A. Jones, J. Ledson, K. McDonnell, N. Duirs, and A.-L. Humphreys, 'A Comparative Study of Cognitive Behavioural Therapy and Shared Reading for Chronic Pain', *Journal of Medical Humanities*, 43.3 (2016), 155–65.
8. T. McEnery and A. Hardie, *Corpus Linguistics: Method, Theory and Practice* (Cambridge: Cambridge University Press, 2012).
9. Note: prior to analysis, the data was 'cleaned' to remove the transcribers' notes, including speakers' names and metalinguistic content (e.g. denoting laughter).
10. P. Baker, *Using Corpora in Discourse Analysis* (London: Continuum, 2006).
11. T. McEnery, R. Xiao, and Y. Tono, *Corpus-Based Language Studies: An Advanced Resource Book* (London and New York: Routledge, 2006).
12. H. Widdowson, *Text, Context, Pretext: Critical Issues in Discourse Analysis* (Oxford: Blackwell, 2004).
13. M. Scott, WordSmith Tools (Version 7) [Computer Software] (Stroud: Lexical Analysis Software, 2016). It should be noted that there is no standard set of procedures in corpus linguistic methodology. Rather, corpus linguistics offers a range of techniques that can be adopted and combined in a variety of ways depending on the research question(s) and type(s) of language being analysed. The techniques we use in this analysis are fairly staple in corpus approaches to discourse analysis. However, for an introduction to the full range of techniques available to corpus linguists, we refer readers to Baker (2006) and McEnery et al. (2006).
14. This is an arbitrary cut-off.
15. The texts read in this session were Edith Wharton's short story 'Mrs Manstey's View' and Norman Nicholson's poem, 'The Pot Geranium'. See Chapter 8.
16. R. Carter and M. McCarthy, *Exploring Spoken English*, 2nd edn (Cambridge: Cambridge University Press, 1997).
17. T. McEnery, *Swearing in English: Bad Language, Purity and Power from 1586 to the Present* (London and New York: Routledge, 2005).
18. Corpus analytical programs like *WordSmith Tools* offer a number of statistical measures for generating and ranking keywords, each of which will produce a slightly different set of keywords which allow the analyst to make different types of claims about their keywords.
19. J. Lave and E. Wenger, *Situated Learning: Legitimate Peripheral Participation* (Cambridge: Cambridge University Press, 1991).
20. A. De Swaan, *The Management of Normality: Critical Essays in Health and Welfare* (London: Taylor & Francis, 1990).
21. D. Biro, *The Language of Pain* (Norton: New York, 2010), p. 16.
22. E. Scarry, *The Body in Pain: The Making and Unmaking of the World* (Oxford: Oxford University Press, USA, 1985), p. 16.
23. M. Kundera, *The Unbearable Lightness of Being* (New York: Harper & Row, 1984), p. 84.

12

Quantitative Methods

Josie Billington, Rhiannon Corcoran, Megan Watkins, Mette Steenberg, Charlotte Christiansen, Nicolai Ladegaard and Don Kuiken

Rhiannon Corcoran, Josie Billington and Megan Watkins, 'Using Standardised Measures to Capture "Non-standard" (Subjective, Personal) Reading Experiences'

This section rises to the challenge posed by health commissioners and public health providers when they require evidence of the benefits of reading according to standard and widely used measures of health and well-being. We report on the experimental approaches we have used and the standard measures we have tested to assess the effect of reading on psychological health.

The original version of this chapter was revised. The incorrect spelling of the author name "Nikolai Ladegaard" has been corrected. The correction to this chapter is available at https://doi.org/10.1007/978-3-030-21762-4_22

J. Billington (✉)
Centre for Research into Reading, Literature and Society,
University of Liverpool, Liverpool, UK
e-mail: jbilling@liverpool.ac.uk

R. Corcoran
Psychology and Public Mental Health, University of Liverpool, Liverpool, UK
e-mail: corcoran@liverpool.ac.uk

M. Watkins
Department of Psychology, University of Liverpool, Liverpool, UK
e-mail: M.C.Watkins@liverpool.ac.uk

J. Billington (ed.), *Reading and Mental Health*,
https://doi.org/10.1007/978-3-030-21762-4_12

Design

Two studies compared reading with a comparator activity or intervention. The first of these sought to tease out the specific and intrinsic components of a specific model of Shared Reading and its benefits to mental health and well-being by comparison with another cultural activity.[1] Participants were recruited from volunteers of UK charity The Reader who were taking part in a UK Big Lottery-funded initiative to involve those at risk of mental health issues and social isolation in meaningful endeavour. Volunteers were based at The Reader's headquarters and then newly housed at Calderstones Mansion in Calderstones Park, Liverpool, which, together with the grounds and immediate parkland, was undergoing reconstruction as an International Centre for Reading and Well-being. The participants were divided into two groups, A and B. In a cross-over design, Group A experienced six Shared Reading sessions (SR) followed by six Built Environment Design Workshops exploring the development of the surrounding parkland (BE); simultaneously Group B experienced six BE sessions followed by six SR sessions. The same literary texts and design activities were used in both groups, and activities were led by trained experts in literature and environmental/architectural design.

Using standard self-report measures of mental health and well-being (detailed separately below), the study found that there was a consistent and statistically significant tendency for involvement in *both* activities to

M. Steenberg
Aarhus University, Aarhus, Denmark
e-mail: mette.steenberg@cas.au.dk

C. Christiansen
Department of Anthropology, School of Culture and Society,
Aarhus University, Aarhus, Denmark
e-mail: cec@cas.au.dk

N. Ladegaard
Department of Depression and Anxiety,
School of Clinical Medicine, Aarhus University, Aarhus, Denmark
e-mail: nicolai.ladegaard@ps.rm.dk

D. Kuiken
Department of Psychology, University of Alberta,
Edmonton, AB, Canada
e-mail: dkuiken@ualberta.ca

be associated with the self-report of more positive than negative affect. The data suggested, however, that involvement in SR prompted the experience of negative affect to a greater extent than involvement in BE. This was consistent with qualitative findings (see Chapter 10) that the intrinsic value of the Shared Reading of literature lies in its capacity to open individuals up to a broader range of emotional states, via vicarious response to characters in the text or the text's bringing to mind analogous personal situations or past events.

A second study compared the effects of SR for people suffering chronic pain with those offered by a more formal, programmatic therapy, cognitive behavioural therapy (CBT), the standard psycho-social treatment for the condition.[2] A CBT and SR group ran in parallel (at the pain clinic of a UK city hospital), with CBT group members joining the SR group after the completion of CBT. Participants kept twice-daily (12-hourly) pain diaries as a measure of physical changes. Pain severity was recorded using a 0–10 rating scale (0 = non-existent, 10 = severe), at 12-hour intervals. Statistical analysis showed the pain rating after the session to be lower than the mean and lower than at two days before and two days after SR. The pain rating two days after was also lower than two days before SR, suggesting the possibility of some prolonged effect, beyond the duration of the group itself. Following CBT, the pain rating was above the mean. There was considerably less evidence here that CBT affected pain and emotion beyond the duration of the group.

The findings correlated strongly with the qualitative and linguistic analysis of the video recordings of both interventions (see Chapters 10 and 11). Where in CBT, participants focused exclusively on their pain with 'no thematic deviation', in SR, by contrast, the literature was a trigger to recall and expression of diverse life experiences—of work, childhood, family members, relationships—related to the entire lifespan, not merely the time period affected by pain. This in itself had a potentially therapeutic effect in helping to recover a whole person, not just an ill one. As one consultant put it, 'When people are in CBT, they are people with pain. When they're in the reading group, they're people with lives' (*Reading and Chronic Pain*, pp. 6, 89; see Chapter 21). Furthermore, where, in CBT, there was a strong emphasis on a sense of diminishment or subtraction—things 'taken away' by chronic pain—in SR, there was frequently a renewed sense of energy and vitality, sometimes of joy and celebration. This was closer to a rediscovery, via the new stimulus of the literary story, of what participants still *did* have (memories, feelings, thoughts, experiences) rather than a rehearsal or repetition of what they no longer had.

Standard Measures

In both studies, a range of standard measures were employed to explore the health and well-being benefits of SR relative to other activities and interventions. This proved a valuable means to test those measures which are most appropriate for capturing the specific aspects of psychological well-being encouraged by reading.

For example, the Warwick-Edinburgh Mental Well-being Scale (WEMWBS)[3] was a measure of choice in both studies as it is a widely used measure in the context of population-level public health evaluation. This general measure of well-being proved a blunt instrument in relation to SR, however, when compared to the more detailed and nuanced instrument offered by the Ryff Scales of Psychological Well-being.[4] Ryff showed that even short involvement in SR produced statistically significant beneficial outcomes in terms of improving an individual's sense of 'purpose in life'. Increased belief in having meaningful life goals and in the significance of past and present life was shown, furthermore, to be an intrinsic benefit of SR, not replicated in the group activity to which it was compared, where distinct psychological effects were reported. (For example, the same participants who scored highly in the 'Purpose in Life' subscale of Ryff when taking part in Shared Reading scored highly on a different subscale, 'Personal Growth', when engaged in the built environment workshops.) This finding has methodological implications pointing to the Ryff scales as a sensitive tool appropriate for further testing in future studies.

Such further testing has been carried out in relation to another standard measure that has proved important to our studies—the Positive and Negative Affect Scale[5]—which was first used in the Shared Reading (SR)/ Built Environment (BE) study to explore participants' affective state immediately following experience of each activity. This scale consists of words describing emotions (10 positives, 10 negatives) and asks participants to write next to each word the extent to which they are feeling each emotion on a scale of 1–5 (1 = not all; 5 = extremely). In addition, participants in the study were asked to write down two words or phrases which best described their experience on each occasion. As noted above, while there was a consistent and statistically significant tendency for involvement in both group activities to be associated with self-report of more positive than negative affect, initial evidence suggested SR produced negative affect to a greater extent than BE, *without this impacting on overall improvement in psychological well-being* (as captured by the Ryff scales). A follow-up use of PANAS in the SR/CBT study likewise showed a tendency for slightly lower negative scores—as well as slightly higher positive scores—in relation to SR and a greater range and intensity of expressed feeling, good and bad, in the two words or phrases which participants recorded after each SR session. This is consistent with the qualitative finding (from linguistic-literary analysis of video-recorded sessions and transcribed interviews, see Chapters 10 and 11) of a far greater diversity of elicited emotion in SR as compared to CBT and an expanded vocabulary for emotional expression. Furthermore, words recorded following CBT tended strongly towards the cognitive ('interesting', 'informative', 'educational') and were narrow in range. SR produced extensive emotional expression *together with,* a more expansive range of cognitive words than was produced by CBT ('intrigued', 'attentive', 'concentrated', 'thoughtful', 'reflective', 'alert', 'determined', 'focussed', 'deep', 'understanding', 'thought-provoking'). This quantifiable evidence gave strong corroboration to the findings emerging from qualitative data analysis that, where CBT encouraged a top-down strategy of mind over matter, SR tended to bring into conscious awareness and verbal explicitness hitherto inarticulate and implicit pain. CBT, that is to say, sought to manage emotions by means of systematic techniques, where SR helped to 'find' (often hidden or buried) pain at its personal-emotional source—as an involuntary rather than intended outcome—and thence to turn passive experience of suffering emotion into articulate contemplation of painful concerns.

Such findings are not only potentially significant for future researchers, but for reading providers and practitioners, and point to areas of further two-way collaboration. The trialing of specific measures in these studies, for example, has strongly influenced The Reader's development of tools for routine evaluation of its Shared Reading model. In consultation with the research team, The Reader has created self-report questionnaires which are nuanced in respect of the reading experience and more specific to particular populations of beneficiaries (dementia sufferers, people with mental health issues, prisoners in the criminal justice system, open community groups, looked-after children). Common to all such questionnaires is the invitation to give 'three words that describe how you feel in the Shared Reading group'. Based on quantitative analysis of the data The Reader is collecting, the research team is currently working on developing a 'reading' measure, a variation on PANAS, which is more sensitive to the individual impact of reading upon emotional experience, expression and articulacy.

Further Research

Recently, the efficacy of weekly Shared Reading for patients at Ashworth Hospital, Merseyside, UK, has been investigated using a 12-month case series design. A case series is a descriptive study that follows a group of patients with a similar diagnosis over a certain period of time. A case series does not test hypotheses but can generate them for future studies.[6]

Ashworth Hospital is a National Health Service hospital in North West England for patients requiring care and treatment in high secure conditions (see Chapters 8 and 14). Participants represented a complex forensic sample with experience of psychosis and a history of self-harm behaviour. Sessions were analysed through discourse analysis, and framework analysis (see Chapter 9) was used to explore participants' interviews about their experience of Shared Reading post-intervention. In addition, questionnaire packs were completed by participants before the intervention, at an interim period of six months and following the intervention. The questionnaire packs comprised tools such as clinical outcome measures, indicators of well-being, perspective taking and impulsivity. Tool selection was orientated around initial hypotheses and considered psychometric properties as well as pragmatic suitability.

Perspective taking was one such outcome of interest given its reported positive effects on communication[7] and negative associations with alexithymia.[8] Perspective taking was quantitatively recorded using the seven-item subscale of the Interpersonal Reactivity Index.[9] The subscale was used in its own right as the full measure is not indicative of total empathy and acceptable psychometric properties of the instrument have been reported.[10]

Impulsivity was also examined due to its link with serious mental distress.[11] In addition, affective impulsivity has been considered a risk factor for self-harm.[12] The 20-item short UPPS-P Impulsive Behavior Scale was employed which accounts for five aspects of impulsive personality: negative urgency, lack of premeditation, lack of perseverance, sensation seeking and positive urgency.[13] Evidence suggests that the instrument is generally comparable to the full measure in terms of internal consistency and inter-scale correlations. The incremental validity of impulsivity traits in predicting non-suicidal self-injury and suicidal behaviour, beyond borderline personality disorder symptoms, has also been demonstrated.[14]

Furthermore, the 18-item Ryff Scale of Psychological Well-being[15] was used to assess psychological well-being more generally. This instrument includes six dimensions: autonomy, positive relations with others, environmental mastery, personal growth, purpose in life and self-acceptance.

The factorial validity of the three-item per scale version has been reported as only just meeting acceptability criteria, but the internal consistency is not as adequate.[16] Fuller versions of the scale evidence more favourable psychometric properties; however, brevity and ease of completion were key factors influencing questionnaire development for this study population.

The quantitative outcome measures described can be used to supplement qualitative data. Examples of this are depicted in case studies of four regular participants, who each attended over sixty per cent of sessions. Participant One's discourse demonstrated a broadening of capacity to consider different interpretations across sessions. This was evident through an increased tendency to use hedging language altering degree of certainty and was reflected quantitatively through a 27% increase in perspective taking scores at six months into the intervention from participant baseline. This appeared largely attributable to stronger endorsement with the item about believing questions have two sides and trying to consider both. The response score for this item was maintained at 12 months.

Participant Two's discourse displayed an increase in self-confidence across sessions, and the participant required fewer prompts from the facilitator to speak and displayed a movement from second person plural pronouns to more first-person singular pronouns. Increased level of ownership over discourse may indicate less discomfort confronting stimuli such as negative emotions. Although total short UPPS-P score showed little change, it is noteworthy that the negative urgency subscale items for this participant mostly decreased from baseline to 6 months which was maintained at 12 months. For example, response to the item which describes saying later regrettable things when feeling rejected changed from 'somewhat agree' to 'strongly disagree'.

Participant Three's initial discourse was characterised by mimicry and alignment with the discourse of others. Mimicry often served to avoid expansion and disagreement and became a less distinguishing feature of discourse in later sessions. In accordance, total Ryff-18 score increased from 75 to 87 in the first six months. Specifically, there was greater endorsement with the autonomy items relating to having confidence in opinions that may differ from the general consensus and not judging the self by the values of others; changes were maintained at 12 months.

In addition, the discourse of Participant Four showed an increase in functionally related adjacency pairs (units of conversation containing one turn each by two speakers, such that the first turn requires a certain type of second turn) and engagement. When interviewed about experience of the intervention, the participant stated they were 'proud… that I pushed myself to do it rather than not'. This sense of satisfaction from completion was mirrored in greater endorsement with the Ryff scale item describing good management of daily responsibilities which progressed from strongly disagreeing before the intervention to somewhat agreeing post-intervention.

Using quantitative outcome measures alone for a study such as this may lead to an overly reductive approach which overlooks the subtleties of individual change. Questionnaire responses, when administered by or in the presence of a researcher or clinician in a psychiatric setting, may be particularly susceptible to the effects of social desirability, demand characteristics, difficulty with introspection and concentration. Triangulation, however, facilitates a more holistic and rigorous examination of the multi-dimensional outcomes of reading and can strengthen qualitative findings.

Mette Steenberg, Charlotte Christiansen, Nicolai Ladegaard, 'Time to Read—A Mixed Method Study of Mental Health Effects of Shared Reading'

'Time to Read' was developed with the purpose of (i) implementing Shared Reading groups for people with mental health vulnerability based on a referral model and (ii) investigating the possible health-related, quality of life (QOL) and cognitive effects of participation. In Chapters 5 and 18, we present the referral model and describe the process of implementation. In this section, we present the design, the quantitative assessment battery and the hypotheses on which the battery was selected. We discuss how mixed method studies can be used to develop improved future research designs in which acquired knowledge in relation to the intervention can feed into and inform the hypothesis on which the assessment battery in turn is selected. We conclude by discussing the difficulties in implementing controlled designs in the field. In the course of the study, we learned that the design and implementation of effect studies are two very different processes with conflicting aims.

Study Design

The aim of the study was to investigate the possible health-related, QOL and cognitive effects of participation in a Shared Reading group intervention, as well as the impact on well-being. Participants were referred by health professionals and included a population of vulnerable adults (see Chapter 18). Vulnerability covered in this case both people with diagnosed mental illness and people with a significantly reduced level of functioning due to mental and/or somatic difficulties, e.g. chronic pain patients. Criteria for exclusion were psychotic illness, drug abuse and apparent suicide risk. In addition, participants had to understand and speak the Danish language. The intervention consisted of 10 sessions in a weekly 1.5-hour Shared Reading group. Group size was 6–8 participants. The reading material comprised excerpts from novels, short stories and poems. The intervention was delivered by librarians trained as reading guides at public libraries (see Chapter 5).

As this was a mixed method study, it involved both ethnographic fieldwork and psychometric methods. The ethnographic method consisted of (ten) participant observation visits in five reading groups, two per group and (four) focus group interviews supplemented by (two) individual interviews with participants. In addition, health professionals involved in referrals to the reading groups were interviewed about their role in the study. Participants were tested at baseline and after 10 weeks of Shared Reading with a follow-up after 3 and 6 months. The specific tests used are discussed below.

Selecting an Assessment Battery on the Basis of a Hypothesis as to What Happens in a Reading Group

The ambition of the study was to establish a data-driven dialogue between the reading process and study outcome measures in order to analyse how active mechanisms of the process relate to effects of participation. The background to the study was a general dissatisfaction with standard designs and methodology within the field of bibliotherapy which very rarely includes data on the reading process. Bibliotherapy is based on the generally accepted thesis that the therapeutic outcome of reading is the result of an identificatory process between a condition suffered and theme treated in the literary work.[17] Nevertheless, studies within the field seldom provide means for analysing the relation between this identificatory process and the therapeutic outcome other than by reference to the originally formulated hypothesis that identification in itself would lead to insight and catharsis.[18]

Perhaps because of this generally accepted hypothesis of the identificatory process, measurements are not selected to test the active mechanisms of the reading process. It is simply assumed that by reading about a condition, whether in literary or non-literary form, a therapeutic process—by means of an unidentified identificatory process not further analysed—'happens'. Assessment batteries are as a result rarely chosen on the basis of a hypothesis of the role of the reading process, but most often on the basis of a hypothesised and desired outcome (weight loss, enhanced self-esteem, etc.).[19]

In order to fill this gap in our current knowledge, a mixed methods design was chosen. By mixed method, we understand a research methodology that collects, analyses and mixes quantitative and qualitative data. Its central premise is that the use of quantitative and qualitative approaches, in combination, provides a better understanding of research problems than either approach alone.[20]

In this study, therefore, the aim was to select an assessment battery, that, although hypothesis-driven concerning the outcome effects of participation, was selected on the basis of previous exploratory (grounded), theory-driven analysis of the processes in Shared Reading groups. This way we were aiming to close the gap between the inductive bottom-up-generated analysis based on observation and top-down-driven hypothesis-testing deductive designs.

Looking across several qualitative studies,[21] we identified three active dimensions that consistently were observed in participatory designs in the reading process as well as reported retrospectively as outcomes by participants through either questionnaires or interviews. These included (1) the social or intersubjective dimension, (2) a sense of meaningfulness of the activity, and (3) feelings of self-growth, development or change. Seeing the consistency of these experiential constructs across qualitative studies of Shared Reading groups, we wanted an outcome measurement that tapped into those three dimensions identified as both active mechanisms of the reading process and outcome measurements.

On this basis, we selected the well-being questionnaire developed by Ryff. As explained above ('Rhiannon Corcoran, Josie Billington and Megan Watkins, "Using Standardised Measures to Capture 'Non-standard' (Subjective, Personal) Reading Experiences"'), Ryff's scale is built around six theoretically constructed dimensions: autonomy, environmental mastery, personal growth (positive), relations with others, purpose in life and self-acceptance (Ryff and Keyes, 1995). The choice of instrument was reinforced by the fact that one of the dimensions of this test—meaningfulness or 'purpose of life'—had been shown to demonstrate significant effects in a cross-over controlled design concerned with the differences between Shared Reading groups and a non-literary group activity (Longden, 2015; see section above).

In relation to the active processes of the reading group, we hypothesised that the emotive and reflective process in the Shared Reading experience of relating to and discriminating one's own thoughts and feelings from those of other participants (social or intersubjective dimension) would enhance both sense of self (relating to the dimensions of change in the qualitative literature, and to aspects of autonomy, self-acceptance and growth in Ryff's model) as well as provide a ground for building (positive) relations with others. We further hypothesised that this process would in itself generate a feeling of meaningfulness and include aspects of personal growth.

We further selected Becks cognitive insight scale (BCIS)[22] to evaluate participants self-reflectiveness and possible overconfidence in interpretations of their own experiences. We were interested in using this scale as it has been suggested that reading can promote both a de-centring, or the ability put oneself in the other's shoes, and self-insight.[23] In addition, possible effect on depressive and anxious symptomatology was assessed by use of The Hospital Anxiety and Depression Scale (HADS).[24] Finally, quality of life was assessed by use of the EQ-5D,[25] a widely used standardised instrument as a measure of health-related quality of life that reflects the patient's own judgement.

The Mode of Literary Reading

Since the hypothesis concerning active mechanisms of the reading group was not based on a thematic driven identificatory process, texts were not selected on the basis of themes relating to depression or psychic vulnerability but on their ability to reflect a variety of complex human experiences relating to existential themes of hope, grief, loss, love, death, loneliness and togetherness from multiple perspectives (children, adults, older people, men and women). The most important criteria for text selection, however, were not thematic but concerned the ambiguity and complexity of texts: the emphasis was upon affording open-ended reflective processes rather than providing definitions or solutions and strategies for how to deal with defined problems. The complexity criterion of literary texts is based on the hypothesis that ambiguity and complexity generate the kind of 'emergent thinking' (Longden, 2015; Davis et al., 2016) or 'liveliness' of the reading process which further allows the processes of reflexivity, inter-subjectivity and growth which are productive of well-being.

Results

Qualitative/Ethnographic Findings

The ethnographic method was inductive, inspired by a grounded theory framework[26] in which the analytical categories were formed on the basis of observation and interviews. In other words, the analysis was not driven from the theoretical categories of Ryff's model but grew out of a descriptive account of what was seen and experienced in the group and what reading group participants explained in interviews.

Three analytical categories of well-being emerged:

1. *The reading group as a social space: Safe and intimate, without being private*

'The reading group', the anthropologist observed, 'becomes a place for individual and social learning processes', where people can practise either taking space themselves or giving space to others. Within the reading group, participants became better over time at navigating the social space and obtained an insight into their own social habits (of talking too little or too much). Participants spoke in the interviews about the joy of building social skills, which had often withered after periods with mental illness. One participant (male aged about 40) said: 'It's been cool, this, just, pulling yourself together to say something in this kind of group, because I, many times, would just sit [...] and say nothing'. The group was also a place to practise the expression of and the insistence on one's own opinion, which was made easier by the repeated assurance that 'there are no right or wrong opinions'. One person said it gave her confidence when she said something out loud and people were still sitting there, listening and accepting her viewpoint, emotion or experience. Subsequently, other participants expressed that they would, as a consequence of participation, dare to interact in social settings with 'ordinary' people.

These observations point to instances of an increased sense of autonomy and environmental mastery and the ability to believe in and hold on to your own perspective, while also becoming aware of the others in the group and their need for expression. This leads to more positive relations to others. One participant's awareness of, and acquired ability to restrain herself from, constant talking and give others space for expression provided the ground for more positive relation between her and other group members.

2. *'The joy of literature'*

Participants spoke of the ability to relate their own personal experiences to the literature and gain insight into how others experience a text. One reader was very affected by reading a story about a boy who was bullied (Cecilie Bødker) and told of her own childhood experiences. This was listened to and accepted as a valuable contribution to the reading.

This personal dimension can be analysed in terms of Ryff's category of 'personal growth', but can again also be seen as a process towards autonomy. One lady said: 'I can feel that I'm positively influenced by it (the reading group). I'm looking forward to it, and it's been a long time since I felt pleasure doing anything. I can feel it touches something inside of me. It touches things that I bring along with me in life. Whether it's a feeling or experience. It gives a perspective'. A common expression was that 'the best part of reading literature together was that it allowed people to share inner experiences'. Although this analytical category related to the joy of reading literature (one spoke of the pleasure of enjoying 'great sentences'), the joy of participating in a Shared Reading group also related actively to categories of self-growth and building positive relations with others.

3. *Creating meaning in everyday life*

Most participants were on sick leave, in job training or early retirement. Many said they would usually sit at home that they needed quietness and were easily drained by social activities or simply couldn't cope with them. 'Because I am an early retirement pensioner I need to find some content in my life and be with other people', one woman (in her 50s) said. Participants talked about a lack of 'meaning in life'. In contrast, they experienced the reading group as an activity that gave them energy; they talked about the weekly reading group as something they were looking forward to.

Meaningfulness was observed in two different dimensions. It was observed as a quality of the engagement in the reading group; they found participation to be a meaningful activity in itself, relating this to the joy of both the personal and social dimensions of reading. And Shared Reading was observed as an activity that provided participants with a purpose in life that they had lacked. One female participant talked about how the reading group had become an inspiration. After years of not coming to the library, she had gone back and started reading some of those books that she had given up on years back: 'I've become, after I've started this, what to say, it has stimulated me to come back to where I used to be'.

For many, it was a positive challenge to join a social setting and find a new community of interest in literature. One elderly man drove with his friend to the weekly reading group and enjoyed it very much, even though reading literature was a completely new activity for him. He even took the texts from the group to his social activity centre and proudly read them aloud for the other users.

For those on sick leave or disability pension, the reading group was one of few communities of interests. For another group, literacy was something they had lost after periods of mental illness, and the reading group was a place to develop and regain reading abilities. Expressions under this category of meaningfulness can be analysed as instances of Ryff's dimension of purpose in life.

Quantitative Results

Depressive and anxious symptom load were found to be statistically significantly lower between baseline and post-intervention. In line with this finding, QOL had significantly increased from baseline to post-intervention. For all measures except depressive symptoms, 6-month follow-up data had dropped to trend level. Depressive symptom load was still significantly better at 6-month follow-up. No changes were found in instruments measuring psychological well-being (PWB) or cognitive insight (CBIS).

The most instructive learning afforded by the mixed method design was the clash between the qualitative and the quantitative data. The qualitative evidence supported our hypothesis that the reading group would enhance well-being, but the quantitative data did not support this. Given the inductively derived categories—(1) the reading group as a social and personal space, (2) the joy of reading, subjectively and intersubjectively, and (3) the meaningfulness of the activity in terms of both the immediate reading experience and the purpose it brought to people's lives—we assumed that the selected assessments of both reflexivity and well-being would be adequate in fulfilling our aim to capture process and outcome and close the gap between the two.

That this was not the case made us return to and reflect on the design in the light of the implementation process. The study was originally designed as a controlled, pre- and post-test research design. We were not able, however, to recruit participants for the control group. From the ethnographic interviews with health professionals, we learned that there was a bias among health professionals towards recruiting for the test group, and when they asked people their reasons for not participating as controls, the reply was that people simply were not motivated to participate in an inactive control.

In fact, we had already made one important design adjustment with such considerations in mind. In the planning phases, the design had originally included a waiting list group. But the necessity of health professionals to offer an activity to our target group, the health issues experienced by the latter, and job market requirements to stand by, made commitment to participation in the study impossible.

We therefore conclude that the aims for delivery of the intervention on the part of health professionals on the one hand, as well as more general societal demands, and the need for scientific scrutiny on the other hand (including a comparison group to control for the active mechanisms of the intervention in relation to the measured effects) are in conflict.

Thus, in hindsight, the ideal design would have been an active control, as in the cross-over design presented in Longden 2015. That would have given us the opportunity to compare Ryff and Beck across different forms of engagement (literary vs. non-literary) in the light of which we might have been able to define differences in the process as they related to dimensions of the Ryff model and offer a meaningful activity for the control group.

Lastly, the non-finding in the statistical material might be due to the sample size or simply the fact that we chose the short version of PWB, which has been known to demonstrate less internal validity (Ryff and Keyes, 1995). This was again a pragmatic choice—based on the need for a questionnaire battery that wouldn't present too much of an obstacle for the target group—that outweighed scientific criteria.

Another factor explaining the non-finding in the quantitative material might have been the length of the interventions. It is likely that 10 weeks of reading group intervention is simply not enough to develop into lasting dimensions of autonomy, self-acceptance and positive relations to others. The issue of how long it takes to build a lasting repertoire of new habits is indicated by other data points in the study. In the demographic section, we had included a question about reading habits and didn't find any significant effect on those; in fact, at follow-up, there seemed to be a reduction in time spent reading. This stands in sharp contrast to the individual case descriptions of people regaining their joy and ability of reading literature or learning to enjoy it for the first time. It also stands in direct conflict with the fact that 90% of participants reported that they would like to continue the activity. This strong response led to an initiative to establish open voluntary-led reading groups in continuation of the 10-week referral period. Although this data falls outside of the present study, we have learned from praxis that at least a third of the participants have continued in a reading group. In the same vein, reading group facilitators' report that in one of the libraries, after the conclusion of the study, some of the most vulnerable participants now participate successfully in an open reading group with a group of 'ordinary' people. In another library, the two referral groups have continued on their own, re-reading the study reading material. Perhaps in these prolonged reading groups, where the subjective and intersubjective dimensions of the reading process grow into life skills and habits, Ryff will prove an adequate measurement. Ryff and Singer[27] stress that 'positive human health' is more about eudaimonia than hedonia. A good life is based on sense of meaningfulness and deep lasting relations, achieved by an acceptance also of difficult and negative emotions. In the time span of the design, and the inability to identify the active process in comparison with a control group, such lasting dimensions were not captured by the assessment battery although indicated by the qualitative data.

This leads us to conclude that research designs have to be designed carefully both with concern to methodology and intervention to capture the 'active' mechanisms of Shared Reading.

Don Kuiken, 'Empirical Phenomenology: Articulating Different Types of Reading Experience'

Phenomenological research involves use of the 'phenomenological reduction' to disclose and explicate the 'essential structure' of moments within lived experience. The 'phenomenological reduction' invites (a) direct reflection on what is pre-reflectively 'given' in a moment of lived experience; (b) fresh disclosure ('thematization') of the concrete attributes of that 'given' moment of lived experience; and (c) articulation of the attributes that make that 'given' experience a moment of a particular kind (or type). Three empirical extensions of the phenomenological approach provide sufficient detail to guide replicable investigative practice: (a) Giorgi's *descriptive phenomenology*;[28] (b) Smith's *interpretive phenomenology*;[29] and (c) Petitmengin's *neurophenomenology*.[30] Each approach distinguishes transcendental phenomenological studies from empirical phenomenological studies and prescribes key aspects of the phenomenological reduction (such as the *epoché*, which involves 'bracketing' pre-reflective presuppositions about the type of experience that is under consideration). However, each fails to develop precisely how the 'eidetic' aspect of the reduction is accomplished, leaving unclear how to explicate the attributes that make an experiential phenomenon the kind (or type) of experience that it is. Stated differently, each fails to describe precisely how to derive empirically the 'essential structure' of selected categories of lived experience (e.g. moments of empathy, moments of deep reading).

An alternative phenomenological approach to the disclosure and explication of essential structures has been proposed.[31] Moreover, this approach has been the point of departure for a research project concerning transformative experiences during literary reading.[32] In that pivotal study, we examined experiential accounts of readers' engagement with Coleridge's *The Rime of the Ancient Mariner*. We (a) compared these experiential accounts to identify recurrent meaning expressions (called constituents); (b) created matrices reflective of the profiles of constituents found in each account; (c) created clusters of accounts according to the similarities in their profiles of constituents; and (d) examined each cluster of accounts to ascertain their more-or-less invariant attributes. Among the six types of experiential moments that were disclosed and explicated, one involved (a) metaphoric and quasi-metaphoric engagement with sensory imagery from the poem; (b) progressive transformation of an emergent affective theme; and (c) metaphoric blurring of boundaries between the reader's and narrator's perspectives. This type of reading, called expressive enactment, contrasted with five other types of experiential accounts that we called: (a) ironic allegoresis (moments in which readers interpreted passages of the poem allegorically by referring to abstract themes embodied in cultural narratives external to the poem); (b) aesthetic feeling (moments in which readers engaged sensuous imagery in the passage without considering its self-relevance); (c) autobiographical assimilation (moments in which readers identified simile-like relations between events in the poem and personal memories that then were their primary focus); (d) autobiographical diversion (moments in which readers were reminded of significant personal 'associations' that were not integral to interpretation of the poem itself); and (e) non-engagement (moments in which readers did not report the themes that were characteristic of the other five clusters, i.e. autobiographical associations, engagement with sensuous imagery and so on). Our study incorporated numeric procedures that, as argued here, also may usefully complement other empirical phenomenological efforts, including descriptive phenomenology, interpretive phenomenology and neurophenomenology.

Eidetic Reduction: In Search of 'Essential Structure'

The eidetic aspects of the phenomenological reduction involve the steps by which thematised attributes of a phenomenon are reflectively considered to determine which, if any, are characteristic of a particular kind (or type) of lived experience. In philosophical investigations, eidetic aspects of the *transcendental* version of the eidetic reduction involve imaginative variation and comparison.[33] Beginning with a moment of lived experience (e.g. perception of a coloured object), the investigator imaginatively varies its attributes (e.g. the object's colour, the object's size) to make explicit the pattern of attributes (and attribute dependencies) that remains the same across these variations (e.g. the dependency of colour on extension). Imaginative variation reveals the necessary attributes of an intentional object's *essential* structure.[34]

However, in empirical phenomenological studies, imaginative variation is insufficient for reasons that are not consistently made clear. Merely generalising the transcendental version of the eidetic reduction is a problem. Doing so has given rise to critiques of phenomenological studies that characterise both transcendental and empirical phenomenology as 'essentialist'. These complaints often presume that phenomenological studies only pursue the articulation of 'exact essences', much like articulating the logico-mathematical 'essence' of geometric figures. Response to this critique requires consideration of Husserl's proposal that *empirical* phenomenological methods do not disclose exact essences but rather what he called 'morphological essences'. However, it is precisely in articulation of this empirical (rather than transcendental) objective that discussions of the eidetic reduction have faltered.

While careful to separate transcendental from empirical investigations, Giorgi (2009, pp. 195–99) puts *imaginative* variations of a phenomenon into 'dialogue' with *empirical* variations to determine which attributes are necessary aspects of the 'general structure' of an experiential category. He acknowledges that the resulting general structure is more than a list of invariant attributes but adds also that its articulation is in some respects 'not too empirical' (p. 200). Similarly, but without reference to imaginative variation, Smith et al. (2009, pp. 106–07) strive for an interpretation that is both general (i.e. based on multiple themes that recur 'across cases') and structured (i.e. involves the 'interconnections between those recurrent…themes'). Like Giorgi, they emphasise that articulation of such a general structure is more than listing recurrent attributes but also that it is not 'too descriptive' (p. 103). Finally, Petitmengin (2017, p. 13) advocates the articulation of 'generic experiential categories', perhaps including subordinate 'clusters'.[35]

However, she provides almost no guidance regarding the procedures required to identify a generic experiential category or to distinguish its subordinate clusters. In short, within contemporary approaches to empirical phenomenology, the procedural steps towards the 'general' or 'essential' structure of morphological essences are, at best, incompletely developed.

A Methodological Alternative

A modified methodological imperative can be derived from the later Husserl's modified discussion of the limits of imaginative variation in phenomenological studies. Often with reference to biological species (e.g. trees, whales), he argued that empirical phenomenological investigations necessarily disclose and explicate 'degrees' of similarity, primarily because the 'extent' of similarity between two or more intentional objects depends upon how many parts of each are, in themselves, similar.[36] Thus, Husserl acknowledged that there is inherent quantification of 'extent' and 'degree' within similarity judgements—and, hence, within the interrogative activities that disclose and explicate morphological essences.

To appreciate this proposal, consider the kind of reading experience that was identified as 'expressive enactment' in the Sikora et al. study. Expressive enactment was found to be a kind of reading moment that *usually* involves metaphoric elaboration of sensory imagery from the poem—but the kind of reading moment called ironic allegoresis also *usually* involved this kind of elaboration of sensory imagery. Furthermore, although the reported presence of this kind of metaphoric elaboration differentiated *both* expressive enactment and ironic allegoresis from autobiographical assimilation, (a) expressive enactment possessed *many* of the *other* attributes typically found in accounts of that type of experiential moment and (b) ironic allegoresis possessed *many* of the *other* attributes typically found in accounts of that type of experience. In this context, imaginatively varying single discrete attributes (e.g. metaphoric elaboration) to identify essential structures of either expressive enactment or ironic allegoresis simply (and in principle) is not viable.

Considerations such as these prompted the later Husserl to circumscribe more tightly the role of imaginative variation. A modified form of the empirical phenomenological reduction involves systematic examination of numerous empirical instances of a phenomenon and articulation of its idealised limits, a process requiring imaginative 'interpolation'—but not the 'comparison' of real and imagined variations—across instances.[37] Such interpolation enables the articulation of the ideal, prototypic limits of the category. This formulation captures the essential structure of an experiential category (i.e. the more-or-less invariant attributes of expressive enactment and the prototypic idealisation of those more-or-less invariant attributes). In doing so, it rescues the notion of essential structure from the strictures of exact essences. It also underscores the distinctive comparative contributions of actual empirical variations to the articulation of morphological essences, a complexity seldom acknowledged in critiques of phenomenology's 'essentialism'. The essential structures of most categorial phenomena within the human sciences (e.g. categories of experiential accounts such as expressive enactment) are almost certainly morphological rather than exact—and amenable to this kind of analysis.

Without sacrificing phenomenological objectives, empirical phenomenological methods in the service of disclosing morphological essences may be articulated as a hybrid 'qualitative-quantitative' endeavour. Formalisation of phenomenological procedures begins by considering the following question: What are the attributes (from $A_1 \ldots A_N$) of an experiential account such that, when jointly present, that experiential account instantiates a chosen category (e.g. expressive enactment)? Formalising these procedures requires that (a) each instance of a category of experiential accounts possesses a *large but unspecified number* of attributes (from $A_1 \ldots A_N$); (b) each category attribute (from $A_1 \ldots A_N$) is an attribute of *many but not all* instances of the category; and (c) no attribute (from $A_1 \ldots A_N$) is an attribute of *every* instance of the category.[38]

a. By virtue of the first criterion, comparison of experiential accounts across attributes ($A_1 \ldots A_N$) discloses a category (type) that possesses a *characteristic* (but not invariant) profile of attributes (e.g. the profile of attributes that constitutes expressive enactment). Several numeric algorithms (e.g. hierarchical cluster analysis) facilitate access to such categories based on similarities between their attribute profiles.[39]
b. By virtue of the second criterion, each attribute of a category of experiential accounts is *more-or-less* invariant—although imaginative extrapolation from *relatively* invariant attributes enables articulation of the ideal ('prototypic') limits of each category as disclosed by the numeric algorithms mentioned above. For example, the metaphoric blurring of boundaries between the reader's and narrator's perspectives in expressive enactment is a *more-or-less* characteristic attribute of expressive enactment that can also be represented as an attribute of an 'idealized' prototype.[40]

c. By virtue of the third criterion, which defeats imaginative variation in its commonly advocated form, no attribute of an experiential account is strictly invariant. Nonetheless, *sometimes* an attribute derived using these numeric algorithms is in fact *empirically* invariant. Such invariance keeps alive the transcendental (ontological) project in empirical phenomenological studies. For example, the type of reading we called aesthetic feeling distinctively and *invariably* involved reader references to synaesthetic imagery, especially cross-modal representations of the narrative setting. Such invariance is rare but in principle possible in empirical psychological studies.

Because the preceding formalisation of morphological essences allows quantitative implementation, the related mode of inquiry has been called numerically aided phenomenology (Kuiken, Schopflocher, and Wild, 1989; Kuiken, Wild, and Schopflocher, 1992; Kuiken and Miall, 2001). Numeric formalisation is one of two primary sources of precision in numerically aided phenomenology; the other, which will not be discussed here, is the process of comparison (including metaphoric 'comparison') that supports expressive nuance in articulation of category attributes (i.e. themes or constituents). Neither of these sources of precision is expendable. Coordination of numeric formalisation with other requirements of the phenomenological reduction (e.g. direct reference, the *epoché*, thematisation and the eidetic reduction) is a work in progress. So, also, is coordination of this formalisation with several other design desiderata, as indicated below.

Concern with Construct Validity

It is commonplace to worry whether first-person experiential accounts are reliable and valid. Thus, in empirical phenomenological studies of literary reading, it is tempting to consider hybrid research designs that allow assessment of the validity of the disclosed and explicated experiential categories.[41] Evidence of construct validity requires examination of correlations between an index of membership in a category of experiential accounts and *theoretically related* self-report, behavioural or physiological indices. However, in phenomenological studies, this research option is, in principle, misguided. Empirical phenomenological methods are designed to facilitate the disclosure and explication of *previously unidentified categories of experience.*

By implication, it is not possible to anticipate which measures are theoretically related to a category that is only articulable *after* the relevant thematisation and numerical algorithms have disclosed heuristically enriched categories.[42] For example, until expressive enactment was disclosed and explicated as an experiential category, it was not possible to explore the correlates of membership in that experiential category. Since the original Sikora et al. (2011) study, the construct validating convergence between expressive enactment and narrative absorption has been examined.[43]

Concern with Disclosure

Emphasis on the disclosure and explication of essential structures remains crucial within numerically aided phenomenological inquiry. To use a biological analogy, rather than going to the Galapagos Islands to determine whether swallowtail butterflies live there, phenomenological investigators go to the Galapagos Islands to disclose and explicate the previously unknown (or perhaps vaguely known) categories (species) of butterflies that live there. Similarly, rather than eliciting experiential accounts to determine whether readers report some preconceived type of engaged reading, phenomenological investigators elicit such experiential accounts to disclose and explicate previously unknown (or perhaps vaguely known) categories of reading engagement. In the Sikora et al. study, expressive enactment and ironic allegoresis were two kinds (or types) of reading moment that were vaguely anticipated but poorly articulated when the study began. Also, the kind of reading moment called aesthetic feeling was vaguely anticipated but certainly not as a separate kind of reading moment. So, we went to the Galapagos Islands and found butterflies, but their several species—with their characteristic attributes—simply could not have been spelled out with empirical concreteness in advance.

Concern with Contrasts

In numerically aided phenomenological studies, the invited sample of experiential accounts extends beyond the range of categories of experience that the investigator (perhaps vaguely) expects to disclose and articulate. This is like going to the Galapagos Islands and collecting what vaguely resemble butterflies *or moths* (even if the investigation is concerned with identifying and describing previously unknown species of *butterflies*). Prior to articulation of their type (species), previously unidentified butterflies may not be differentiable from previously unidentified moths. Openness to contrast with moths is like openness to the contrast between expressive enactment and ironic allegoresis (neither of which was a clearly articulated category of reading moments until the Sikora et al. study was complete). Such over-inclusive sampling underscores that category disclosure and explication involve more than identification of the attributes of certain target construct(s). Experiential categories are often identifiable by virtue of comparison with the other *contrasting* experiential categories. Besides the attributes experiential categories demonstrably *do* possess (but others do not), experiential categories are often identifiable by virtue of attributes they *do not* possess (i.e. attributes that identify another experiential categories). It may matter, for example, that attention to auditory imagery and phonetic features of the text was not characteristic of moments of aesthetic feeling but was characteristic of moments of expressive enactment. Such results motivate further consideration of the sense in which expressive enactment involves auditory/phonetic aspects of readers' resonance with the text—and how that differs from the attention to synesthetic imagery that is characteristic of moments of aesthetic feeling.

Deferring Causal Explanation

Besides putting into abeyance unexamined preconceptions and presuppositions, the phenomenological *epoché* requires putting aside causal explanations for a freshly disclosed and explicated phenomenon. The authors of empirical phenomenological approaches concur that causal induction is separable from and complementary to empirical phenomenological description. The objective of empirical phenomenology is to bring to coherent clarity the full complexity of different types or kinds of lived experience (morphological essences). With all the refinement and nuance that language will allow, and with the support of selected numeric algorithms, the aim is to disclose and articulate the general structure of these morphological experiential categories—prior to their causal explanation. The Sikora et al. phenomenological projects *subsequently* led to development of a model of expressive reading[44] in which (a) openness to experience supports (or enables) expressive enactment and (b) expressive enactment mediates the relationship between openness to experience and aesthetic reading outcomes (e.g. sublime feeling, being moved). Specifying these causal relations depended upon prior articulation of expressive enactment—and their specification may, in turn, motivate more refined phenomenological investigation.

Notes

1. P. Davis, J. Billington, R. Corcoran, V. Gonzalez-Diaz, S. Lampropoulou, G. Farrington, F. Magee, and E. Walsh, 'Cultural Value: Assessing the Intrinsic Value of The Reader Organization's Shared Reading Scheme' (University of Liverpool: Centre for Research into Reading, Literature and Society [CRILS], 2015); E. Longden, P. Davis, J. Billington, S. Lampropoulou, G. Farrington, F. Magee, E. Walsh, and R. Corcoran, 'Shared Reading: Assessing the Intrinsic Value of a Literature-Based Health Intervention', *Journal of Medical Humanities*, 41.2 (2015), 113–20.
2. J. Billington, G. Farrington, S. Lampropoulou, K. McDonnell, J. Lingwood, A. Jones, James Ledson, A.-L. Humphreys, and N. Duirs, 'A Comparative Study of Cognitive Behavioural Therapy and Shared Reading for Chronic Pain' (University of Liverpool: CRILS, 2016); J. Billington, G. Farrington, S. Lampropoulou, J. Lingwood, A. Jones, J. Ledson, K. McDonnell, N. Duirs, and A.-L. Humphreys, 'A Comparative Study of Cognitive Behavioural Therapy and Shared Reading for Chronic Pain', *Journal of Medical Humanities*, 43.3 (2016), 155–65.
3. R. Tennant, L. Hiller, R. Fishwick, S. Platt, S. Joseph, S. Weich, J. Parkinson, J. Secker, and S. Stewart-Brown, 'The Warwick-Edinburgh Mental Well-Being Scale (WEMWBS): Development and UK Validation', *Health and Quality of Life Outcomes*, 5.63 (2007), 1–13.
4. C. D. Ryff, 'Happiness Is Everything, or Is It? Explorations on the Meaning of Psychological Well-Being', *Journal of Personality and Social Psychology*, 57.6 (1989), 1069–81.
5. D. Watson, L. A. Clark, and A. Tellegen, 'Development and Validation of Brief Measures of Positive and Negative Affect: The PANAS Scale', *Journal of Personality and Social Psychology*, 54.6 (1988), 1063–70.
6. J. Sim and C. Wright, *Research in Health Care: Concepts, Designs and Methods* (Andover: Cengage Learning, 2000).
7. R. M. Krauss and S. R. Fussell, 'Perspective-Taking in Communication: Representations of Others' Knowledge in Reference', *Social Cognition: A Journal of Social, Personality, and Developmental Psychology*, 9.1 (1991), 2–24.
8. H. Guttman and L. Laporte, 'Alexithymia, Empathy, and Psychological Symptoms in a Family Context', *Comprehensive Psychiatry*, 43.6 (2002), 448–55.
9. M. H. Davis, 'A Multidimensional Approach to Individual Differences in Empathy', *JSAS Catalog of Selected Documents in Psychology*, 10 (1980), 85.
10. M. H. Davis, 'Measuring Individual Differences in Empathy: Evidence for a Multidimensional Approach', *Journal of Personality and Social Psychology*, 44.1 (1983), 113–26; A. M. Fernández, M. Dufey, and U. Kramp, 'Testing

the Psychometric Properties of the Interpersonal Reactivity Index (IRI) in Chile: Empathy in a Different Cultural Context', *European Journal of Psychological Assessment*, 27.3 (2011), 179–85.

11. P. Nanda, N. Tandon, I. T. Mathew, J. L. Padmanabhan, B. A. Clementz, G. D. Pearlson, J. A. Sweeney, C. A. Tamminga, and M. S. Keshavan, 'Impulsivity Across the Psychosis Spectrum: Correlates of Cortical Volume, Suicidal History, and Social and Global Function', *Schizophrenia Research*, 170.1 (2016), 80–86.
12. J. Rawlings, M. Shevlin, R. Corcoran, R. Morriss, and P. J. Taylor, 'Out of the Blue: Untangling the Association Between Impulsivity and Planning in Self-Harm', *Journal of Affective Disorders,* 18.4 (2015), 29–35.
13. M. A. Cyders, A. K. Littlefield, S. Coffey, and K. A. Karyadi, 'Examination of a Short English Version of the UPPS-P Impulsive Behavior Scale', *Addictive Behaviors*, 39.9 (2014), 1372–76.
14. D. R. Lynam, J. D. Miller, D. J. Miller, M. A. Bornovalova, and C. W. Lejuez, 'Testing the Relations Between Impulsivity-Related Traits, Suicidality, and Nonsuicidal Self-Injury: A Test of the Incremental Validity of the UPPS Model', *Personality Disorders: Theory, Research and Treatment*, 2.2 (2011), 151–60.
15. C. D. Ryff and C. M. Keyes, 'The Structure of Psychological Well-Being Revisited', *Journal of Personality and Social Psychology*, 69.4 (1995), 719–27.
16. D. van Dierendonck, 'The Construct Validity of Ryff's Scales of Psychological Well-Being and its Extension with Spiritual Well-Being', *Personality and Individual Differences*, 36.3 (2004), 629–43.
17. G. Katz and J. Watt, 'Bibliotherapy: the Use of Books in Psychiatric Treatment', *Canadian Journal of Psychiatry*, 37.3 (1992), 173–78.
18. Caroline Schrodes, 'Reading and the Emotions', *The Reading Teacher*, 9.1 (1955), 24–29.
19. J. T. Pardeck and J. A. Pardeck, *Bibliotherapy: A Clinical Approach for Helping Children*, vol. 16 (Langhorne, PA: Gordon and Breach Science Publishers, 1993); R. S. Lenkowsky, 'Bibliotherapy: A Review and Analysis of the Literature', *Journal of Special Education*, 2.2 (1987), 123–32; L. I. Silverberg, 'Bibliotherapy: The Therapeutic Use of Didactic and Literary Text in Treatment, Diagnosis, Prevention and Training', *Journal of the American Osteopathic Association*, 103.3 (2003), 131–35.
20. J. W. Creswell and V. L. Plano Clark, *Designing and Conducting Mixed Methods Research*, 2nd edn (Thousand Oaks, CA: Sage, 2011).
21. Longden et al. (2015); Billington et al. (2016); Gray et al. (2016) (see Chapter 9); M. Steenberg, 'Literary Reading as a Social Technology: An Exploratory Study on Shared Reading Groups', in *Plotting the Reading Experience: Theory/Practice/Politics*, ed. by P. M. Rothbauer, K. I. Skjerdingstad, L. McKechnie, and K. Oterholm (Waterloo, ON: Wilfrid Laurier University Press, 2016), pp. 183–98.

22. A. T. Beck, E. Baruch, J. M. Balter, R. A. Steer, and D. M. Warman, 'A New Instrument for Measuring Insight: The Beck Cognitive Insight Scale', *Schizophrenia Research*, 68.2–3 (2004), 319–29.
23. K. Oatley, 'Fiction: Simulation of Social Worlds', *Trends in Cognitive Sciences,* 20.8 (2016), 618–28. See also Chapter 15.
24. A. S. Zigmond and R. P. Snaith, 'The Hospital Anxiety and Depression Scale', *Acta Psychiatrica Scandinavica*, 67.6 (1983), 361–70.
25. T. E. Group, 'EuroQol: A New Facility for the Measurement of Health-Related Quality of Life', *Health Policy*, 16.3 (1990), 199–208.
26. A. Strauss and J. M. Corbyn, *Basics of Qualitative Research: Techniques and Procedures for Developing Grounded Theory* (Thousand Oaks, CA: Sage, 1998).
27. C. Ryff and B. H. Singer, 'The Contours of Positive Human Health', *Psychological Inquiry*, 9.1 (1998), 1–28; C. Ryff and B. H. Singer, 'Know Thyself and Become What You Are: A Eudaimonic Approach to Well-Being', *Journal of Happiness Studies*, 9.13 (2008), 13–39.
28. A. Giorgi, *Phenomenology and Psychological Research* (Pittsburgh, PA: Duquesne University Press, 1985); A. Giorgi, *The Descriptive Phenomenological Method in Psychology* (Pittsburgh, PA: Duquesne University Press, 2009).
29. J. A. Smith, 'Beyond the Divide Between Cognition and Discourse: Using Interpretative Phenomenological Analysis in Health Psychology', *Psychology & Health*, 11.2 (1996), 261–71; J. A. Smith, P. Flowers, and M. Larkin, *Interpretative Phenomenological Analysis: Theory, Method, and Research* (London: Sage, 2009).
30. C. Petitmengin, 'Enaction as a Lived Experience', *Constructivist Foundations*, 12.2 (2017), 139–47; M. Bitbol and C. Petitmengin, 'Neurophenomenology and the Micro-Phenomenological Interview', in *The Blackwell Companion to Consciousness*, ed. by S. Schneider and M. Velmans (Chichester, UK: Wiley, 2017), pp. 726–39.
31. D. Kuiken, D. Schopflocher, and T. C. Wild, 'Numerically Aided Methods in Phenomenology: A Demonstration', *Journal of Mind and Behavior*, 10.4 (1989), 373–92; D. Kuiken and D. S. Miall, 'Numerically Aided Phenomenology: Procedures for Investigating Categories of Experience', *Forum Qualitative Sozialforschung / Forum: Qualitative Social Research Online Journal*, 2.1 (2001). Available at: http://www.qualitative-research.net/index.php/fqs/article/view/976.
32. D. Kuiken, D. S. Miall, and S. Sikora, 'Forms of Self-Implication in Literary Reading', *Poetics Today*, 25.2 (2004), 171–203; and S. Sikora, D. Kuiken, and D. S. Miall, 'An Uncommon Resonance: The Influence of Loss on Expressive Reading', *Empirical Studies of the Arts*, 28.2 (2010), 135–53; S. Sikora, D. Kuiken, and D. S. Miall, 'Expressive Reading: A Phenomenological Study of Readers' Experience of Coleridge's "The Rime

of the Ancient Mariner"', *Psychology of Aesthetics, Creativity, and the Arts*, 5.3 (2011), 258–68.

33. It is not possible here to consider other crucial features of the phenomenological reduction (departure from the 'natural attitude', 'direct reference' to the pre-reflective 'sense' of a phenomenon, etc.).
34. The 'intentional object' in phenomenological investigations is neither an external object nor an internal act, but rather an integrated subject/object (noetic/noematic) structure. Thus, first-person experiential accounts do not derive from either 'interoception' or 'introspection' but rather from reflection on this integrated structure.
35. Compare: A. Lutz, J.-P. Lachaux, J. Martinerie, and F. J. Varela, 'Guiding the Study of Brain Dynamics by Using First-Person Data: Synchrony Patterns Correlate with Ongoing Conscious States during a Simple Visual Task', *Proceedings of the National Academy of Sciences*, 99.3 (2002), 1586–91.
36. E. Husserl, *Experience and Judgment*, trans. by J. S. Churchill and L. Eley (Evanston, IL: Northwestern University Press, 1973), p. 193.
37. The phenomenological perspective supports differentiation between the descriptive activities that articulate empirical categories (types, species) and the development of hypotheses that identify the causal relations between such categories. The prestige of causal explanation, the devaluation of 'mere' description and inadequately developed conceptions of abduction continue to detract from the clear formulation of qualitative methods (cf. D. Kuiken, T. C. Wild, and D. Schopflocher, 'Positivist Conceptions of Induction and the Rejection of Classificatory Methods in Psychological Research', in *Positivism in Psychology*, ed. by C. W. Tolman [New York, NY: Springer, 1992], pp. 47–56; P. F. Bendassolli, 'Theory Building in Qualitative Research: Reconsidering the Problem of Induction', *Forum Qualitative Sozialforschung / Forum: Qualitative Social Research*, 14.1 [2013], 1851).
38. M. Beckner, *The Biological Way of Thought* (New York: Columbia University Press, 1959).
39. An earlier generation of such algorithms relied upon Q-type factor analysis, as implemented in isolated studies of literary reading (cf. W. Stephenson, 'Applications of Communication Theory: II. Interpretations of Keats' "Ode on a Grecian Urn"', *The Psychological Record*, 22.1 [1972], 177–92). Increasingly accessible neural network models provide a formal mode of access to types (rather than continua) that depends not only on profiles of first-level attributes but also upon higher order interactions among these first-level attributes (cf. D. Borsboom, M. Rhemtulla, A. O. J. Cramer, H. L. J. van der Maas, M. Scheffer, and C. V. Dolan, 'Kinds Versus Continua: A Review of Psychometric Approaches to Uncover the Structure of Psychiatric Constructs', *Psychological Medicine*, 46.8 [2016], 1567–79). We are currently exploring use of these algorithms in studies of literary reading.

40. A prototypic attribute is not an average but an extrapolation that may *not* be represented in the original 'sample'; nonetheless, it is an attribute of an empirically 'grounded' ideal type (cf. K. D. Bailey, *Typologies and Taxonomies: An Introduction to Classification Techniques* [Newbury Park, CA: Sage, 1988], pp. 17ff).
41. K. Slaney, *Validating Psychological Constructs: Historical, Philosophical, and Practical Dimensions* (London: Palgrave Macmillan, 2017).
42. On the other hand, assessing sources of bias (e.g. socially desirable responding) or deficiency (e.g. the inability to construct a narrative) may be useful when such measures pertain to first-person experiential accounts *in general* (rather than to any specific—and perhaps not yet known—experiential category).
43. D. Kuiken and S. Douglas, 'Forms of Absorption that Facilitate the Aesthetic and Explanatory Effects of Literary Reading', in *Narrative Absorption*, ed. by F. Hakemulder, M. M. Kuijpers, E. S. Tan, K. Bálint, and M. M. Doicaru (Amsterdam: John Benjamins Publishing Company, 2017), pp. 217–49.
44. Kuiken and Douglas 2017; D. Kuiken and S. Douglas, 'Living Metaphor as the Site of Bidirectional Literary Engagement', *Scientific Study of Literature*, 8.1 (2018), 47–76; and M. M. Kuijpers, S. Douglas, and D. Kuiken, 'Personality Traits and Reading Habits That Predict Absorbed Narrative Fiction Reading', *Psychology of Aesthetics, Creativity, and the Arts*, 13.1 (2018), 74–88.

13

Reading: Brain, Mind and Body

Philip Davis, Rhiannon Corcoran, Rick Rylance, Adam Zeman, David Kidd and Christophe de Bezenac

Philip Davis, Rhiannon Corcoran, Rick Rylance, Adam Zeman, 'Brain-Imaging and the Reading Mind'

The first part of this chapter is concerned with several groundbreaking neuroscientific studies of the reading brain coming out of the Centre for Research for Reading, Literature and Society (CRILS) at the University of Liverpool and out of the University of Exeter.

Davis and Corcoran, University of Liverpool

The first CRILS' experiment in this area examined the effect on brain activity of Shakespeare's literary invention and syntactic complexity.[1] Specifically, the study considered Shakespeare's dramatic transformation of one part of

P. Davis (✉)
Centre for Research into Reading, Literature and Society,
University of Liverpool, Liverpool, UK
e-mail: phildav@liverpool.ac.uk

R. Corcoran
Psychology and Public Mental Health,
University of Liverpool, Liverpool, UK
e-mail: corcoran@liverpool.ac.uk

J. Billington (ed.), *Reading and Mental Health*,
https://doi.org/10.1007/978-3-030-21762-4_13

speech into another grammatical mode. For example, 'To *lip* a wanton in a secure couch' (*Othello*, IV.i.70); 'He *childed* as I fathered' (*King Lear*, III.vi.103); 'I shall see/Some squeaking Cleopatra *boy* my greatness/I' the posture of a whore' (*Antony and Cleopatra*, V.ii.215–17).[2] The movement (in these instances) of noun into verb ('lip', 'childed', 'boy') is what modern-day linguists call functional shift or word-class conversion. It is what the Elizabethan critic George Puttenham called 'enallage or the figure of exchange' when the poet did not change one word for another but with powerful economy 'kept the word and changed the shape of him only'.[3] Functional shift (FS) was chosen as the focus for the study because it offers powerfully compressed instances of Shakespeare's rapid movement from one sense to another in the sudden creation of metaphor. It is the epitome of live literary thinking. It is also localisable: you can point to it in a sentence, target it in an experiment. Such localisation has no necessary relation to reductivism,[4] only to specificity. It offers a place where the mind may get some hold on itself and its own processes.

Using electroencephalography (EEG), the study measured the electrical activity in the brain produced by sentences in which FS occurs relative to control sentences. Thus, the neural processing of, for example, Shakespeare's

(a) A father and a gracious aged man: him have you **madded** (*King Lear*)

was compared to that of three equivalent sentences in which the critical word was replaced by:

a correct grammatical equivalent which might be semantically expected (i.e. the control with no semantic or grammatical violations):

(b) A father and a gracious aged man: him have you **enraged**;

R. Rylance
University of London, London, UK

A. Zeman
Cognitive and Behavioural Neurology,
University of Exeter, Exeter, UK

D. Kidd
Harvard Graduate School of Education, Cambridge, MA, USA
e-mail: david_kidd@gse.harvard.edu

C. de Bezenac
University of Liverpool, Liverpool, UK
e-mail: cedb@liverpool.ac.uk

a grammatically correct but semantically incongruent word:

(c) A father and a gracious aged man: him have you **poured**;

a semantically and grammatically unsuitable word:

(d) A father and a gracious aged man: him have you **charcoaled**.

In EEG, an increase in the amplitude of the P600 wave signals the violation of the *syntactic* structure of a sentence (peaking 600 milliseconds after the word which upsets grammatical integrity); an increase in the N400 wave (occurring 400 milliseconds after the triggering word) takes place when the *semantic* integrity of a sentence seems disrupted in defiance of meaningfulness. In this experiment, P600, as predicted, was significantly increased in relation to (a), yet crucially with no N400 effect (the negative wave modulation occurring after meaning is disrupted, and only if it is disrupted, was not significantly increased).

What does this mean? That the brain can still recognise fundamental sense amidst the electric surprise of 'madded' which meanwhile creates a suddenly raised level of attention and a newly primed alertness to difficulty. Or to put it another way, while the brain accepts the violation with ease at one level, it is excited by the oddity it is experiencing at another. This is a positive use of prediction error,[5] but here there is no error, neither mistake by the poet nor incapacity in the reader. Instead, by the baulking of simple automaticity—adjective, noun, verb travelling all too easily left to right—functional shift forces the mind away from knowing in advance into enlivened search for pathways to meaning.

This sudden electrical excitement is the neural equivalent of readers' powerfully involuntary responses, triggered by a poem or story, which were witnessed in Chapter 10. Here, it is possible to *see* the revitalising effect upon mental life as the brain lights up and makes powerful interconnections in the scanner, not simply going along with an explanatory language but short-circuiting it, getting closer to the very roots of sudden mental-verbal formulation.

In a second experiment, now using functional magnetic resonance imaging (fMRI) to investigate brain activation in relation to functional shift,[6] it was found that sentences featuring functional shift elicited significant activation beyond regions classically activated by typical language task. There was a shift in activation from traditional left hemisphere structures to right hemisphere additional networks usually involved in processing non-literal aspects of language. This indicated functional shift's recruitment of non-verbal or visualised access to conceptual knowledge. It is as if Shakespeare's language, thus engaging multiple levels of brain activity, creates a three-dimensional space behind the eyes, a theatre of the mind.

These preliminary findings have potentially crucial implications for the role of literature in mental health and in the support of fluid, adaptive forms of intelligence that can support us through the everyday uncertainty of life. Literary reading, these studies suggest, involves the immersion of attention in a dense medium that holds back the mind from superficial, over-speedy decisions or habitual biases. It is a mode of attention which encourages the tolerance and use of complexity and which supports the emergence of novel connections and flexible thinking necessary to navigate uncertainty and advance a repositioning of the self in the world.

In order further to test this hypothesis, the most recent CRILS fMRI brain-imaging experiments[7] asked twenty-four individual participants to read in the scanner 16 four-line texts, half of them from poems, half being more prosaic paraphrases and acting as controls. Across both types, half the stimuli developed linearly in terms of expected meaning, but half consisted of a fourth line—what was called the 'a-ha' moment of shift and surprise, negative or positive—that gave rise to an overall meaning that could not have been anticipated prior to it and thus invoked a drive to reappraise. It was found that with both poetic and control 'a-has' there was increased activity in the inferior temporal gyrus (updating meaning) and the hippocampus (consolidating new meaning). But with the poetic 'a-has' the left caudate nucleus was also activated (as it is with Shakespeare's functional shift). The left caudate nucleus recognises prediction errors (at top, dorsal) and creates a sense of reward (at tail, ventral). This finding suggests that a willingness and ability to update expectancies/thoughts/beliefs on the basis of new evidence are related to a greater awareness of what is poetic and what is not. In many clinical disorders, rigid beliefs fail to be updated even when dis-confirmatory evidence is presented. The area that provided a sense of reward (left caudate) in this activation study is known to be particularly under-activated in those suffering from depression. Thus, it is conceivable that repeated experience of excited 'a-ha!' moments—naturally experienced through the sustained reading of poetry and literature with poetic effects—might enrich the ability to challenge rigid expectancies and fixed understandings of life through the intrinsically rewarding process of reappraisal of meaning and acceptance of fresh meanings.

Rylance (University of London) and Zeman (University of Exeter)

The authors share an interest in the role of the imagination in how humans function and how they adapt (or mal-adapt) to their circumstances, sometimes transforming them. One of us (Rylance) is a humanist with a background in English and the history of psychology.[8] The other (Zeman) is a clinical neurologist whose work focuses on disorders of memory and sleep.[9] We are both committed to interdisciplinary explorations of the wonder of human cognition.

In our study of what happens in the brain when people read complex literary language, we asked volunteers with an expert background in literature (university staff or postgraduates) to read chosen texts in an fMRI scanner. They were also asked to choose texts of their own which they found personally evocative (this was similar to experiments done by others on pieces of music).[10]

The texts were in poetry and prose and were rated to be 'functional' (e.g. the Highway Code), demanding at a middle level of 'literariness', and very demanding under the same criterion. The poems were all sonnets (Shakespeare or Wilfred Owen, for example), and the prose passages, many from novels (Dickens, Lawrence Durrell, etc.), were cut to size. Practical considerations determined this. Readers need to keep their heads very still in an fMRI scanner, and in any case, the task-specific duration of a 'clean' signal is around a minute. The brain is a busy beast and soon multitracks its attention. We needed focus, and for this, we needed short texts.

The passages were read on a conventionally sized computer screen suspended above the reclining reader who wears thick ear defenders against the pulsing noise. He or she controlled the transition from one passage to the next. The sequence of poetry and prose and their different orders of difficulty were randomly distributed. Afterwards, readers completed a qualitative questionnaire on their experiences including questions relating to such things as the emotional power of each passage and relative levels of literary difficulty. These were correlated with the findings from the scanner.

fMRI works by detecting small changes in oxygen levels related to changes in neuronal activation. It therefore tracks the networks of activity in the brain under stimulus from the reading. Much of the research on language and the brain has focused on small units (words or phrases) and not on larger ones. But larger units are crucial to the experience of literature and are a reason why it carries greater emotional depth and sense of meaningfulness than more functional writing, we suppose. (This is not to deny the power of local effects, as shown by CRILS' studies (see above), at the level of the impacts of the literary phrase especially as it deviates from language norms.) It is tempting to correlate this with the complex patterns of excitation observable from the scanner. It has long been observed that language processing in the brain is a function of networked activity. But complex, literary writing evokes responses across a greater variety of those parts of the brain associated with, for example, visual as well as semantic functions, and personal memory. Its literariness may lie in its distributed variety.

Among our conclusions from this experiment are these: texts of every kind engaged the previously identified 'reading network', as we expected; more emotional passages activated a set of regions associated with the brain's response to emotionally resonant music, echoing the thought that poetry involves the musical use of language; favourite poems, selected by our participants, strongly excited areas linked to memory, as if they were being recollected rather than read. These were our strongest findings. There were other, more tentative, but suggestive results. In particular, we were intrigued by a relationship we observed between the reading of poetry and activation of the brain's so-called default network, a set of areas that become especially active when external demands fall away. It is the supposed locus for autobiographical memory and daydreaming and may be one of the neural keys to our sense of personal identity.

It can be a habit of humanists to draw large inferences from slender data. We can only indicate fields of interest from this work that excite investigation. Among them are these. In terms of clinical benefit, reading may help us recover a valuable sense of connection with our past selves when identity is threatened by trauma or dementia. For literary thinkers, there may be an opportunity to develop a better sense of what constitutes 'literariness', a powerful notion launched by Russian theorists a century ago and still potent. And, beyond these, there is the temptation of an old question: why is culture good for our well-being? Maybe it is because, through relationship with wide-ranging brain networks including the default, it substantiates our sense of self, enriches memory and sustains our potential.

David Kidd, 'Investigating the Psychological Importance of Literary and Popular Genre Fiction'

The literary scholar William Deresiewicz concludes a review of two histories of the novel with the observation that 'the novel rose with modern selves because the novel, classically, relates the story of an individual attempting to create herself against existing definitions'.[11] The notion of a self defined, as Mikhail Bakhtin puts it, in terms of 'his social position, the degree to which he is sociologically or characterologically typical, his habitus, his spiritual profile and even his very physical appearance' was supplanted by one in which the self is given meaning by 'the significance of these features for the hero himself, for his self-consciousness'.[12] Of course, self-consciousness is not a recent innovation and modern selves do not always challenge existing definitions. The emphasis placed on subjectivity in much of literature, though, is hard to miss.

Taking note of modern fiction's apparent preoccupation with characters' inner lives, psychologists have begun to investigate how reading habits relate to individual differences in the psychological processes involved in understanding other's mental states in the real world. Mar and his colleagues[13] gave this line of research initial empirical traction with two studies designed to test whether exposure to fiction would positively predict performance on an advanced test of mental-state understanding, or Theory of Mind (ToM). ToM was assessed using the Reading the Mind in the Eyes Test[14] which requires that participants correctly identify complex mental states (e.g. contemplative, confident) shown in images of actors' eyes. Familiarity with fiction was measured with the Author Recognition Test (ART). The ART consists of a list containing names of authors and non-authors, and participants are asked to select those they recognise as authors. Participants who select more authors are more likely to prefer reading, report reading regularly[15] and include fiction on an online shopping wishlist.[16] Results of both studies showed that familiarity with fiction (ART score) was positively related to performance on the test of ToM (RMET score), even after accounting for exposure to non-fiction, age, gender, general intelligence, self-reported empathy and openness to experience. These results show that exposure to fiction, at least as indicated by high ART scores, positively correlates with a critical sociocognitive ability.

The correlational evidence offered by Mar et al. (2006, 2009) is consistent with claims about the ability of fiction to prompt readers to engage with the unique experiences of other people, and it is particularly notable given the well-documented tendency of people to process social information in superficial and schematic ways. Swencionis and Fiske[17] draw on decades of psychological research on stereotyping and prejudice to argue that a strong motivation to understand another person is critical to prompting perceivers to build upon and revise their initial impressions. Like Swencionis and Fiske (2013), Fiebich and Coltheart[18] propose that multiple processes are at play in social perception, and that perceivers are prone to adopt the least costly approach, which typically involves reliance on stereotypes associated with a particular social identity. Only when these efficient heuristic processes fail to yield coherence or adequate information are perceivers likely to turn to more effortful processes of theorising about the other's mental states or simulating them to arrive at an understanding of the other as an individual. That is, the mere presence of social content is insufficient to fully engage advanced mentalising, or ToM.

Like perceivers in the real world, readers are likely able to navigate the social worlds of many fictional texts with little recourse to demanding sociocognitive processes, such as ToM. Cognitive literary theorists have argued that formulaic social situations and stock characters capitalise on readers' schematic social knowledge and familiarity with genre conventions, facilitating quick and easy construction of the story's social world.[19] Information about a character's social identity and role, rather than attention to their particular subjective experiences, can serve as the primary foundation for the reader's representation of that character.

Since the processes of social categorisation and stereotype application tend to be efficient and often the default (Swencionis and Fiske, 2013), it is unsurprising that audiences readily respond to fictional works with characters who are easily understood in such terms. These guilty pleasures, beach reads or airplane novels may be exciting, immersive and emotionally evocative, but their characters are often fairly simple, easily understood and even stereotypic.[20] Yet, ordinary readers also seek out fiction that celebrates ambiguity and complex characters[21] suggesting that easy processing is not key to reader engagement.

Although the alignment is a bit rough, these two types of reading correspond with the distinction between popular genre fiction and literary fiction. In popular genre fiction, characters are more likely to be defined by genre-specific roles or social stereotypes, while those in literary fiction tend to be more fully developed as unique individuals.[22] Readers seem to be attuned to this distinction, seeking literary fiction when interested in complex characters, multiple perspectives and ambiguous meanings (Miesen, 2004).

Thus, fiction, though nearly always preoccupied with social content,[23] can promote distinct ways of processing social information. In the case of more literary fiction, readers may be prompted more often to rely extensively on their capacity for advanced ToM to make and update inferences about psychologically complex characters. By contrast, more formulaic genre fiction might be more easily understood in terms of existing schema. This theoretical approach yields empirically testable hypotheses. First, reading literary fiction will lead to improved performance on a subsequent test of ToM by more fully recruiting ToM processes. Second, people who read more literary fiction over their lifetime will perform better on tests of ToM than those who read less. Although clearly related, each hypothesis makes distinct assumptions about reading literary fiction. In the first case, the claim is that ToM processes are more fully engaged by literary than popular genre fiction.

In the second, the claim is that habitual engagement of ToM in fictional worlds helps develop the capacity and makes it more readily deployed in the real world.

The initial empirical evidence in support of the first hypothesis, namely that reading literary fiction would lead to improved performance on a ToM test, comes from a series of five experiments.[24] In four of these experiments, participants were randomly assigned to read a short work (or excerpt) of award-winning literary fiction or to read a work of popular genre fiction before completing a test of ToM.[25] Each condition (literary fiction, popular genre fiction) was represented by at least three different texts (10–15 pages) in every experiment in order to reduce the impact of the unique features of the texts in each category. In all but one of these experiments, the primary measure of ToM was the same as that used in Mar et al.'s (2006, 2009) correlational studies, the RMET (Baron-Cohen et al., 2001). Across these four experiments, participants assigned to read literary fiction performed better on the RMET than those assigned to read popular genre fiction.

However, these findings were challenged by the results of subsequent replication efforts[26] that showed no difference in ToM performance between participants assigned to read literary fiction and popular genre fiction. In the case of Panero et al. (2016), the null finding appeared to be at least partially attributable to a failure to ensure that participants read their assigned texts and variations in protocols across multiple research sites.[27] Nonetheless, these failed replication attempts clearly indicated the need for additional research to evaluate the hypothesis that reading literary fiction improves Theory of Mind performance. Consequently, three high-powered pre-registered replications of the final experiment in Kidd and Castano (2013) were conducted.[28] The first of these experiments yielded evidence of a moderated effect, with only relatively experienced readers demonstrating improved performance in the literary fiction condition. The second showed no support for the hypothesis, but also did not conclusively support the null hypothesis. The third experiment clearly replicated the initial finding. As these findings were being reviewed, an independent research group[29] published the results of another successful replication of the fifth experiment in Kidd and Castano (2013). As noted in Kidd and Castano (2018), the effects observed in the successful replications, though small, are consistent with those reported in Kidd and Castano (2013), suggesting that, at least in the short term, reading literary fiction evokes ToM more fully than reading popular genre fiction.

The experiments reported in Kidd and Castano (2018) were also designed to more directly test the key premise that readers perceive characters in literary fiction as less stereotypic and predictable than those in popular genre fiction. To do this, a Character Clarity Scale (CCS) was developed. The construct of character clarity was informed by both cognitive literary theory (e.g. Culpeper, 2001) regarding schema-based characterisation and psychological theories of essentialism[30] that describe inflexible ways of thinking about others. This construct was operationalised by asking participants to respond on a sliding scale to four items addressing the character's stereotypicality and predictability. In addition, they rated a main character on a brief personality inventory and a brief semantic differential questionnaire. These personality ratings themselves were not analysed. Instead, after responding to each set of questions, participants were asked to rate their confidence in their answers. These two confidence ratings were averaged with the other four items to form a measure of character clarity.

As expected, character clarity scores were substantially lower in the literary fiction condition compared to the popular genre fiction. There was only weak evidence that this effect was moderated by prior familiarity with fiction, suggesting that, in general, ordinary readers are well-attuned to the depth of characterisation in fiction. It is important to note that readers were not aware of the genre or author of their assigned short stories, so differences in their ratings of character clarity can be clearly linked only to affordances of the texts themselves. Though perhaps unsurprising to literary scholars and ordinary readers, these findings empirically demonstrate that literary fiction, as operationalised in these experiments, engages readers with more nuanced characters than popular genre fiction.

These experimental findings lend important support to the theoretical distinction between literary and popular genre fiction. However, these studies investigated only immediate effects, leaving open the question of how regularly engaging ToM to make sense of the complex social worlds in literary fiction might contribute to stable changes in social cognition. To gain a better understanding of the more general long-term effects of reading literary and genre fiction, Kidd and Castano[31] analysed responses to a measure of familiarity with authors, an author recognition test and RMET scores from over 2400 adult participants. Participants in this study completed an updated version of the Author Recognition Test[32] that includes 130 names, 65 of which are those of authors of fiction. A factor analysis of ART responses yielded two factors easily interpreted as reflecting familiarity with literary and popular genre fiction.[33]

Consistent with the experimental work, analyses across three large samples indicated that familiarity with literary fiction positively predicted performance on the RMET, the test of ToM, but familiarity with popular genre fiction did not. This relation could not be accounted for by differences in gender, age, undergraduate major, educational attainment or self-reported trait empathy. This pattern was also clearly replicated in each of the three studies reported in Kidd and Castano (2018), attesting to their reliability. These results are consistent with the hypothesis that, over time, reading literary fiction may cultivate advanced ToM, or mentalising. However, as with previous correlational findings (e.g. Mar et al., 2009), it is possible that the relation is caused by greater interest in literary fiction among individuals with higher ToM test scores, or that a combination of these effects is reflected in this finding. Nonetheless, these findings suggest that the robust relation between exposure to fiction and ToM performance[34] may be primarily driven by literary fiction.

The experimental and correlational research described above generally supports the psychological importance of the lay and scholarly distinction between literary and popular genre fiction. The findings converge to suggest that literary fiction engages readers with greater sociocognitive complexity and may contribute to the development or greater deployment of advanced ToM. This research constitutes only a narrow slice of the work currently being conducted to better understand the interplay of reading fiction and social cognition, and, more broadly, to investigate the role of cultural engagement in cultivating psychological capacities and dispositions.

However, conclusions drawn from these studies, particularly the experiments, should be tempered by their methodological limitations and the generally small effects detected. Advances in psychological methods, including obtaining sufficient statistical power, pre-registering protocols and analyses, and making data available to other researchers, should be incorporated into future research to provide a stronger empirical basis for understanding the impacts of fiction on social cognition. In addition, extant findings in this domain, particularly those based on single studies, should be evaluated in replication studies to help arrive at clearer estimates of their magnitude and reliability.

Christophe de Bezenac, 'Physiological Measures of Emotional Processing in Reading Experiences'

Introduction

In what follows, I outline quantitative methods that I have been developing and testing within our research group (CRILS) to investigate explicit and implicit processes that take place in Shared Reading contexts. The aim of this research is to contribute to an evidence-based understanding of whether reading experiences have a measurable impact on psychological and interpersonal function and to establish the conditions and mechanisms through which such changes take place. However, this type of research comes with unique challenges. In most experimental settings, data can be segmented and then contrasted based on the timings of known conditions or states. In contrast, there is often no obvious ground-truth or gold standard procedure that allows researchers to distinguish salient from non-salient moments during reading experiences and how these eventually relate to particular outcomes. Readers themselves are often not consciously aware of the dynamic cognitive and emotional interplay that determines their experiences. The effect of reading literature is likely to involve complex processes that take place 'behind the scenes' and that neither readers nor researchers have access to. This can lead to an over-reliance on inferences that can result in inaccurate research interpretations. Below I propose ways that these challenges can be addressed in the light of methodological and technological advances and, more specifically, by examining physiological signals alongside other sources of available data.

Heart Rate Variability

Body signals such as heart rate (HR) and skin conductance response (SCR) can provide a window into both conscious and unconscious emotional processing.[35] Signals reflect the interplay between sympathetic and parasympathetic mechanisms that are crucial to stress regulation response.[36] The sympathetic system has been associated with a 'fight/flight' mode linked to increased HR and sweat production, while the parasympathetic system facilitates homeostasis of the body, a 'rest/digest/socialise' mode characterised by reduced HR with more variability (HRV).[37]

Heartbeats are not completely regular, but vary slightly over time depending on physiological and environmental factors. The extent to which HR varies over time is also thought to reflect the level of emotional and cognitive arousal that we experience. For example, increased HRV has been associated with an enhanced ability to recognise and regulate our own as well as other's emotions[38] and better cognitive functioning particularly in stressful situations.[39] In a recent study, the emotional state of participants was predicted with 85% accuracy based on HR measures alone.[40] HRV has also been found to decrease under conditions of reduced physical and mental health, elevated state anxiety and emotional strain.[41]

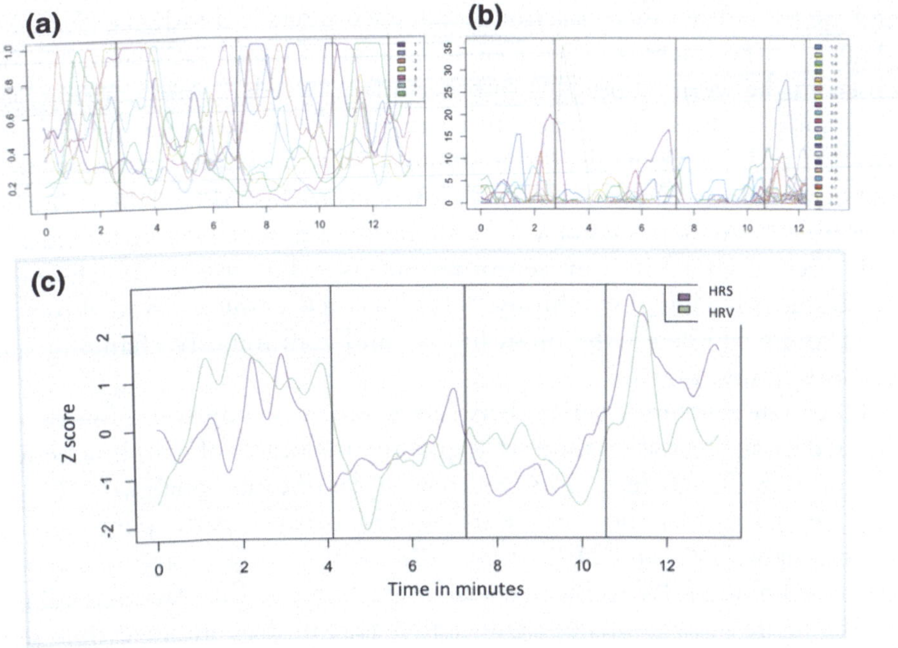

Fig. 13.1 (a) HRV for each participant in a Shared Reading session. (b) HRS between each participant pair (c) mean HRS (purple line) and HRV (green line)

In developing new methods for research into reading experience, we carried out a series of preliminary tests. These took the form of filmed Shared Reading sessions involving five to eight individuals wearing wristbands capable of detecting HR, SCR, body temperature and movement. Change of HRV throughout the session was calculated using recurrence quantification analysis over consecutive/sliding time windows. This is shown for each participant in Fig. 13.1a, with averaged HRV across all group members shown in (c) (green line). Elevated group HRV levels (c) are apparent in the first and last quarter of the session (c). To understand what this tells us about participant reading experience, however, physiological observations of this sort need to be triangulated with and examined in relation to other forms of evidence (see below).

Heart Rate Synchrony

In a Shared Reading context, useful information may also emerge from physiological and behavioural relationships between individuals in the group. We voluntarily and involuntarily synchronise our brains, heart rate and bodies with others during social encounters.[42] Evidence for physiological entrainment and associated feelings of social cohesion has been observed between couples,[43] mother-infant dyads[44] and during joint behaviours such as dance and music-making.[45] Interpersonal synchrony is thought to be a mechanism that supports fluid social interactions, prosocial behaviour and affiliation,[46] with lower values linked to deficits in social cognition.[47] At a physiological level, interbrain synchronisation has not only been observed in joint sensorimotor tasks, but also in the absence of detectable behavioural synchrony.[48] This may reflect our evolved ability and need to quickly detect the often hidden and continuously changing states of those around us.

Heart rate synchrony (HRS) between members of a dyad or group can be assessed using analysis methods that quantify the degree of coupling between two or more signals (e.g. cross-recurrence quantification analysis). The purple line in Fig. 13.1 shows the level of HRS between participant pairs (b). Interestingly, HRV and HRS seem to broadly co-vary in accordance with evidence linking HRV to fluent social interaction (c). The black vertical lines on the figure show points of significant change in the combined time series (multivariate change point analysis). These subsections can be examined in relation to data extracted from audiovisual recordings of the session (see Chapter 10), with the aim of understanding how group-level changes in HR within and between individuals relate to behaviour and participant experience throughout the duration of the session.

Skin Conductance Response

Skin conductance response (SCR)—a property of the human body that causes continuous variation in the electrical characteristics of the skin—is thought to be a psychophysiological index of bodily arousal and closely associated with emotional, attentional and cognitive states.[49]

SCR was collected and analysed for the test Shared Reading sessions. An example of results may be seen in (b) of Fig. 13.2, where vertical lines indicate when a significant response occurred during the session for 7 participants. For example, the data suggest that highest arousal for participant 1 occurred towards the end of the session. Given that SCR data collected during reading sessions are not explicitly related to events or conditions (as is the case in most experimental paradigms), physiological observations of this sort need to be examined in the context of temporally related events, interactions and experiences. This is particularly important

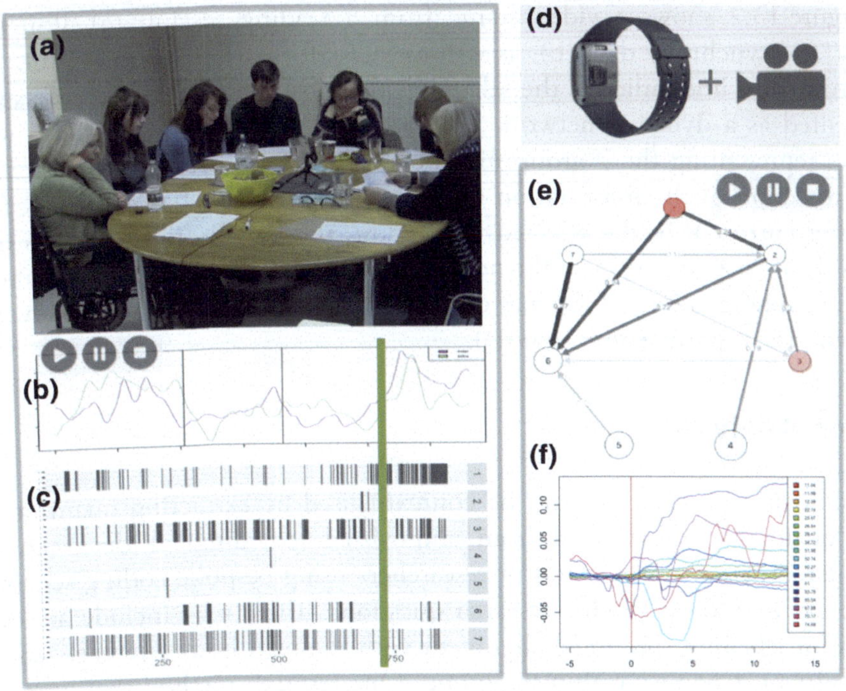

Fig. 13.2 (a) Video recording of a reading session with (b) group HRV and HRS data, as well as (c) SCR for participants 1–7. The green line shows the current video position. (d) The devices used in tests, including a Empatica E4 wristband and camera. (e) A dynamic network showing transfer of information between participants' HR. SCR occurs during the selected time window for participants 1 and 3, as indicated by the colour red. (f) Skin conductance level 5 seconds prior to, and 15 following button presses indicating 'significant/salient' moment for one participant during a Shared Reading session

with SCRs, given that the measure provides limited information about whether increased arousal is related to positively or negatively valenced stimuli.

Another approach that our research group has explored is to ask participants to label personally 'significant/salient' moments during the session using the button included on the wristband that allows time-stamps to be added to the data. Observations around these time points can then be examined. Figure 13.2f shows skin conductance level variation 5 seconds before and 15 seconds after one participant's button presses (0). This type of set-up could be used to structure qualitative interviews with the aim of gathering descriptive data related to moments of high physiological arousal.

Figure 13.2 shows a video frame from a reading session (a) alongside HRV and synchrony data (b), as well as SCRs for participants 1–7 (c). The green vertical line indicates the selected video position. HR data can also be presented as a dynamic network time locked to the video recording, with nodes representing the 7 group members and edges indicating the strength and direction of the information flow between members based on HR (i.e. transfer entropy). In the selected time point, the visualisation suggests that the HR of participant 6 is influenced by a number of other group members. In this representation, SCRs that occur within the selected time window are shown in red (participants 1 and 3).

Video Analysis

Physiological observations can be contextualised by extracting quantitative and qualitative information from audiovisual recordings. Videos can be annotated by participants and/or researchers using bespoke coding schemes designed to address specific research questions. These may include annotations for labelling emotional alignment with the text, body language, social attitudes or dynamics within the group. One research method that we have tested (described in detail in Chapter 10) is using a multidisciplinary group of researchers made up of psychologists, linguists and literature experts to rate video clips of Shared Reading sessions on continuous measure of 'salience' over time. Initial tests indicate a high degree of rating agreement between researchers. Continuous ratings of this sort can then be used to predict variation in the physiological observations discussed above. Time-aligned qualitative data can also be collected and examined in relation to body signals through techniques such as 'stimulated recall', which uses video sequences to help participants remember the thoughts that they were having throughout the session.

Computer vision—which aims to extract high-level understanding from digital images or videos[50]—can be used for automatic annotation. For example, it is possible to detect and track objects and people in a video sequence and extract information such as the degree of participant movement over time. With adequate camera positioning, video-based monitoring of vital signs such as patterns of HR and breathing is also becoming a possibility,[51] as is the detection of basic emotions (anger, contempt, disgust, happiness, sadness, surprise, fear, neutral) from facial features. Figure 13.3 shows findings from an emotion categorisation analysis of a filmed debate between two individuals (c).

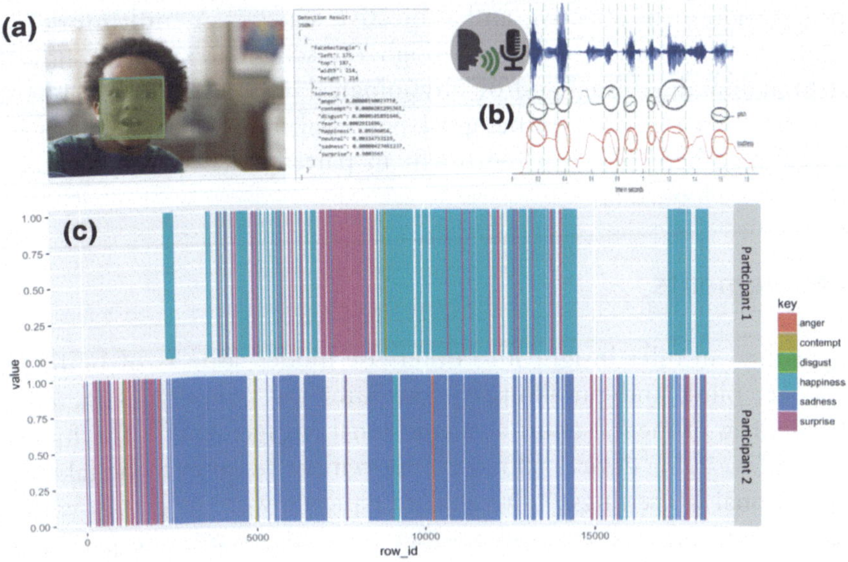

Fig. 13.3 (a) Sample results for the facial emotions analysis of one video frame. (b) Representation of an emotional prosody analysis. (c) Results of facial emotions analysis for a complete video recording of a debate between two individuals

Speech Analysis

Auditory information can also provide meaningful information about the mental processes of a speaker.[52] Prosody refers to rhythmic and melodic aspects of speech, the silences, the stress patterns, the dynamics of intonation that can implicitly specify affective states sometimes hidden from view (i.e. absent in the speakers' concurrent facial expressions) (Fig. 13.3b). Acoustic features implicated in emotion detection include changes in fundamental frequency, intensity, segment and pause duration, tempo and voice quality. These also play an important role in linguistic communication, providing cues for syntax and pragmatics.[53]

In the context of research into Shared Reading experiences, I have been exploring diarisation algorithms able to automatically distinguish between different speakers in an audio recording. Valence and arousal levels can then be determined from the acoustic features of each participant's voice. Though accuracy level can still be an issue, participant contributions can also be transcribed with associated timings for each spoken word. Generated text can then be put through text mining procedures described below, including sentiment analysis which uses computational linguistics to study variation in affective and subjective states.[54] A multimodel analysis that compares what is said (through transcribed text) with how it is said (through audio, visual and/or physiological data) is then possible, with mismatches between the two being of potential interest. For example, the degree of alignment between sentiment in participants' vocal features and the text can be looked at.

Eye Movements

Eye-tracking can offer insight into otherwise hidden aspects of brain function. Gaze, blink and pupillometry measures are typically extracted and used as indices of mental effort and emotional engagement.[55] The increased accuracy of wearable devices allows eye movement research to be taken outside traditional lab settings.[56] Devices are typically worn as glasses with one camera focused on each eye and another directed towards the participant's field of view. Multiple devices in the context of Shared Reading sessions can be used to explore patterns of social and emotional processing during face-to-face interaction.

Our research group has also examined eye movement characteristics during the act of reading. Though eye-tracking studies of reading tend to examine low-level visual and lexical processing of text, there is evidence that eye movements are influenced by higher-order comprehension and the process of deriving meaning.[57] These type of data have the potential to provide a moment-to-moment indication of a reader's information-seeking strategies that allow us to make tentative inferences about emotional and cognitive engagement with the written word. For example, in a recent fMRI study, we showed a series of poetic and prosaic texts to participants while eye movement behaviour was tracked.[58] In addition to contrasting largely unfamiliar poetic and matched prosaic pieces, the final line in half of the texts was unexpected, prompting a semantic reappraisal that allowed us to also examine the effects of semantic model updating on patterns of eye movement. In relation to gaze, we found that poetry and the need for reappraisal of meaning was related to longer eye fixations and less linear gaze paths through the text (more regressions) (Fig. 13.4). With low-level textual features such as word length and frequency accounted for, these findings may reflect increased emotional and cognitive engagement commonly associated with the experience of reading literature. This can be taken a step further by identifying parts of the text likely to be key to the search for meaning and then examining eye movement behaviour in relation to these predictions.

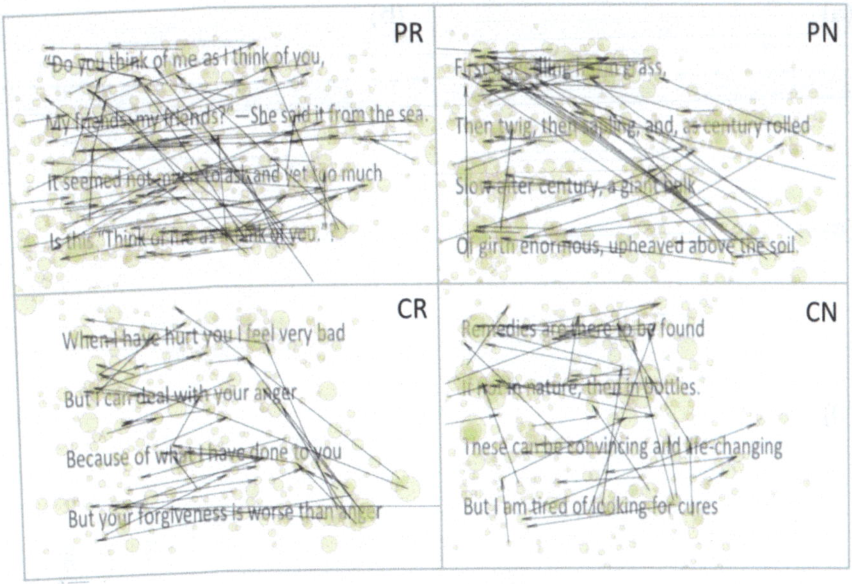

Fig. 13.4 Text stimuli sample with eye movement parameters for each of the 4 conditions (P=poetic; C=control/prosaic; R=reappraisal; N=no reappraisal). Circles indicate fixation positions for all participants with size representing fixation duration. Arrows show the origin and destination of fixations classified as regressions for all participants

Text/Transcription Analysis

Text derived from transcriptions of Shared Reading sessions has potential to also contribute to understanding reading experiences. In addition to information gleaned from the qualitative analysis of transcriptions, algorithms capable of automatically extracting textual data made significant advances in recent years. The aim of text mining is to discover hidden patterns and connections in text to uncover new meaningful information.[59] Algorithms include natural language processing (NLP) techniques such as parts of speech tagging, syntactic parsing and entity extraction (e.g. names of people or places); text summarisation procedures able to identify keywords and concepts; unsupervised learning methods such as clustering or topic modelling that explore hidden structure in text; supervised learning methods that allow models to be trained manually, for example, based on the results of a qualitative analysis; dynamic social network procedures based on the patterns of turn-taking or content similarities between participants or sessions; and text-based sentiment analysis which allows attitudes behind

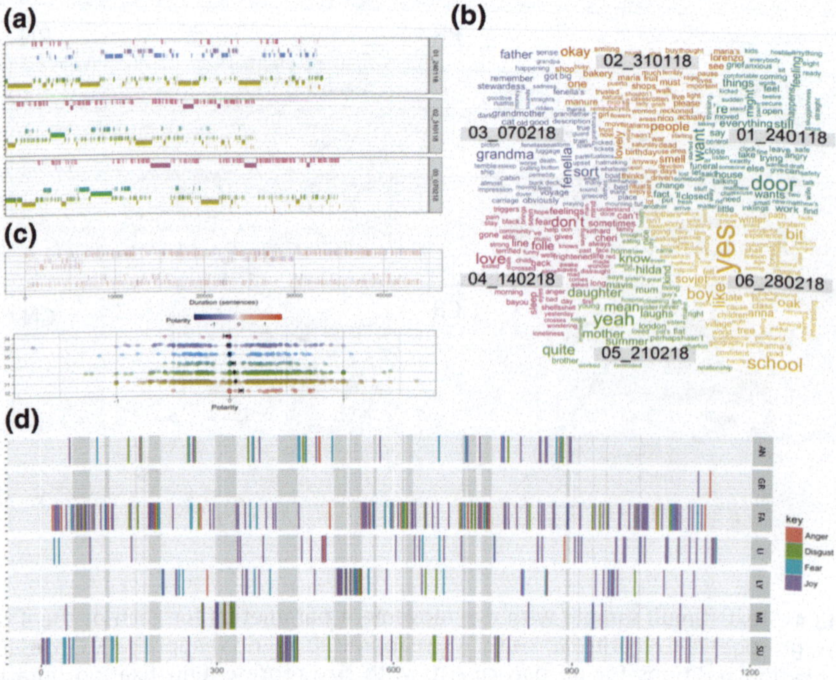

Fig. 13.5 Examples of text mining possibilities 1. (a) Participant contributions across 3 sessions; (b) word frequency comparison cloud for six sessions; (c) sentiment analysis for one session by participant (polarity: blue = negative; red = positive); and (d) emotion classification for one session for each participant, with grey segments indicating reading moments

contributions to be detected, including overall valence (positive, negative or neutral) and emotion classification (e.g. anger, disgust, fear, happiness, sadness and surprise).

To give the reader a flavour of available possibilities, Figs. 13.4 and 13.5 show a number of text mining procedures that I tested on transcriptions of Shared Reading sessions. In Fig. 13.5, participant contributions are shown for 3 different sessions (a), along with a word frequency comparison cloud for six sessions (b). Results of a sentiment analysis applied to one session are shown in (c), with negative contributions represented in blue and positive contributions in red. Participants overall sentiment across the session can be seen below ordered from most negative to most positive. Text-based emotion classification analysis results for one session are visualised for each participant in (d), with grey sections representing reading (as opposed to discussion) moments. The ability to distinguish reading material from participant discussion makes it possible to explore alignment changes that occur

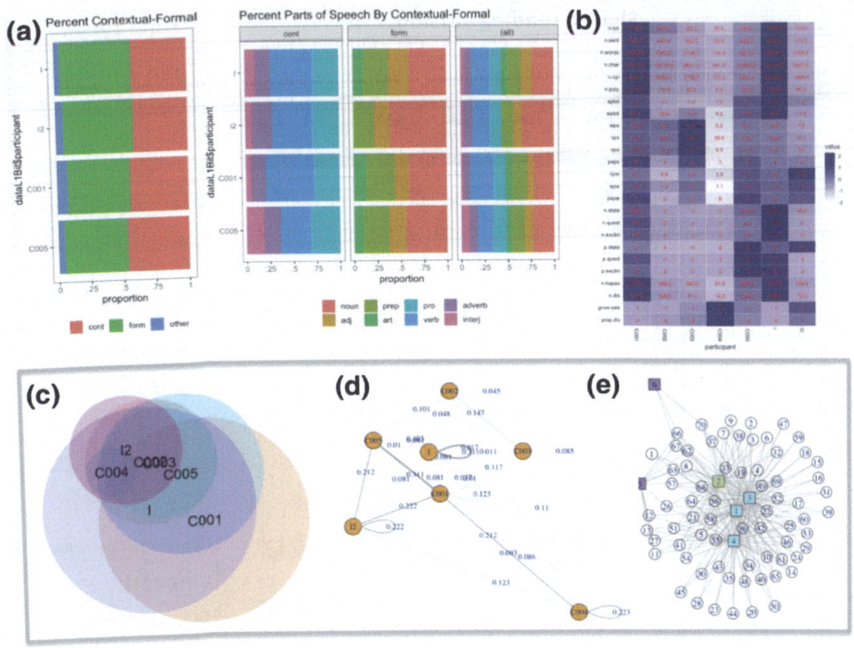

Fig. 13.6 Examples of text mining possibilities 2. (a) NLP parts of speech analysis results for each participant for one session; (b) additional stats derived from that session; (c) Venn diagram showing participant overlap based on the semantic similarity of contributions; (d) semantic similarity network (nodes = participants; edges = connection strength); (e) patterns of turn-taking during one session (participants shown as coloured squares)

between the two both within and across sessions. Figure 13.6 shows the outcome of a NLP (parts of speech) analysis of one transcribed session (a) as well as examples of other stats that can be extracted from text (b). The Venn diagram in (c) represents the overlap between participants based on semantic similarities in participant contributions. This can also be visualised as a network with nodes representing individuals and edges the strength of the connections between them (d). Patterns of turn-taking during a session are shown in (d), where participants (represented as coloured squares) may be seen as more or less central to the discussion. All of the above mentioned textual features can be used to compare participants and examine changes across multiple sessions. This extra layer of quantitative analysis can thus statistically measure the degree to which the literary text is the catalyst for change over longer periods of time. However, the real potential of applying text mining to transcriptions of reading experiences is to explore temporal relationships with physiological signals within sessions (see Fig. 13.7).

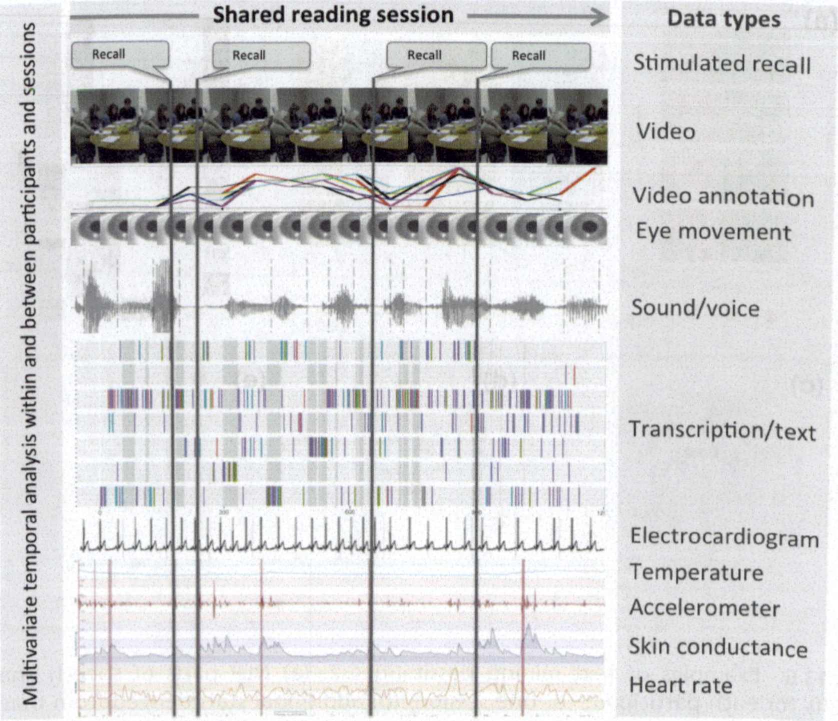

Fig. 13.7 Summary of the sources of data that can be combined to provide a more complete picture of mechanisms underlying Shared Reading experiences

A Holistic Approach

Many methods traditionally employed to understand complex psychological processes can be defined as reductionist, in that the focus is on understanding the function of each part of a system separately. Only a fraction of available information is used at any one time. Despite the utility of this approach for redefining complex problems into manageable chunks, it is not always the most effective way of understanding the emergent properties of a system, particularly in contexts where gaps of information are common. In contrast, more holistic, top-down approaches use the simultaneous observation and analysis of multiple sources of evidence to more directly understand the dynamics of the system as a whole.

Methodological advances in quantifying physiological and behavioural signals as multivariate phenomena provide new possibilities for addressing the inherent challenges of research into reading experiences. The hope is that a more complete picture can emerge by looking for temporal relationships/

co-occurrences in data from different modalities. For example, to understand why a sharp increase in HR synchrony between group members occurred towards the end of a session, it may be necessary to examine information available in the audiovisual recording, for example, the quality of a speaker's voice, the content or topic of discussion, the relationships between participant body movements or the reported quality of subjective experience before and during the observed swell in HRS. Figure 13.7 summarises measures reviewed above that, examined together, provide a greater chance of understanding both conscious and unconscious mechanisms related to Shared Reading experiences. In brief, these include synchrony and variation in heart rate between and within participants, skin conductance response, movement detection, emotion recognition of vocal or textual features, and variation in facial expressions and eye movements. By setting up analysis frameworks that allow relationships between such data to be examined alongside qualitative experiential descriptions, it may be possible to uncover latent or hidden states that correspond to the lived cognitive and emotional experiences of shared readers. This area of study can provide a test bed for an interdisciplinary, more integrative approach to research, where quantitative and qualitative methods are seen as complementary rather than conflicting,[60] and where practices from different research environments come together to probe the inner workings of the mind.

Conclusion

In conclusion, collecting and comparing multi-modal sources of evidence from the body can promote the development of a rich, robust and comprehensive picture of Shared Reading experiences, with the aim of understanding putative contributions to psychological and interpersonal change.

Notes

1. P. Davis, G. Thierry, N. Roberts, and V. Gonzalez-Diaz, 'Event-Related Potential Characterisation of the Shakespearean Functional Shift in Narrative Sentence Structure', *NeuroImage*, 40 (2008), 923–31. (NB. All studies represented here received ethical approval.)
2. W. Shakespeare, *The Complete Works*, ed. by Stanley Wells and Gary Taylor (Oxford: Oxford University Press, 1998), pp. 842, 929, 1034.
3. G. Puttenham, *The Arte of English Poesie* (1589), ed. by Frank Whigham and Wayne A. Rebhorn (Ithaca, NY: Cornell University Press, 2007), pp. 3, 15. See also above, Chapter 2.

4. The classic humanist objection to neuroscience is that the localisation of functions is inherently reductive and leads only to a travesty of understanding. 'We tend to overlook the complexity of the most ordinary aspects of our lives when we think about the supposed neurophysiological basis of consciousness. Neuromythology – which claims that neuroscience can explain far more than it can – seems halfway plausible only if it is predicated upon a desperately impoverished account of our many-layered, multi-agendaed, infinitely folded but wonderfully structured and organized selves.' Raymond Tallis, *The Infinite Kingdom of Space: A Fantastical Journey Around Your Head* (London: Atlantic Books, 2008), p. 160. The literary interest here, however, is in sudden dramatic and dynamic movement within complexity between the mobile shifting of layer and fold.
5. It is generally assumed that the human brain is set up as a prediction/Bayesian system to reduce uncertainty and enable safe management of our lives (hence the human tendency to reason by analogy, live by routines): see J. B. Tenenbaum et al., 'Theory-Based Bayesian Models of Inductive Learning and Reasoning', *Trends in Cognitive Sciences*, 10.7 (2006), 309–18.
6. P. Davis, J. L. Keidel, and V. Gonzalez-Diaz, 'How Shakespeare Tempests the Brain: Neuroimaging Insights', *Cortex*, 48 (2012), 21–64.
7. N. O'Sullivan, P. Davis, J. Billington, V. Gonzalez-Diaz, and R. Corcoran, '"Shall I Compare Thee": The Neural Basis of Literary Awareness, and Its Benefits to Cognition', *Cortex*, 73 (2015), 144–57.
8. R. Rylance, *Literature and the Public Good* (Oxford: Oxford University Press, 2016); R. Rylance, *Victorian Psychology and British Culture 1850–1880* (Oxford: Oxford University Press, 2000).
9. A. Zeman: 'Neurology Is Psychiatry—And Vice Versa', *Practical Neurology*, 14.3 (2014), 136–14; A. Zeman and C. Butler, 'Transient Epileptic Amnesia', *Current Opinion in Neurology*, 23.6 (2010), 610–16; A. Zeman, *A Portrait of the Brain* (Yale University Press, 2008).
10. A. Zeman, F. Milton, A. Smith, and R. Rylance, 'By Heart: An fMRI Study of Brain Activation by Poetry and Prose', *Journal of Consciousness Studies*, 20.9–10 (2013), 132–58.
11. W. Deresiewicz, 'How the Novel Made the Modern World', *The Atlantic*, 17 June 2014.
12. M. Bakhtin, *Problems of Dostoevsky's Poetics*, trans. by C. Emerson (Minneapolis, MN: University of Minnesota Press, 1984), p. 48.
13. R. A. Mar, K. Oatley, J. Hirsh, and J. B. Peterson, 'Bookworms Versus Nerds: Exposure to Fiction Versus Non-fiction, Divergent Associations with Social Ability, and the Simulation of Fictional Social Worlds', *Journal of Research in Personality*, 40.5 (2006), 694–712; R. A. Mar, K. Oatley, and J. B. Peterson, 'Exploring the Link Between Reading Fiction and Empathy: Ruling Out Individual Differences and Examining Outcomes', *Communications*, 34.4 (2009), 407–28.

14. S. Baron-Cohen, S. Wheelwright, J. Hill, Y. Raste, and I. Plumb, 'The "Reading the Mind in the Eyes" Test Revised Version: A Study with Normal Adults, and Adults with Asperger Syndrome or High-Functioning Autism', *Journal of Child Psychology and Psychiatry*, 42.2 (2001), 241–51.
15. K. E. Stanovich and A. E. Cunningham, 'Studying the Consequences of Literacy Within a Literate Society: The Cognitive Correlates of Print Exposure', *Memory & Cognition*, 20.1 (1992), 51–68; K. E. Stanovich, R. F. West, and M. R. Harrison, 'Knowledge Growth and Maintenance Across the Life Span: The Role of Print Exposure', *Developmental Psychology*, 31.5 (1995), 811–26.
16. M. Rain and R. A. Mar, 'Measuring Reading Behaviour: Examining the Predictive Validity of Print-Exposure Checklists', *Empirical Studies of the Arts*, 32.1 (2014), 93–108.
17. J. K. Swencionis and S. T. Fiske, 'More Human: Individuation in the 21st Century', in *Humanness and Dehumanization*, ed. by P. Bain, J. Vaes, and J-Ph. Leyens (New York: Psychology Press, Taylor & Francis, 2013), pp. 276–93.
18. A. Fiebich and M. Coltheart, 'Various Ways to Understand Other Minds: Towards a Pluralistic Approach to the Explanation of Social Understanding, *Mind & Language*, 30.3 (2015), 235–58.
19. J. Culpeper, *Language and Characterisation: People in Plays and Other Texts* (London: Longman, 2001); R. Schneider, 'Toward a Cognitive Theory of Literary Character: The Dynamics of Mental-Model Construction, *Style*, 35.4 (2001), 607–39.
20. S. Keen, 'Readers' Temperaments and Fictional Character', *New Literary History*, 42.2 (2011), 295–314.
21. H. Miesen, 'Fiction Readers' Appreciation of Text Attributes in Literary and Popular Novels: Some Empirical Findings', *International Journal of Arts Management*, 7.1 (2004), 45–56.
22. F. Hakemulder, *The Moral Laboratory: Experiments Examining the Effects of Reading Literature on Social Perception and Moral Self-Concept* (Amsterdam: John Benjamins Publishing Company, 2000).
23. R. A. Mar and K. Oatley, 'The Function of Fiction Is the Abstraction and Simulation of Social Experience', *Perspectives on Psychological Science*, 3.3 (2008), 173–92.
24. D. C. Kidd and E. Castano, 'Reading Literary Fiction Improves Theory of Mind', *Science*, 342.6156 (2013), 377–80.
25. In the first experiment in Kidd and Castano (2013), participants were assigned to read either non-fiction or literary fiction. However, the effect in this study was not replicated in a large-scale replication project (C. F. Camerer, A. Dreber, F. Holzmeister, T. H. Ho, J. Huber, M. Johannesson, … and A. Altmejd, 'Evaluating the Replicability of Social Science Experiments in Nature and

Science Between 2010 and 2015', *Nature Human Behaviour*, 2.9 (2018), 637), suggesting that it is not reliable under the original experimental conditions.
26. M. E. Panero, D. S. Weisberg, J. Black, T. R. Goldstein, J. L. Barnes, H. Brownell, and E. Winner, 'Does Reading a Single Passage of Literary Fiction Really Improve Theory of Mind? An Attempt at Replication', *Journal of Personality and Social Psychology*, 111.5 (2016), e46–e54; D. Samur, M. Tops, and S. L. Koole, 'Does a Single Session of Reading Literary Fiction Prime Enhanced Mentalising Performance? Four Replication Experiments of Kidd and Castano (2013)', *Cognition and Emotion*, 32.1 (2018), 130–44.
27. D. C. Kidd and E. Castano, 'Panero et al. (2016): Failure to Replicate Methods Caused the Failure to Replicate Results', *Journal of Personality and Social Psychology*, 112.3 (2017), e1–e4.
28. D. Kidd and E. Castano, 'Reading Literary Fiction and Theory of Mind: Three Preregistered Replications and Extensions of Kidd and Castano (2013)', *Social Psychological and Personality Science* (2018). https://doi.org/10.1177/1948550618775410.
29. I. van Kuijk, P. Verkoeijen, K. Dijkstra, and R. A. Zwaan, 'The Effect of Reading a Short Passage of Literary Fiction on Theory of Mind: A Replication of Kidd and Castano (2013)', *Collabra: Psychology*, 4.1 (2018), 7.
30. B. Bastian and N. Haslam, 'Psychological Essentialism and Stereotype Endorsement', *Journal of Experimental Social Psychology*, 42.2 (2006), 228–35.
31. D. Kidd and E. Castano, 'Different Stories: How Levels of Familiarity with Literary and Genre Fiction Relate to Mentalizing', *Psychology of Aesthetics, Creativity, and the Arts*, 11.4 (2017), 474–86.
32. D. J. Acheson, J. B. Wells, and M. C. MacDonald, 'New and Updated Tests of Print Exposure and Reading Abilities in College Students', *Behavior Research Methods*, 40.1 (2008), 278–89.
33. M. Moore and P. C. Gordon, 'Reading Ability and Print Exposure: Item Response Theory Analysis of the Author Recognition Test', *Behaviour Research Methods*, 47.4 (2015), 1095–109
34. M. Mumper and R. Gerrig, 'Leisure Reading and Social Cognition: A Meta-analysis', *Psychology of Aesthetics, Creativity, and the Arts*, 11.1 (2017), 109–20.
35. M. D. Tooley, D. Carmel, A. Chapman, and G. M Grimshaw, 'Dissociating the Physiological Components of Unconscious Emotional Responses', *Neuroscience of Consciousness*, 2017.1 (2017), nix021.
36. J. L. Andreassi, *Psychophysiology: Human Behavior and Physiological Response* (London: Psychology Press, 2010).
37. Y. M. Ulrich-Lai and J. P. Herman, 'Neural Regulation of Endocrine and Autonomic Stress Responses', *Nature Reviews Neuroscience*, 10.6 (2009), 397.
38. R. A. Fabes, N. Eisenberg, and L. Eisenbud, 'Behavioral and Physiological Correlates of Children's Reactions to Others in Distress', *Developmental*

Psychology, 29.4 (1993), 655; D. Quintana, A. Guastella, T. Outhred, I. Hickie, and A. Kemp, 'Heart Rate Variability Is Associated with Emotion Recognition: Direct Evidence for a Relationship Between the Autonomic Nervous System and Social Cognition', *International Journal of Psychophysiology*, 86.2 (2012), 168–72.
39. A. L. Hansen, B. H. Johnsen, and J. F. Thayer, 'Relationship Between Heart Rate Variability and Cognitive Function During Threat of Shock', *Anxiety, Stress, & Coping*, 22.1 (2009), 77–89.
40. M. Nardelli, G. Valenza, A. Greco, A. Lanata, and E. Scilingo, 'Recognizing Emotions Induced by Affective Sounds Through Heart Rate Variability', *IEEE Transactions on Affective Computing*, 6.4 (2015), 385–94.
41. A. J. Grippo, 'Opinion: "Heart Rate Variability, Health and Well-Being: A Systems Perspective" Research Topic', *Frontiers in Public Health*, 5 (2017), 246.
42. J. M. Ross and R. Balasubramaniam, 'Physical and Neural Entrainment to Rhythm: Human Sensorimotor Coordination Across Tasks and Effector Systems', *Frontiers in Human Neuroscience*, 8.1 (2014), 576.
43. E. Ferrer and J. L. Helm, 'Dynamical Systems Modeling of Physiological Coregulation in Dyadic Interactions', *International Journal of Psychophysiology*, 88.3 (2013), 296–308.
44. S. Atzil, T. Hendler, and R. Feldman, 'The Brain Basis of Social Synchrony', *Social Cognitive and Affective Neuroscience*, 9.8 (2014), 1193–202.
45. V. Müller and U. Lindenberger, 'Cardiac and Respiratory Patterns Synchronize Between Persons During Choir Singing', *PloS One*, 6.9 (2011), e24893.
46. G. Knoblich, S. Butterfill, and N. Sebanz, 'Psychological Research on Joint Action: Theory and Data', in *Psychology of Learning and Motivation*, vol. 54 (London: Academic Press, 2011), pp. 59–101.
47. K. L. Marsh, R. W. Isenhower, M. J. Richardson, M. Helt, A. D. Verbalis, R. C. Schmidt, and D. Fein, 'Autism and Social Disconnection in Interpersonal Rocking', *Frontiers in Integrative Neuroscience*, 7 (2013), 4.
48. G. Dumas, J. Nadel, R. Soussignan, J. Martinerie, and L. Garnero, 'Inter-brain Synchronization During Social Interaction', *PloS One*, 5.8 (2010), e12166; J. Llobera, C. Charbonnier, S. Chagué, D. Preissmann, J. P. Antonietti, F. Ansermet, and P. J. Magistretti, 'The Subjective Sensation of Synchrony: An Experimental Study', *PloS One*, 11.2 (2016), e0147008.
49. H. Critchley, 'Review: Electrodermal Responses: What Happens in the Brain', *The Neuroscientist*, 8.2 (2002), 132–42; W. Boucsein, *Electrodermal Activity* (Springer Science & Business Media, 2012).
50. T. Morris, *Computer Vision and Image Processing (Cornerstones of Computing)* (London: Palgrave Macmillan, 2004).
51. L. Tarassenko, M. Villarroel, A. Guazzi, J. Jorge, D. A. Clifton, and C. Pugh, 'Non-contact Video-Based Vital Sign Monitoring Using Ambient Light and Auto-regressive Models', *Physiological Measurement*, 35.5 (2014), 807.

52. G. Fairbanks and W. Pronovost, 'Vocal Pitch During Simulated Emotion' *Science*, 88.2286 (1838), 382–83; A. Wennerstrom, *The Music of Everyday Speech: Prosody and Discourse Analysis* (Oxford: Oxford University Press, 2001).
53. See K. R. Scherer, 'Vocal Communication of Emotion: A Review of Research Paradigms', *Speech Communication*, 40.1–2 (2003), 227–56.
54. M. V. Mäntylä, D. Graziotin, and M. Kuutila, 'The Evolution of Sentiment Analysis—A Review of Research Topics, Venues, and Top Cited Papers', *Computer Science Review*, 27 (2018), 16–32.
55. M. K. Eckstein, B. Guerra-Carrillo, A. T. M. Singley, and S. A. Bunge, 'Beyond Eye Gaze: What Else Can Eyetracking Reveal About Cognition and Cognitive Development?', *Developmental Cognitive Neuroscience*, 25 (2017), 69–91.
56. J. J. MacInnes, S. Iqbal, J. Pearson, and E. N. Johnson, 'Wearable Eye-Tracking for Research: Automated Dynamic Gaze Mapping and Accuracy/Precision Comparisons Across Devices', *bioRxiv* (2018), 299925.
57. K. Rayner, K. H. Chace, T. J. Slattery, J. Ashby, 'Eye Movements as Reflections of Comprehension Processes in Reading', *Scientific Studies of Reading*, 10.3 (2006), 241–55.
58. N. O'Sullivan, P. Davis, J. Billington, V. Gonzalez-Diaz, and R. Corcoran, '"Shall I Compare Thee": The Neural Basis of Literary Awareness, and Its Benefits to Cognition', *Cortex*, 73 (2015), 144–57.
59. M. Allahyari, S. Pouriyeh, M. Assefi, S. Safaei, E. D. Trippe, J. B. Gutierrez, and K. Kochut, 'A Brief Survey of Text Mining: Classification, Clustering and Extraction Techniques', *arXiv* (2017) Preprint arXiv:1707.02919.
60. C. Jones, 'Quantitative and Qualitative Research: Conflicting Paradigms or Perfect Partners?', in *Networked Learning 2004: A Research Based Conference on E-learning in Higher Education and Lifelong Learning: Proceedings of the Fourth International Conference on Networked Learning*, ed. by S. Banks, P. Goodyear, V. Hodgson, C. Jones, V. Lally, D. McConnell, and C. Steeples (Lancaster: Lancaster University, 2004), pp. 106–12.

Part IV

Towards a Theoretical Understanding of Reading and Health

14

Reading and Psychiatric Practices

David Fearnley and Grace Farrington

The Context

Mersey Care NHS Mental Health Trust is a specialist provider of mental health and learning disability services. Serving a population of one million across Merseyside, Mersey Care is one of only three trusts of its kind in the UK providing the entire range of specialist mental health services. Typically, the Trust serves people living with mood disorders and experience of psychosis, dementia and brain injury, personality disorders and alcohol and drug addiction, in inpatient and community, as well as in medium and high secure care. Mersey Care has a strong track record of working with non-NHS agencies to encourage social inclusion and to promote the rights, needs and aspirations of people with mental health difficulties, challenging the stigma attached to mental distress. The Trust's mission is to enable people with mental health difficulties and their carers to optimise their health by enriching their life experience in the broadest possible sense.

In 2007, Mersey Care took the bold step of commissioning a Shared Reading programme for inpatients.[1] In the first experiment of its kind, the

D. Fearnley (✉)
Mersey Care NHS Foundation Trust, Liverpool, UK
e-mail: david.fearnley@nhs.net

G. Farrington
The Reader, Liverpool, UK
e-mail: graceframe@thereader.org.uk

J. Billington (ed.), *Reading and Mental Health*,
https://doi.org/10.1007/978-3-030-21762-4_14

Trust funded a full-time Reader in Residence, trained by The Reader, to grow a reading group culture at Mersey Care, in part by training and supporting the Trust's own staff. This has become the precedent for The Reader's current international volunteer model.

A Different Kind of Engagement

One key element of the Shared Reading programme is that a reading group runs every week for an hour or two, with the book taken up again from where it was left off. This model ensures protected, uninterrupted time for staff and patient contact, which is an invaluable achievement in itself, and potential catalyst for promoting change, in an often austere organisational culture. A number of psychiatrist colleagues at Mersey Care have welcomed in particular the opportunity to put to one side their professional knowledge and expertise, and to enter into a different kind of mental space with the people with whom they are reading. One psychiatrist, for example, who works in a hospital setting commented that she does not take any of her 'therapy skills' into the reading group. This kind of approach allows the reading group to become a space that would not be found elsewhere within the hospital, and that exists on different terms from those of the institution, even momentarily transcending it. (One member of a group that meets in a prison confirmed this idea: the reading group, she said, was 'something the prison couldn't touch',[2] see Chapter 9.) Another psychiatrist who runs a reading group for service users referred by the community mental health team commented on what differentiates the reading group from her habitual therapeutic practice. The first focus is not on 'interpreting' individual responses—which is where the work of the therapist begins, in seeking explanation. Rather, the reading group leader must concentrate on being able to sense the 'power' of the poem as 'that thing in the room that you want to make come through'. This included its coming through the group participants at the level of thoughtful feeling, individual and shared: *performing it, not so much explaining it*, is how the psychiatrist put it, in shorthand. This is a different type of engagement, a different type of experience. It fills a gap between the staff and the patients, for whom it's entirely new to find medical staff contributing their own experiences and being on the same plane within the shared present moment.

More, the reading *material* is as much a part of this democratisation as the act of reading itself. The groups tackle a wide range of literature, from Emily Brontë's *Wuthering Heights*, through short stories by Anton Chekhov, to the work of Doris Lessing, George Orwell and John Wyndham, in addition to poetry by, for example, C. Day Lewis, Ted Hughes and W. B. Yeats. There is always the sense that the book or poem deserves respect, that it deserves time. Everyone involved—both group leader and participants—is primed by the very presence of the book for 'this is something significant'. When a psychiatrist sits down with patients on a one-to-one basis or in group psychotherapy, he or she is paid to have all the answers, or at least to be able to plot out the path towards them. But together in the reading group, we all respect that the writer is somebody else coming in with their own point of view. The book, not the psychiatrist, becomes the expert.

The power of such shifts is not to be underestimated, especially in those parts of the Trust where the culture might be most austere. The experience of high secure patients at Ashworth Hospital—in whom self-esteem tends to be low and the sense of isolation and self-stigma often high—represents the extreme end of urgent patient needs which exist throughout the Trust. In an environment where patients in some services can be detained under the Mental Health Act 1983 for lengthy periods, there is a necessity for the kind of relevant and reparative pursuit that is vital in encouraging a sense of hope and recovery potential. To bring any kind of cultural activity into a such a health setting will often produce a benign shock to the system and routine, and is likely to be of benefit simply by providing a link with the normal, unconstrained habits of a human community. For long-stay patients, for whom boredom and loneliness are acute problems, reading together offers genuinely meaningful activity and authentic engagement under conditions of cultural austerity. A challenging book promotes discussion about serious life issues, develops self-expression and encourages mutual tolerance and peer support. Above all, reading engages the whole person, not just the ill part. Reading is not a typical prison/hospital experience. It is not obviously therapy. It hasn't been sanitised or processed as an evidence-based programme. Perhaps, it is because the ward is such an unusual or unreal environment, by giving people a bit of the real world, you see a bit more of the real person.

Connections

Sharing and Community

What distinguishes the practice of Shared Reading from traditional book clubs or individual reading habits is the reading *aloud* of the literature. This creates, with each reading and within each new group of people, a fresh starting point and a dynamic presence for what follows. The literature is now re-experienced as a live happening in which the reader is invited to participate, by attending not only to the words on the page but to the human voice in which those words are being made present. It is an embodied and performed realisation of the potential that literature offers as the container of a sharable human event. In ordinary public experience, the achievement of a sense of community and commonality between people is often dependent upon an agreement or acceptance of certain shared norms for a particular purpose. This may limit both the depth and the reach of such community as well as the place that the individual is able to occupy within it. But a non-reductive literary language works beneath conventional defaults and allows the reader, out of an immediate sense of being personally moved, to relate both to the literature and to the other responsive readers. The reading aloud creates a present moment in time and an imaginative space within which a personal response is called for.

Connecting Across Time

The literature is inclusive not only of a wide range of persons in the group but also of a wide range of experiences throughout different ages of time. What is often striking in a reading group is how the literature might allow readers to connect with the experiences of men and women down the generations and across history. Carl Jung's thinking on archetypes is relevant here. 'It is sufficient to know', Jung wrote, 'that there is not a single important idea or view that does not possess historical antecedents. Ultimately they are all founded on primordial archetypal forms whose concreteness dates from a time when consciousness did not *think*, but only *perceived*'.[3] It is as though the fiction and poetry we read are subtly reminding us of this collective humanity and its ancient common experience. The literature and reading involve a kind of emotional archaeology. Like a fossil, the emotion was experienced long ago, but a reader can experience it as present.

The reading group leader has a key role to play in holding this 'package' of emotional experience for as long as possible. He or she responds to the other readers in the same way as he or she responds to the literature: attentive to inarticulate gestures towards meaning and to matter that is as yet implicit or unstated. The concern is neither exclusively with the individual nor with the group, but with the source place of resonant feeling and with keeping that resonance alive.

For some people, taking part in the reading group means crossing the first threshold of emotional expression. It is a step that must not be underestimated. Lapsing back into default attitudes or potentially divisive personal opinion, or just benign chat, would be all too easy. And this is not an issue exclusive to Mersey Care service users. In an age when people are as concerned to preserve their digital life as their emotional life, and when life expectancy is much higher than it was even a century ago, we have lost the urgency to verbally express the things that really matter. The opening up of the kind of profundity preserved in literature is very rare in Western culture in general. Whilst such 'resting-places' were common in ancient human practices, they are more often forced upon the modern individual as Charles Dickens recounts when describing Arthur Clennam's imprisonment in the Marshalsea towards the close of *Little Dorrit*: 'a stop in the whirling wheel of life … comes with sickness, it comes with sorrow, it comes with the loss of the dearly loved, it is one of the most frequent uses of adversity'.[4] In taking time and care over the reading itself, pausing for reflection on what has been read, Shared Reading recreates a lost habit not only of community but of contemplation.

Connecting Within and Before

The performative 'liveness' of the literature in Shared Reading is critical too. When a poem or story is read aloud, making every word and every line a close, vocal-emotional presence, the reader's response is likely to be situated in the body, as the biological substrate of an emotion, before it ever reaches mental awareness or consciously understood meaning. The primary emotion involved in literary response will almost inevitably be closer to earlier life. Reading is a form of emotional archaeology in this sense too: that it can take a person back to early experiences before adult stress patterns took hold or hardened into ill health. It can get underneath habitual categories and frames, those of identity as well as of medical condition.

Reading's operation at pre-linguistic and preverbal levels distinguishes it from the majority of therapies, which are deliberately focused on the use and analysis of words from the perspective of trying to alter badly formed linguistic patterns or to create new ones. Cognitive behavioural therapy, itself rooted in the ancient tradition of stoic philosophy,[5,6] is the most widely practised therapy in clinical settings. The danger of CBT's rationalist approach, critics argue, is that it concentrates on the removal of 'surface' symptoms rather than tackling the 'underlying structures' which the symptom inarticulately expresses.[7] Talking therapies, working before or after the event in cases of repeated distress or trauma, 'too often bypass the emotional-engagement system, encoded in visceral sensation, that is the foundation of who we are and instead focus narrowly on correcting "faulty thinking" and on suppressing unpleasant emotions and troublesome behaviours'.[8] The literature's non-targeted approach allows connections to be made at a point of need which may be more primary and more personally relevant than formal diagnosis and treatment, or the individuals themselves could consciously locate or touch off.

This is a deep model of 'recovery' where, in the re-emergence of lost memories, feelings, faculties or beliefs, adult default frames can be refreshed and people can begin to know things anew. The possibility that the literature can reach back to a period or condition prior to trauma, before damage set in—as if not everything has to be destroyed by what subsequently happened in life's narrative—is a version of the restoration of a state prior to the Fall, as in Elizabethan poetics (see Chapter 3 above). The sonnet was once called 'the alphabet of the human heart'[9] for including in its tight, well-wrought form the disparate matter of the human universe. It offers (as we might now say) a common DNA structure of human experience. It is a clue as to why literature is highly transportable into human situations of trouble and distress, if only we can create the right space for it.

Notes

1. For a fuller account of the development of this experiment, see J. Billington, P. Davis, and G. Farrington, 'Reading as a Participatory Art: An Alternative Mental Health Therapy', *Journal of Arts and Communities*, 5.1 (2013), 25–40.
2. See also J. Billington, '"Reading for Life": Prison Reading Groups in Practice and Theory', *Critical Survey*, Special Issue, 'Reading and Writing in Prisons', 23.3 (2012), 67–85.
3. C. G. Jung, *The Archetypes and the Collective Unconscious* (Collected, 1959), trans. by R. F. C. Hull (Princeton University Press, 1969), p. 33.
4. C. Dickens, *Little Dorrit* (1855–1857), ed. by Harvey Peter Sucksmith (Oxford: Oxford University Press, 1999), p. 752.

5. D. Robertson, *The Philosophy of Cognitive-Behavioural Therapy (CBT): Stoic Philosophy as Rational and Cognitive Psychotherapy* (London: Karnac, 2010).
6. J. Evans, *Philosophy for Life and Other Dangerous Situations* (London: Rider, 2012).
7. D. Leader, *The New Black: Mourning, Melancholia and Depression* (London: Penguin Books, 2009), pp. 18–19.
8. B. van der Kolk, *The Body Keeps the Score: Mind, Brain and Body in the Transformation of Trauma* (London: Penguin Books, 2015), p. 349.
9. W. Davies, 'The Sonnet', *The Quarterly Review*, 134 (1873), 186–204 (p. 186).

15

Reading and Psychology I. Reading Minds: Fiction and Its Relation to the Mental Worlds of Self and Others

Rhiannon Corcoran and Keith Oatley

Introduction

One may think of mental health as the absence of such states as depression, anxiety, psychosis or addiction, but if one were to put it more positively, how would this be? Might it be living a life of purpose and interaction with others, a life of meaning? This distinction is important, not least, because it frames mental wellbeing and mental distress outside the pathological and inside the public health domain where it can exist beside less stigmatised policy concerns such as loneliness and lack of social integration as articulated in movements such as the UK's 'Campaign to End Loneliness'. Personal wellbeing can be thought of as functioning well; the wider determinants of sustainable wellbeing are currently the topic of both international

See https://www.campaigntoendloneliness.org.

R. Corcoran (✉)
Psychology and Public Mental Health, University of Liverpool, Liverpool, UK
e-mail: corcoran@liverpool.ac.uk

K. Oatley
Department of Applied Psychology and Human Development,
University of Toronto, Toronto, ON, Canada
e-mail: keith.oatley@utoronto.ca

J. Billington (ed.), *Reading and Mental Health*,
https://doi.org/10.1007/978-3-030-21762-4_15

research and policy-making. Evidence is often drawn together by national organisations such as the Office for National Statistics and the What Works Centre for Wellbeing.[1] Recent research indicates that reading, perhaps especially the reading of fiction, can be helpful in improving aspects of what is commonly referred to as psychological wellbeing where purpose and meaning in life are the aspirations, rather than mere pursuit of pleasure (this latter is often referred to as hedonic wellbeing). It has been suggested that while the pursuit of pleasure is unsustainable, draining of long-term resources of both individuals and communities, the search for meaning and purpose sustains humankind through the life-course and provides the means to resilience and growth through adversities that life delivers. This argument is famously expressed by Viktor Frankl in *Man's Search for Meaning*,[2] which chronicles the author's experience in Auschwitz, and demonstrates how his response to these experiences provided the foundation for the form of psychotherapy that he developed.

Reading and Psychological Wellbeing: Some Evidence

Let us start with two pieces of research on reading generally. First is the extended range of studies by Stanovich and West (1995)[3] on the value of reading. These researchers found that the more people read, the better are their general knowledge, their verbal skills and their ability to reason in most kinds of ways. Second is a study of 3635 participants in a health and retirement cohort by Bavishi et al. (2016).[4] After adjusting for factors that included age, sex and education, they found that, as compared with those who did not read or who read only newspapers and magazines, those who read books lived an average of 23 months longer. In a follow-up of Stanovich et al.'s study, Mar and Rain (2015)[5] found that by far the largest effect of reading on verbal skills came from reading fiction. It is likely, also, that it was the reading of books of fiction that had the largest effect on longevity, found by Bavishi et al.

Although one might have the idea that readers of fiction curl up in corners and do not interact with others, Mar et al. (2006)[6] found the opposite. As compared with people who primarily read non-fiction, they were more likely to take part in social interactions and had better social support, one of the most fundamental contributors to mental health.[7]

The Special Thing That Reading Does

The work of Tomasello and colleagues shows that we human beings are distinguished from other animals not just in our language, but in the means by which language could come about and be sustained: our ability to cooperate with each other.[8] Though human infants are much the same as chimpanzees at physical tasks such as looking to find where something was hidden, they are superior in their social skills. They can, for instance, perceive when a person has a plan, then if that plan goes wrong or cannot be accomplished, make moves to help that person in an appropriate way. In some ways, chimpanzees are on the edge of this, but on the whole, this is not an ability they have.

Tomasello (2014, 2016)[9] proposes that in our separation from our evolutionary cousins, this new trait came about in two stages. The first is that humans began to cooperate in joint activities, in which a shared goal is agreed, and is given priority over individual goals. The second is what we now generally call morality, in which members of a community agree with each other about how to act and interact, for instance, to be fair, and share with others. Influenced by the research of Tomasello and his colleagues, Oatley (2018)[10] has argued that a transformation is taking place in psychology to be not just about the individual as it has been in the past, not even about sociality, but about how people interact in their cooperative activities. We cooperate in our friendships and sexual relationships, in our roles as parents and children, in our activities with colleagues at work. All forms of culture and technology depend on cooperation. Even buying something in a shop, walking along the street or driving a car are cooperative. The deeper issues of mental health and wellbeing, then, are about how we accomplish this fundamental kind of activity, in a human way. To cooperate, one needs to understand other people. Even in conflict, one needs such understanding. As we show, below, this understanding is increased by certain kinds of reading.

Empirical Effects of Reading Fiction and Literature

In school and university education in the West, there has been a tendency to emphasise skills of science and technology and to phase out the humanities. But to do this puts the matter the wrong way round. All science and technology depend on cooperation, so understanding others comes first.

This is part of why recent findings that certain kinds of reading enable social understanding to improve are important.

Two kinds of effect have been found. The first effect is on people's social understanding. Starting with Mar et al. (2006), it was found that the more fiction a person reads and has read, in day-to-day life, the better are that person's empathy and understanding of others (theory of mind or mind-reading). The main outcome measure used in this study was the Mind in the Eyes Test (Baron-Cohen et al., 2001).[11] This effect has now been replicated by the original researchers and by others (Oatley, 2016; Mar, 2018).[12] Although in such studies other variables have been controlled for, a difficulty has been that these studies were at first correlational [i.e. a link between reading and empathy was established but not a causal one]. To deal with this limitation, experiments have been performed, starting with Kidd and Castano (2013) (see Chapter 13) in which researchers found that as compared with reading an essay, reading a fictional short story prompted an increase in empathy and social understanding.[13] Kidd and Castano's experiments were short term, with effects being measured after reading a single short story or essay. Experiments have also been performed over a week or more. Bal and Veltkamp (2013)[14] found that people who were more involved with a story they read were found to be more empathic one week later, whereas those who remained uninvolved did not. Koopman (2015)[15] also worked over a week and compared people who read three kinds of text about grief and depression. As compared with those who read a different kind of text, those who read a life narrative were more empathic and made more donations to a charity that worked with people of the kind they had read about. Koopman (2016)[16] found that those who read a text that was literary became more empathic than those who read the same text that had its literary elements removed (see also Koopman, 2018[17]). Pino and Mazza (2016)[18] asked people to read a book, which was a literary autobiographical memoir, or a work of science fiction, or a work of expository non-fiction. Those who read the literary work improved their empathy and theory-of-mind scores on a number of validated and widely used tests of these attributes. Other research on this issue includes the books of Nunning (2014)[19] and of Hakemulder et al. (2017).[20] Two meta-analyses of effects of reading fiction have been published, by Mumper and Gerrig (2017)[21] and by Dodell-Feder and Tamir (2018).[22] Both showed a small and positive effect of reading fiction on empathy and theory-of-mind.

The second effect is that reading a piece of literary art can enable a person to change some aspects of themselves, to change their personality. Djikic et al. (2009a)[23] compared effects of reading a short story by Chekhov ('The Lady with the Toy Dog', translated into English at 6367 words) and reading a control text, a non-fictionalised version of the story of the same length that contained the same information, that was at the same level of reading difficulty, and that readers found just as interesting. As compared with those who read the control text, those who read the Chekhov story changed their personality by small amounts, not all in the same direction, as occurs with persuasion, but with each person changing in her or his own individual way. The amount of the change was mediated by the amount of emotion people reported experiencing while reading the story. In a different analysis of the same experiment, Djikic et al. (2009b)[24] found a direct effect of reading on mental health. This study explored the effect of reading different texts on people who had an attachment style that predisposed them to avoid close relationships, keep to themselves and to mistrust others. The avoidantly attached individuals who read the Chekhov story were enabled to feel more emotions than the avoidantly attached people who read the control text. In a follow-up study, Djikic et al. (2012)[25] compared reading one of eight fictional stories with reading one of eight essays that were literary but that were non-fiction. The finding was that genre (fiction as compared with essay) had no effect of personality change but readers who judged the text that they read (short story or essay) to be literary changed their personality in an idiosyncratic way, in the same manner that had been found for those who read the Chekhov story as compared with its non-fictionalised control version. In a different analysis of the results of this study, an effect of fiction was, however, seen: Djikic et al. (2013)[26] found that people who read a fictional story, as compared with those who read an essay, decreased their need for cognitive closure expressed as needing to 'keep their minds closed', an effect of which has been found to inhibit creativity.

These findings, and others like them, demonstrate that literary fiction enables people to expand their minds in a way that makes them more socially adaptable and so able to make the most of opportunities and to successfully navigate the challenges of our social world in cooperative ways. This demonstrable effect could be put to use psychotherapeutically with the reading of literature potentially very valuable for people experiencing social isolation, loneliness and/or mental distress. But what will it mean for wellbeing and are there any circumstances under which such benefits could be maximised?

Reading Communities: Exploring Together and Finding Purpose

One traditional kind of reading community is that of book clubs in which people, who typically are middle-class neighbours, come together in a host's home to discuss a book they have all read as individuals.[27] This practice is enjoyed and is likely to confer benefits to wellbeing for its members.[28] A variation on this practice is a programme called Changing Lives Through Literature founded by a professor of English literature, Robert Waxler, and a judge, Robert Kane, in which people convicted of a criminal offence could be sentenced to probation rather than jail on condition that they attended a seminar on literature.[29] Provisional results of this practice are that people who took the seminar were less likely to reoffend. In Toronto, in 2000, Jo Altilia founded Literature for Life (based on a model that started in Chicago) which runs book clubs for women aged 15 or so, who have become pregnant. Reading books about circumstances similar to their own and discussing them with others can be transformative and can enable these women to understand others and themselves better and to talk about problems in a safe environment. Many participants say they read more often on their own after joining a book group. Altilia has reported that book club members 'experience an increase in perspective-taking, empathy, and problem-solving as a result of their participation'.[30]

The method of Shared Reading is somewhat different. It has been found best to start at an early age, with parents reading to their children. Reading by parents of picture books with their children, and discussing them, is not only enjoyable, but enables parents to feel closer to their children, for the children to acquire better understanding of others and to develop their language more quickly and fully. Then, they themselves come to read more. Children who read more tend to have better mental health and to be less aggressive as adolescents and adults.[31]

This idea of Shared Reading has been extended to adults in a programme pioneered by UK charity The Reader and delivered by sister organisations in Europe (see Part II, Practices) in which literature is opened up even to those whose literacy may be limited, those who feel under-confident or to those who simply do not regard themselves as readers. The model is one where literary material is read aloud, in the beginning usually by a facilitator but as the group progresses, increasingly by the individual members but without pressure to do so. The live reading is interspersed with talk and discussion focused on the book as if the book's characters are members of the group.

The unlocking of, often demanding, literary material in a social setting that is strictly non-educational brings it within the capacity of everyone to enjoy. This can have profound effects on confidence and sense of mastery as people learn that they actually can identify with fictional characters and 'get' what Jane Austen or George Eliot 'were on about'.

What happens in the best of these sessions is a process that psychologists refer to as inductive or analogical reasoning whereby the experiences of the character and their inner thoughts about these experiences as they are expressed in the book are taken in, absorbed, compared, contrasted and likened to the experiences of the reader. What's more the group setting means that the minds of all of the readers meet and are exposed in relation to the questions and issues set out in the prose or the poem. Sustained life beliefs and choices can be challenged—as prompted by the plot or the characters in the literature—or opened up and discussed within a focused and supportive environment. As such the practice has various potential benefits for the readers and, importantly, those benefits will accrue most significantly to those whose lives, for whatever reasons, have not afforded the enjoyment of literature before. As such, and in contrast to the book club, adult Shared Reading has potential to become an intervention within the public mental health sphere whose benefits are stacked in favour of those at the disadvantaged end of the health inequity spectrum.

Several chapters in Parts II, III and V of this book show the adaptability of Shared Reading to a range of mental health settings. What do we know about the measurable benefits of Shared Reading? In a study with two small groups of volunteers, half of whom came from vulnerable backgrounds, Longden et al. (2015)[32] examined this question using a cross-over design in which Shared Reading was compared to another active, arts-based non-reading intervention involving co-design solutions for the built environment. Using a detailed measure of psychological wellbeing (Ryff et al., 1989),[33] the authors found that the group scores on the psychological wellbeing pathway of Purpose in Life improved following Shared Reading in a way that was not seen in relation the built environment co-design activity which itself seemed to have more of an effect on personal growth (see Chapter 12). The quantitative findings were reinforced by qualitative data showing the contrast between the two activities in terms of emotionality, introspective load, the 'open' nature of the thinking and discussion that took place in the Shared Reading context along with its ability to trigger live induction—the use of past or others' experiences to re-think present challenges.[34]

The Mechanism of Change and Key Ingredients of Shared Reading

So far, we have argued that the reading of literature and particularly the Shared Reading of literature can affect a shift from sometimes habitual socio-emotional thinking styles to more considered and sensitive positions. What the reading of literature does is to allow the time and the intrapersonal and, in the case of Shared Reading, the interpersonal context in which to think about human challenges and complex, day-to-day human situations, a luxury that is not typically afforded by pressured, busy and demanding lives but which is invaluable as an underpinning life resource to enhance sustainable psychological wellbeing. There seem to be two key essential ingredients which support this: the language of literature and the Shared Reading context.

Many years ago one of us was involved in an early brain imaging study that examined the processing of novel metaphors where many of the stimuli were taken from literary sources (Bottini et al., 1994).[35] The findings emphasised the role of the right hemisphere in processing these figures of speech where the brain is engaged imaginatively in an 'as-if' mode of processing so that literal interpretations are forsaken in favour of a broader, associative thinking style. While metaphors and similes are not the only linguistic tools that can induce this style of thinking, they are the form most clearly associated with literary material and these vehicles serve to keep us in the literary 'as-if' mode. This mode supports new thinking and re-thinking by opening up the mind to the possibility of alternatives even as life's challenges might press into close us down. These tools, supported by thick description of scenes, circumstances and characters bring about an active reading mode that primes learning and adaptability. The idea that the literary mind may be one that is more flexible, aware of its processing and tolerant of alternative possibilities was reinforced by the findings of a much later fMRI study exploring short pieces of poetic versus prosaic text (O'Sullivan et al., 2015).[36]

When this literary language processing is undertaken with friendly and supportive others during a devoted time and within a contained and comfortable space, there is the opportunity for significant additional human value. Your mind bounces off and relays to other minds in the room.[37] Your experiences are shared and compared with others' experiences. New alternatives are explored together, bounded by the literary material. It is in such contexts that we might begin to understand the practice as a form of implicit therapy.

Reading as Mentalisation-Based Therapy

Mentalising is a term that has emerged from the literature on theory of mind. It refers to a level of awareness where there is the capacity to think about thinking. Its formulation as a therapy is aimed at helping us to consider our own and others' feeling, thoughts, beliefs and intentions in ways that can help us make sense of our own and others' actions and behaviours. As some mental health conditions seem to be characterised by difficulties in this domain and because mentalising is something we rely on every minute of every day, it has taken off, in recent years, as a particular form of psychological therapy. While evidence supports the benefits of mentalisation-based therapy particularly for borderline personality disorders,[38] formalised therapy will never be available to everyone. A voluntary Shared Reading group in which mentalisation is combined with literacy, mastery and social benefits and with the outcome of increasing sense of purpose in life must be considered as having wide potential societal benefit. While its practitioners rightly argue that this practice should never be labelled therapy, they acknowledge and record its benefits for wellbeing with one recent evaluation showing improvements in the psychological wellbeing pathway of Purpose in Life, replicating Longden et al., while also demonstrating improvement in Positive Relations with Others.[39]

Conclusion

We have argued, supported by a range of evidence, that reading literary fiction is good for us. It actively engages the brain in an imaginative 'as-if' mode that is not so readily accomplished during our everyday waking lives. When we read with others in this way, it delivers a sense of purpose and can support better interpersonal relationships. Shared Reading, used as a public health intervention, has the potential to work preferentially to benefit those most affected by health inequality, whose lives are dominated by the most important social determinants of health in ways that limit the control they can have over their own health and wellbeing. In addressing human challenges within a cooperative, safe and comfortable venture, it can make the most out of the best of our human capacities.

Notes

1. See https://www.ons.gov.uk and https://whatworkswellbeing.org.
2. V. Frankl, *Man's Search for Meaning: An Introduction to Logotherapy*, first published 1959, trans. by I. Lasch (Boston: Beacon Press, 1973).
3. K. E. Stanovich, R. F. West, and M. R. Harrison, 'Knowledge Growth and Maintenance Across the Life Span: The Role of Print Exposure', *Developmental Psychology*, 31.5 (1995), 811–26.
4. A. Bavishi, M. D. Slade, and B. R. Levy, 'A Chapter a Day: Association of Book Reading with Longevity', *Social Science and Medicine*, 164.1 (2016), 44–48.
5. R. A. Mar and M. Rain, 'Narrative Fiction and Expository Nonfiction Differentially Predict Verbal Ability', *Scientific Studies of Reading*, 19.6 (2015), 419–33.
6. R. A. Mar, K. Oatley, J. Hirsh, J. dela Paz, and J. B. Peterson, 'Bookworms Versus Nerds: Exposure to Fiction Versus Non-fiction, Divergent Associations with Social Ability, and the Simulation of Fictional Social Worlds', *Journal of Research in Personality*, 40.5 (2006), 694–712.
7. G. W. Brown and T. O. Harris, *Social Origins of Depression: A Study of Psychiatric Disorder in Women* (London: Tavistock, 1978); Z. Wang, L. Cai, J. Qian, and J. Peng, 'Social Support Moderates Stress Effects on Depression', *International Journal of Mental Health Systems* (2014), 8.
8. E. Herrmann, J. Call, M. V. Hernandez-Lloreda, B. Hare, and M. Tomasello, 'Humans Have Evolved Specialized Skills of Social Cognition: The Cultural Intelligence Hypothesis', *Science*, 317.5843 (2007), 1360–66.
9. M. Tomasello, *A Natural History of Human Thinking* (Cambridge, MA: Harvard University Press, 2014); M. Tomasello, *A Natural History of Human Morality* (Cambridge, MA: Harvard University Press, 2016).
10. K. Oatley, *Our Minds, Our Selves: A Brief History of Psychology* (Princeton, NJ: Princeton University Press, 2018).
11. S. Baron-Cohen, S. Wheelwright, J. Hill, Y. Raste, and I. Plumb, 'The "Reading the Mind in the Eyes" Test Revised Version: A Study with Normal Adults, and Adults with Asperger's Syndrome or High-Functioning Autism', *Journal of Child Psychology and Psychiatry*, 42.2 (2001), 241–51. See also Chapters 9 and 13.
12. K. Oatley, 'Fiction: Simulation of Social Worlds', *Trends in Cognitive Sciences*, 20.8 (2016), 618–28; R. A. Mar, 'Evaluating Whether Stories Can Promote Social Cognition: Introducing the Social Processes and Content Entrained by Narrative (SPaCEN) Framework', *Discourse Processes*, 55.5 (2018), 454–79.
13. D. C. Kidd and E. Castano, 'Reading Literary Fiction Improves Theory of Mind', *Science*, 342.6156 (2013), 377–80. In contrast, Panero et al. (2016)

found in several tests that this short-term effect of reading brief short stories did not replicate. (M. E. Panero, D. S. Weisberg, J. Black, T. R. Goldstein, J. L. Barnes, H. Brownell, and E. Winner, 'Does Reading a Single Passage of Literary Fiction Really Improve Theory of Mind? An Attempt at Replication', *Journal of Personality and Social Psychology*, 111.5 (2016), e46–e54.) It may be that this short-term effect was due to priming, an implicit learning or memory effect that, in the short term, makes responses to certain stimuli quicker or more likely and which is known to produce variable results. (See Chapter 13, for Kidd's discussion of the Panero et al. study.)

14. P. M. Bal and M. Veltkamp, 'How Does Fiction Reading Influence Empathy? An Experimental Investigation on the Role of Emotional Transportation', *PLoS One*, 2013, 8.1 (2013), e55341.
15. E. M. E. Koopman, 'Empathic Reactions After Reading: The Role of Genre, Personal Factors and Affective Responses', *Poetics*, 50.1 (2015), 62–79.
16. E. M. E. Koopman, 'Effects of "Literariness" on Emotions and on Empathy and Reflection After Reading', *Psychology of Aesthetics, Creativity, and the Arts*, 10.1 (2016), 82–98.
17. E. M. E. Koopman, 'Does Originality Evoke Understanding? The Relation Between Literary Reading and Empathy', *Review of General Psychology*, 22.2 (2018), 169–77.
18. M. C. Pino and M. Mazza, 'The Use of "Literary Fiction" to Promote Mentalizing Ability', *PLoS One*, 11.8 (2016), e0160254.
19. V. Nunning, *Reading Fictions, Changing Minds: The Cognitive Value of Fiction* (Heidelberg: Universitätsverlag Winter, 2014).
20. F. Hakemulder, M. Kuijpers, E. S. Tan, K. Balint, and M. M. Doicaru, eds., *Narrative Absorption* (Amsterdam: Benjamins, 2017).
21. M. J. Mumper and R. J. Gerrig, 'Leisure Reading and Social Cognition: A Meta-Analysis', *Psychology of Aesthetics, Creativity, and the Arts*, 11.1 (2017), 109–20.
22. D. Dodell-Feder and D. I. Tamir, 'Fiction Reading Has a Small Positive Impact on Social Cognition: A Meta-Analysis', *Journal of Experimental Psychology General*, 147.11 (2018), 1713–27.
23. M. Djikic, K. Oatley, S. Zoeterman, and J. Peterson, 'On Being Moved by Art: How Reading Fiction Transforms the Self' *Creativity Research Journal*, 21.1 (2009a), 24–29.
24. M. Djikic, K. Oatley, S. Zoeterman, and J. B. Peterson, 'Defenceless Against Art? Impact of Reading Fiction on Emotion in Avoidantly Attached Individuals', *Journal of Research in Personality*, 43.1 (2009b), 14–17.
25. M. Djikic, K. Oatley, and M. Carland, 'Genre or Artistic Merit: The Effect of Literature on Personality', *Scientific Study of Literature*, 2.1 (2012), 25–36.

26. M. Djikic, K. Oatley, and M. Moldoveanu, 'Opening the Closed Mind: The Effect of Exposure to Literature on the Need for Closure', *Creativity Research Journal*, 25.2 (2013), 149–54.
27. J. Hartley, *The Reading Groups Book* (Oxford: Oxford University Press, 2002); Z. Todd, 'Talking About Books: A Reading Group Study', *Psychology of Aesthetics, Creativity, and the Arts*, 2.4 (2008), 256–63; and J. Swann and Daniel Allington, 'Reading Groups and the Language of Literary Texts: A Case Study in Social Reading,' *Language and Literature*, 18.3 (2009), 247–64.
28. J. Robinson, S. Hodge, and P. Davis, 'Reading Between the Lines: The Experiences of Taking Part in a Community Reading Project', *Medical Humanities*, 33.1 (2007), 100–04; J. Shipman and L. McGrath, 'Transportations of Space, Time and Self: The Role of Reading Groups in Managing Mental Distress in the Community', *Journal of Mental Health*, 25.5 (2016), 416–21; and O. Walwyn and J. Rowley, 'The Value of Therapeutic Reading Groups Organized by Public Libraries', *Library & Information Science Research*, 33.4 (2011), 302–12.
29. J. R. Trounstine and R. Waxler, *Finding a Voice: The Practice of Changing Lives Through Literature* (Ann Arbor, MI: University of Michigan Press, 2005).
30. Quoted in K. Oatley, *Such Stuff as Dreams: The Psychology of Fiction* (Oxford: Wiley-Blackwell, 2011), p. 186.
31. See, for example, G. J. Whitehurst, D. S. Arnold, J. N. Epstein, A. L. Angell et al., 'A Picture Book Reading Intervention in Day Care and Home for Children from Low-Income Families', *Developmental Psychology*, 30.5 (1994), 679–89; J. E. Vance, G. Fernandez, and M. Biber, 'Educational Progress in a Population of Youth with Aggression and Emotional Disturbance: The Role of Risk and Protective Factors', *Journal of Emotional and Behavioral Disorders*, 6.4 (1998), 214–21; and S. H. Colmar, 'A Parent-Based Book-Reading Intervention for Disadvantaged Children with Language Difficulties', *Child Language Teaching and Therapy*, 30.1 (2014), 79–90.
32. E. Longden, P. Davis, J. Billington, S. Lampropoulou, G. Farrington, F. Magee, E. Walsh, and R. Corcoran, 'Shared Reading: Assessing the Intrinsic Value of a Literature-Based Health Intervention', *Journal of Medical Humanities*, 41.2 (2015), 113–20.
33. C. D. Ryff, 'Happiness Is Everything, or Is It? Explorations on the Meaning of Psychological Well-Being', *Journal of Personality and Social Psychology*, 57.6 (1989), 1069–81.
34. For a fuller description of the design, findings and implication of this study, see Chapters 10, 11, 12.
35. G. Bottini, R. Corcoran, R. Sterzi, E. Paulesu, P. Schenone, P, Scarpa et al., 'The Role of the Right Hemisphere in the Interpretation of Figurative

Aspects of Language: A Positron Emission Tomography Activation Study', *Brain*, 117.6 (1994), 1241–53.
36. N. O'Sullivan, P. Davis, J. Billington, V. Gonzalez-Diaz, and R. Corcoran, 'Shall I Compare Thee: The Neural Basis of Literary Awareness, and Its Benefits to Cognition', *Cortex*, 73.1 (2015), 144–57. See Chapter 13 for a fuller account of this study.
37. P. Davis, J. Billington, R. Corcoran, V. Gonzalez-Diaz, S. Lampropoulou, G. Farrington, F. Magee, and E. Walsh, *Cultural Value: Assessing the Intrinsic Value of The Reader Organization's Shared Reading Scheme* (University of Liverpool: Centre for Research into Reading, Literature and Society, 2015).
38. A. Bateman and P. Fonagy, 'Randomized Controlled Trial of Outpatient Mentalization-Based Treatment Versus Structured Clinical Management for Borderline Personality Disorder', *American Journal of Psychiatry*, 166.12 (2009), 1355–64.
39. C. Davies and R. Corcoran, 'Reading from the Same Page: An Evaluation of the Efficacy of Shared Reading to Improve Wellbeing', Unpublished Undergraduate thesis (School of Psychology, University of Liverpool, 2017).

16

Reading and Psychology II. Metaphoricity, Inexpressible Realisations and Expressive Enactment

Don Kuiken

In the earliest stages of my career, I was guided towards an expressive mode of literary reading by a mentor who was a trained actor and clinical psychologist. He taught me how to guide groups of young adults towards the use of literary narratives (e.g. *The Odyssey*, *Hamlet*) as sources of categorial interpersonal imagery. In that spirit, I remain acquainted with individuals who live the shape-shifting of Proteus and the oratory of Polonius. More recently, I began training that would prepare me to guide the literary reading of people who had experienced trauma (e.g. physical assault, traumatic loss). I studied briefly with a clinical psychologist who shared my confidence that, for example, performative reading of Raskolnikov's dream of the mare (in Dostoevsky's *Crime and Punishment*) might afford expression of the survivor shame that is at trauma's core. Throughout these ventures, the language of 'expression' in use has seemed not only coarse but disturbing. The depth of literary reading seems precariously balanced between enlivening enactment and dissociative reliving.

For some time, I have tried to articulate empirically what is expressive about literary reading. The theoretical framework I now endorse identifies (a) the evocative intimations that are the experiential origin of expression (i.e. inexpressible realisations); (b) the kind of attention that facilitates responsive 'listening' to the implicit meanings of such realisations (i.e. open

D. Kuiken (✉)
Department of Psychology, University of Alberta,
Edmonton, AB, Canada
e-mail: dkuiken@ualberta.ca

J. Billington (ed.), *Reading and Mental Health*,
https://doi.org/10.1007/978-3-030-21762-4_16

reflection); (c) a mode of explicative reflection that supports disclosure of what is implicit in inexpressible realisations (i.e. expressive enactment); and (d) the joint transformation of reader and text that occurs through expressive enactment.

Precursors to the present theoretic account have been provided by Dilthey, Collingwood, Merleau-Ponty and others within the Romantic tradition. Psychologically informed discussions have also been offered in more recent volumes by Jenefer Robinson[1] and Charles Taylor.[2] What may be distinctive here is reliance on a few selected phenomenological precepts and—where possible—empirically warranted argument.

Emotional Expression

To clarify how expression occurs, it is useful to begin by considering *emotional* expression. According to one common formulation, bodily manifestations of emotion are *ipso facto* expressions of emotion. The flicker of a smile, an inadvertent shrug or an unwittingly raised voice expresses an emotion regardless of whether the relevant bodily states and events are accessible as explicitly conscious content. According to a second formulation—a mundane version of William James' classic account[3]—bodily manifestations of emotion become accessible as *explicitly conscious* states and events that are retrospectively construed as feelings. A smile, shrug or raised voice is noticed and then retrospectively understood as a feeling ('I guess I feel bemused [indifferent, excited]'). By this account, the transition from explicitly conscious bodily manifestations of an emotion to their reflective construal as an explicitly conscious feeling is a moment of expression.

Neither of the preceding formulations addresses the tacit—and yet accessible—bodily manifestations of emotion that characterise emotional expression. According to a third formulation—a subtler neo-Jamesian account—manifestations of emotion become initially accessible as implicit bodily intimations of feeling that, through reflection, become explicitly understood as a conscious feeling. A smile, shrug or raised voice is at first accessible as a vaguely 'sensed' bodily feeling; then, during reflection, this 'sense' becomes explicitly articulated as feeling of a particular kind (bemusement [indifference, excitement]). Consistent with this account, empirical studies indicate that the bodily manifestations of emotion can precipitate explicitly conscious feelings[4] even when the feeling's underlying bodily origins are not accessible in consciousness. The transition from *pre-reflectively sensed* bodily states and events to *reflectively articulated* feeling constitutes expression.

More Than Emotion

The neo-Jamesian conception of emotional expression requires modification depending on the kind of feeling expressed. Although the term 'feeling' is used in notoriously varied ways, distinctions that are especially relevant for a theory of expression involve (a) visceral feelings, (b) emotional feelings and (c) existential feelings.

Visceral feelings provide a global sense of the homeostatic processes that facilitate organismic directedness—but not intentional aboutness.[5] Organismic directedness is evident as feelings related to basic drives, needs and motives either in the short term (e.g. tension, excitement) or long term (e.g. vitality, lethargy). Visceral feelings become evident during reflection on the body-as-a-whole, especially on a tacit complex of autonomic changes (e.g. raised heartbeat, accelerated respiration, sweating, trembling) and hormonal changes (e.g. estrogen, testosterone, norepinephrine, serotonin).[6]

In contrast, emotional and existential feelings involve bodily manifestations of intentionality (referential 'aboutness'). That is, even though regularly intertwined with the directedness of visceral feeling, both become evident during reflection on *tacitly intentional* acts (e.g. orienting postural adjustments, manipulative movements, communicative gestures, reaching-touching-grasping). And yet, an emotional feeling involves a relatively short-term intentional relation with (e.g. felt fear *of…*) *a specific object* (e.g. the cougar in my backyard); an existential feeling involves a long-term intentional relation with (e.g. estrangement *from…*) *a global situation* (e.g. everyone around me).[7]

Because of their shared reliance on tacitly intentional acts—and despite their contrasting (specific or global) intentional objects—emotional feelings and existential feelings regularly co-occur. Their influence on each other is mutual. On the one hand, existential feelings (e.g. a global sense of estrangement) often are enabling conditions for certain categories of emotional feeling (e.g. pangs of sadness); that is, existential feelings are selectively attuned to specific situations—or aspects of situations—that involve bodily congruent emotional feelings. On the other hand, reflection on specific emotional feelings (e.g. specific moments of fear) often migrates towards global existential feelings (e.g. pervasive dread). In fact, when they do *not* do so (e.g. during reflection on fearful emotional feelings in the aftermath of traumatic events), efforts towards their expression are often intense but also fixed, repetitive and ruminative.[8]

Self-Finding

Perhaps especially because of the potential for migration from emotional to existential feelings, some investigators[9] have been especially determined to clarify a foundational mode of self-finding that Heidegger (1953/1996) called *Befindlichkeit*. Besides involving a long-term relation with a global situation, *Befindlichkeit* is an implicit mode of intentionality that integrates (a) a mood (*Stimmung*); (b) an understanding (*Verstehen*); and (c) the potential for speaking (*Rede*). In this formulation, an implicitly conscious mood is not just a diffuse long-lasting feeling (e.g. a bad mood); instead, it is a tacit affective *attunement* guided by an equally tacit understanding that seems sayable but not yet said.[10]

Two aspects of this formulation are pivotal. First, that language is implicitly involved in existential feelings broadens the relevant bodily manifestations to include feeling-specific bodily manifestations of language use. There is now considerable evidence that a broad range of linguistic representations involves re-activation of the multi-modal sensorimotor cortical regions that overlap with (or are adjacent to) regions activated during first-hand bodily engagement with the represented object.[11] These multi-modal sensorimotor aspects of linguistic representation are tacitly accessible even when their words are not explicitly spoken. This possibility clarifies why, during explication of an emotional or existential feeling, some words or phrases just feel 'right' or feel 'wrong'. Feelings of rightness or wrongness during reflection depend upon the tacit activation of relevant embodied language.

Second, existential feelings are fundamentally temporal; roughly, they involve integration of a retained past, a present impression and a projected future. Such temporal integrations may constitute either brief feelings (e.g. a fleeting moment of fear) or prolonged feelings (a lengthy period of grief), and the global character of existential feelings suggests that they involve the latter. So, rather than integration of the temporal flux of local impressions that comprise an *enduring entity* (e.g. the streaming system of perspectives that coherently constitute perception of a tree; the streaming system of perspectives that coherently constitute a moment of fear), existential feelings require integration of the temporal flux of impressions, memories, feelings, judgements and anticipations that comprise what Goldie has called a *perduring process* (e.g. the streaming system of heterogeneous moments that coherently constitute 'taking a vacation'; the streaming system of heterogeneous moments that coherently constitute 'living through grief').[12]

More Than Narrative

Goldie (2012) suggested that perduring feelings are accessible as narratives, especially as narratives that facilitate juxtaposition of the narrator's external perspective on the narrated world and a character's internal perspective on the narrated world. Goldie emphasises the 'ironic' character of these perspectival juxtapositions. However, an alternative view is that perduring feelings are implicitly structured as a stream of heterogeneous moments that are *not quite* narratives[13] and *more like* the stream of heterogeneous moments that constitute the 'involuntary poetry' of dreams.[14] This approach shifts the emphasis from irony to metaphor; the understandings that implicitly structure existential feelings are metaphoric structures—in the same way that dreams are metaphoric structures.

In dreams, such metaphoricity functions at two levels. The first involves noun-noun compounds (B-*ish* A) that are implicitly nominal metaphors (A *is a* B). For example, a child who '...dreamed [she] was in [a] bathtub asleep'[15] may have dreamed a compound bed(ish)-bathtub that was implicitly a nominal metaphor ('My bathtub *is* a bed'). The fusions described in Freud's (1900/1953) classic account of condensation (especially 'collective images') take this form—and their prevalence has been substantiated by empirical studies of dream anomalies.[16] At a higher level of syntactic complexity, dream fusions involve entire episodes (roughly, a setting, an initiating event, a character action and action consequences). Available evidence indicates that dreams regularly place familiar people or objects in unfamiliar settings[17] as though the fusion of two discontinuous narrative episodes (B-*ish* A) is implicitly metaphoric (episode A *is* episode B).

The present proposal is that the tacit structure of existential feelings is dream-like in this way. That is, the expression of existential feelings is grounded in sensed fusions of implicitly metaphoric noun-noun and episode-episode semantic structures. To extend this analogy, intimations of existential feeling are analogous to content-less dream recall, i.e. awakening from sleep, being aware of having dreamed, but not remembering dream content.[18] Empirical studies indicate that such 'unremembered' dreams nonetheless influence post-awakening thoughts and feelings.[19] Just as these forms of metaphoric fusion are such stuff as the 'unremembered' intimations of dream feelings are made on, they are also such stuff as the 'unremembered' intimations of existential feeling are reflectively made on.[20]

Direct Reference and Open Reflection

During literary reading, the expression of existential feeling *becomes possible* when textual metaphoric 'fusions' elicit (and enfold) the dreamy metaphoric 'fusions' of the reader's existential feelings. The subsequent transition from passively elicited metaphoric structures to evocative intimations involves *direct reference*.[21] Direct reference is an attentional gesture oriented towards a bodily 'present' (but conceptually tacit) sense of 'the same' within the unspoken fusions that comprise this complex structure. Direct reference to this sense of 'the same' produces an evocative intimation, an *inexpressible realisation*, that motivates subsequent (and potentially expressive) explication of this sensed 'sameness'.[22]

In Collingwood's oft-cited portrayal of this referential turn,[23] the transition from passive elicitation to reflective explication *begins* by becoming '… conscious of having an emotion but not conscious of what that emotion is'. Lyotard goes further when he identifies an initial reflective turn towards:

> The unstable state and instant of language wherein something which must be able to be put into phrases cannot yet be. This state includes *silence*, which is a negative phrase, but it also calls upon phrases which are in principle possible. This state is signaled by what one ordinarily calls a *feeling*: 'One cannot find the words,' etc. A lot of searching must be done to find new rules for forming and linking phrases that are able to express the differend disclosed by the feeling. (my italics)[24]

Within the silence of a feeling, finding what might be but has not been said resembles listening closely within acoustic silence for the farthest sound. Such listening is not active search for particular sounds but rather receptive openness to the coming and going of sounds within silence. Similarly, within the silence of a feeling, listening is not active search for particular words or phrases but rather the onset of receptive openness to the coming and going of words that seem to 'come from' the feeling. The more effectively silence is realised, the more noticeable previously unheard sounds (or words) become. Sounds (or words) come from and return to silence through time; their waxing and waning embody and make salient the passage of time.[25]

During reading, receptive attunement within the silence of existential feeling is two-sided. On the one hand, it involves sustained concentration (i.e. persistent attention to feeling-relevant words or phrases and resistance to distraction by feeling-irrelevant words or phrases). On the other hand, it also involves attentional reorienting (i.e. persistent readiness to disengage from currently focal feeling-relevant words or phrases and redirect attention to *unexpected* feeling-relevant words or phrases).[26] Thus, the integration of sustained concentration and sustained readiness to reorient does not facilitate 'task switching' but rather 'salience monitoring'. While the former has been implicated in the evaluation of creative ideas, the latter has been implicated in their generation.[27]

The integrated function of sustained concentration and readiness to shift attention defines the open reflection that supports subsequent explication.[28] While sustained concentration has been addressed in studies of deeply engaged reading,[29] sustained readiness to shift attention has not. However, a recently developed instrument, the Absorption-like States Questionnaire (Kuiken and Douglas, 2017), includes scales that measure both sustained concentration (resisting personal distraction, resisting task-related distraction) and attentional reorienting (shift to narrative time, altered sense of time). Recent studies (Kuiken and Douglas, 2017, 2018) indicate that a composite of these scales predicts inexpressible realisations, i.e. vaguely sensed understandings that exceed what can be said (e.g. 'I began to understand something that could not be put into words') (Kuiken, Campbell, and Sopčák, 2012).

Expressive Explication

When direct reference (open reflection) changes tacit and passively elicited metaphoric structures to evocative intimations, the result is that their explication potentially provides disclosure of the *emergent meaning* of those metaphoric structures. However, fraught with difficulty the conception of emergent meaning may be, *some* empirical clarity is possible. The emergent meaning of a metaphoric representation traditionally refers to the disclosure of category attributes that were not previously considered attributes of either the metaphoric vehicle or topic considered in isolation.[30] Some empirical studies of such metaphorically generated emergent meaning in this sense are available for simple nominal metaphors.[31]

In addition, there have been attempts to articulate empirically the *kind of reflection* that follows direct reference—and potentially involves disclosure of the emergent meaning of 'poetic' metaphors. Often the relevant mode of reflection is understood as inferential interpretation, i.e. identification of a plausible cause or a projected outcome of the object of direct reference (e.g. 'In reaction to your ironic remark, I feel bemused'; 'My bemusement with your remark strengthens my affection for you'). This explanatory mode of reflection contrasts with reflective explication of the particular kind of feeling that is present in experience (e.g. identifying what it is like to feel bemused). Roughly, reflective—and potentially expressive—explication addresses 'how' (rather than 'why') a feeling presents itself in experience (e.g. 'I feel bemused—but not disturbed—by your irony').

The theoretical contrast between explanatory and explicative reflection has been substantiated empirically,[32] but its articulation in phenomenological philosophy is perhaps more precise. Specifically, Husserl's (1973) account of explanatory reflection posits an implicit (pre-reflective) 'unity of presence' (simultaneous 'retention' in awareness of multiple intentional objects) as the foundation for articulating the non-categorial 'relations' (e.g. larger or smaller, before or after, enable or cause) that constitute 'situations'.[33] In contrast, his account of explicative reflection also posits an implicit (pre-reflective) 'unity of presence' but, in this case, as the foundation for articulating 'relations of likeness and similarity' (p. 183).

A reader's 'choice' between explanatory and explicative modes of reflection occurs repeatedly during reading. As a common example, one relevant choice point is a moment of emotional contagion. Emotional contagion occurs when involuntary imitation of another's bodily manifestations of emotion (e.g. fist clenching while viewing another in a fist fight) is followed by explicit awareness of such feeling in oneself (e.g. an acknowledged hint in oneself of the other's anger). During literary reading, emotional contagion can occur when the text elicits in the reader involuntary imitation of the bodily manifestations of the emotions of text personae. So, a reader may find herself 'short of breath' while reading the last scene from Poe's *The Tell-tale Heart* and immediately recognise that 'this' is an involuntary echo of the narrator's shortness of breath. This moment of unarticulated resonance is a choice point that may lead either towards explanatory attributions (e.g. 'Oh, my feeling is a response to the narrator's feelings about confinement') or towards explicative construal of the kind of feeling that is 'given' (e.g. 'Oh, a pause; a hint of arrest; that is what it is like when you feel like this about confinement').[34]

Besides open reflection, the Absorption-like States Questionnaire (Kuiken and Douglas, 2017) assesses these two modes of reflective engagement: integrative comprehension and expressive enactment. Integrative comprehension involves explanatory reflection, i.e. interpretation of the causal relations, background states (emotions, attitudes), author motives, etc. (p. 375) that comprise a coherent 'situation model'.[35] In contrast, expressive enactment involves reflective explication of a vaguely sensed textual object, iterative re-expression of what that vaguely sensed object 'is like', and perhaps category-shifting 'realization' of the kind of object it is.[36] Kuiken and Douglas (2017, 2018) found that, integrative comprehension distinctively mediates the effects of open reflection on the comprehension of *conventional nonliterary* metaphors (e.g. 'Genes are blueprints'). In contrast, expressive enactment distinctively mediates the effects of open reflection on the comprehension of *unconventional literary metaphors* (e.g. 'Death is a fat fly'). Evidence that these effects on the comprehension of unconventional literary metaphors involve emergent meanings is indirect; clarification of that hypothesis remains an important research objective.

Movingly Sublime Disclosure

One reason it remains plausible that expressive enactment culminates in disclosure of the emergent meaning of 'poetic' metaphoric structures is that it facilitates the self-reported transformation of existential feelings. Gendlin calls the disclosive transition from an inexpressible realisation to a moving self-relevant disclosure a *felt shift*.[37] A felt shift marks the transition from a vaguely realised feeling to a compellingly realised felt understanding; it is a moment that moves from words that seem not to 'fit' to words that compellingly 'fit' an existential feeling.

Kuiken and Douglas (2017, 2018) found that reflectively open expressive enactment (but not reflectively open integrative comprehension) predicted not only inexpressible realisations and enhanced comprehension of poetic metaphors, but also sublime disquietude (Kuiken, Campbell, and Sopčák, 2012). Sublime disquietude is defined as the *interactive combination* of (a) inexpressible realisations (i.e. understandings that cannot be put into words), (b) self-perceptual depth (sensitivity to aspects of life usually ignored, reconsidered personal commitments) and (c) acute disquietude (feeling deeply disturbed or profoundly ill at ease). Moreover, Kuiken and Douglas (2017, 2018) found that reflectively open expressive enactment (but not reflectively open integrative comprehension) predicted 'being moved' (e.g. moved to tears).[38]

The metaphoric grounding of expressive enactment—and the movingly sublime disquietude it supports—entails a subtle epistemic 'risk'. In studies of reflective openness, this epistemic risk is warily addressed by some investigators as potential 'dissociation'[39] and sympathetically addressed by others as potential 'self-transcendence'.[40] The epistemic risk in expressive enactment is made salient by research indicating that reflective expression leads to sublime disquietude among readers reporting traumatic and separation distress, especially among those reporting dissociation.[41] Perhaps reflectively open and expressively engaged literary reading entails implicit feelings and metaphoric disclosures that are epistemically risky reminders of emotionally significant 'endings'.[42] For these reasons, the expressive power of literary reading still seems to me precariously balanced between enlivening and expressive enactment and dissociative and repetitive reliving of those metaphoric structures.

Notes

1. J. Robinson, *Deeper Than Reason: Emotion and Its Role in Literature, Music, and Art* (Oxford, New York: Oxford University Press, 2005).
2. C. Taylor, *The Language Animal: The Full Shape of the Human Linguistic Capacity* (Cambridge, MA: Belknap Press of Harvard University Press, 2016).
3. William James, *The Principles of Psychology* (1890), 2 vols. (Cambridge, MA: Harvard University Press, 1983), vol. 2, Chapter 25.
4. T. Fuchs and S. C. Koch, 'Embodied Affectivity: On Moving and Being Moved', *Frontiers in Psychology*, 6.5 (2014), 508.
5. P. Goldie, 'Emotions, Feelings and Intentionality', *Phenomenology and the Cognitive Sciences*, 1.3 (2002), 235–54.
6. A. R. Damasio, *The Feeling of What Happens: Body and Emotion in the Making of Consciousness* (London: Vintage, 2000).
7. M. Ratcliffe, 'The Feeling of Being', *Journal of Consciousness Studies*, 12.8–10 (2005), 43–60.
8. C. McCarroll, *Remembering from the Outside: Personal Memory and the Perspectival Mind* (Oxford: Oxford University Press, 2018).
9. E. T. Gendlin, 'Heidegger and the Philosophy of Psychology', *Review of Existential Psychology and Psychiatry*, 16.1–3 (1978), 43–71; Ratcliffe (2005).
10. M. Ratcliffe, 'Why Mood Matters', in *The Cambridge Companion to Heidegger's 'Being and Time'*, ed. by M. A. Wrathall (Cambridge: Cambridge University Press, 2013), pp. 157–76.
11. L. Meteyard, S. R. Cuadrado, B. Bahrami, and G. Vigliocco, 'Coming of Age: A Review of Embodiment and the Neuroscience of Semantics', *Cortex*, 48.7 (2012), 788–804.
12. P. Goldie, *The Mess Inside: Narrative, Emotion, and the Mind* (Oxford: Oxford University Press, 2012).
13. T. Nielsen, D. Kuiken, R. Hoffmann, and A. Moffitt, 'REM and NREM Sleep Mentation Differences: A Question of Story Structure?' *Sleep and Hypnosis*, 3.1 (2001), 9–17.

14. B. O. States, *Seeing in the Dark: Reflections on Dreams and Dreaming* (New Haven: Yale University Press, 1997), Chapter 8.
15. D. Foulkes, *Children's Dreaming and the Development of Consciousness* (Cambridge, MA: Harvard University Press, 1999).
16. For example: A. Revonsuo and K. Tarkko, '"Binding in Dreams": The Bizarreness of Dream Images and the Unity of Consciousness', *Journal of Consciousness Studies*, 9.7 (2002), 3–24.
17. E. Dorus, W. Dorus, and A. Rechtschaffen, 'The Incidence of Novelty in Dreams', *Archives of General Psychiatry*, 25.4 (1971), 364–68.
18. D. B. Cohen, 'Presleep Mood and Dream Recall', *Journal of Abnormal Psychology*, 83.1 (1974), 45–51.
19. D. Kuiken, A. Porthukaran, K. A. Albrecht, S, Douglas, and M. Cook, 'Metaphoric and Associative Aftereffects of Impactful Dreams', *Dreaming*, 28.1 (2018), 59–83 (pp. 63–64).
20. D. Kuiken, 'A Theory of Expressive Reading', in *Directions in Empirical Literary Studies: Essays in Honor of Willie van Peer*, ed. by S. Zyngier, M. Bortolussi, A. Chesnokova, and J. Auracher (Amsterdam: John Benjamins Publishing Company, 2008), pp. 49–68; D. Kuiken and S. Douglas, 'Living Metaphor as the Site of Bidirectional Literary Engagement', *Scientific Study of Literature*, 8.1 (2018), 47–76.
21. E. T. Gendlin, *Experiencing and the Creation of Meaning: A Philosophical and Psychological Approach to the Subjective* (Evanston, IL: Northwestern University Press, 1962/1997).
22. D. Kuiken, P. Campbell, and P. Sopčák, 'The Experiencing Questionnaire: Locating Exceptional Reading Moments', *Scientific Study of Literature*, 2.2 (2012), 243–72; D. Kuiken and S. Douglas, 'Forms of Absorption That Facilitate the Aesthetic and Explanatory Effects of Literary Reading', in *Narrative Absorption*, ed. by F. Hakemulder, M. M. Kuijpers, E. S. Tan, K. Bálint, and M. M. Doicaru (Amsterdam: John Benjamins Publishing Company, 2017), vol. 27, pp. 217–49.
23. R. G. Collingwood, *The Principles of Art* (New York: Oxford University Press, 1958), p. 27.
24. J.-F. Lyotard, *The Differend: Phrases in Dispute* (Minneapolis: University of Minnesota Press, 1988), p. 13.
25. D. Ihde, *Listening and Voice: Phenomenologies of Sound*, 2nd ed. (Albany: State University of New York Press, 2007), p. 111.
26. S. E. Petersen and M. I. Posner, 'The Attention System of the Human Brain: 20 Years After', *Annual Review of Neuroscience*, 35.1 (2012), 73–89.
27. M. Ellamil, C. Dobson, M. Beeman, and K. Christoff, 'Evaluative and Generative Modes of Thought During the Creative Process', *Neuroimage*, 59.2 (2012), 1783–94.
28. E. Koopman and F. Hakemulder similarly suggest that the 'slowing down of readers' perceptions of the fictional world' creates moments of 'stillness'

['Effects of Literature on Empathy and Self-Reflection: A Theoretical-Empirical Framework', *Journal of Literary Theory*, 9.1 (2015), 79–111]. However, their unidimensional conception of stillness differs from the *integrated* function of sustained concentration and readiness to reorient attention proposed here.

29. For example: R. Busselle and H. Bilandzic, 'Measuring Narrative Engagement', *Media Psychology*, 12.4 (2009), 321–47; M. M. Kuijpers, F. Hakemulder, E. S. Tan, and M. M. Doicaru, 'Exploring Absorbing Reading Experiences: Developing and Validating a Self-Report Scale to Measure Story World Absorption', *Scientific Study of Literature*, 4.1 (2014), 89–122.
30. Compare, C. Cazeaux, *Metaphor and Continental Philosophy: From Kant to Derrida* (New York: Routledge, 2007).
31. For example: A. H. Becker, 'Emergent and Common Features Influence Metaphor Interpretation', *Metaphor and Symbol*, 12.4 (1997), 243–59; Z. Estes and T. B. Ward, 'The Emergence of Novel Attributes in Concept Modification', *Creativity Research Journal*, 14.2 (2002), 149–56; A. Terai and R. L. Goldstone, 'An Experimental Examination of Emergent Features in Metaphor Interpretation Using Semantic Priming Effects', *Proceedings of the Thirty-Fourth Annual Conference of the Cognitive Science Society*, 2012, pp. 2399–404; R. Tourangeau and L. Rips, 'Interpreting and Evaluating Metaphors', *Journal of Memory and Language*, 30.4 (1991), 452–72.
32. R. P. Spunt and R. Adolphs, 'Validating the Why/How Contrast for Functional MRI Studies of Theory of Mind', *NeuroImage*, 99 (2014), 301–11; R. P. Spunt and M. D. Lieberman, 'Dissociating Modality-Specific and Supramodal Neural Systems for Action Understanding', *Journal of Neuroscience*, 32.10 (2012), 3575–83.
33. E. Husserl, *Experience and Judgment: Investigations in a Genealogy of Logic*, trans. by L. Landgrebe (Evanston: Northwestern University Press, 1973), p. 248ff.
34. This generalizing form of second person pronoun use may refer to the narrator, the reader, and unspecified 'others'. This locution has been observed in recent studies of the metaphoric kind of identification that is evident during expressive literary reading (D. Kuiken, D. S. Miall, and S. Sikora, 'Forms of Self-Implication in Literary Reading', *Poetics Today*, 25.2 (2004), 171–203; D. Kuiken, D. S. Miall, and S. Sikora, 'Expressive Reading: A Phenomenological Study of Readers' Experience of Coleridge's *The Rime of the Ancient Mariner*', *Psychology of Aesthetics, Creativity and the Arts*, 5.3 (2011), 258–68).
35. A. C. Graesser, M. Singer, and T. Trabasso, 'Constructing Inferences During Narrative Text Comprehension', *Psychological Review*, 94.101 (1994), 371–95; R. A. Zwaan, 'Situation Models: The Mental Leap into Imagined Worlds', *Current Directions in Psychological Science*, 8 1 (1999), 15–18.
36. R. Ingarden, 'Aesthetic Experience and Aesthetic Object', *Philosophy and Phenomenological Research*, 21.3 (1961), 289–313; M. A. Natanson,

The Erotic Bird: Phenomenology in Literature (Princeton, NJ: Princeton University Press, 1998).

37. E. T. Gendlin, *Focusing-Oriented Psychotherapy: A Manual of the Experiential Method* (New York: Guilford Press, 1998).
38. W. Menninghaus, V. Wagner, J. Hanich, E. Wassiliwizky, M. Kuehnast, and T. Jacobsen, 'Towards a Psychological Construct of Being Moved', *PloS One*, 10.6 (2015), e0128451.
39. For example: D. Simeon, T. Giesbrecht, M. Knutelska, R. J. Smith, and L. M. Smith, 'Alexithymia, Absorption, and Cognitive Failures in Depersonalization Disorder: A Comparison to Posttraumatic Stress Disorder and Healthy Volunteers', *The Journal of Nervous and Mental Disease*, 197.7 (2009), 492–98.
40. E. Cardeña and D. B. Terhune, 'Hypnotizability, Personality Traits, and the Propensity to Experience Alterations of Consciousness', *Psychology of Consciousness: Theory, Research, and Practice*, 1.3 (2014), 292–307.
41. D. Kuiken and R. Sharma, 'Effects of Loss and Trauma on Sublime Disquietude During Literary Reading', *Scientific Study of Literature*, 3.2 (2013), 240–65; S. Sikora, D. Kuiken, and D. S. Miall, 'An Uncommon Resonance: The Influence of Loss on Expressive Reading', *Empirical Studies of the Arts*, 28.2 (2010), 135–53.
42. M. Heidegger, *Being and Time*, trans. by J. Stambaugh (Albany, NY: State University of New York Press, 1953/1996).

17

Reading and Psychoanalysis
Adam Phillips in interview with Philip Davis

Adam Phillips and Philip Davis

The interview was conducted in January 2018 at Adam Phillips's office and consulting room in Notting Hill, London, in a room lined with bookshelves; volumes of novels and poetry also lying in scattered piles on the floor. The psychoanalyst and essay writer likes to have his books around him. As he wrote in the Preface to Promises, Promises (2000) in favour of what he calls a 'literary' psychoanalysis: 'I think that reading what used to be called Literature is probably a better preparation for the practice of psychoanalysis than the reading of anything else'.[1]

I started by going back to an interview Adam Phillips gave me for The Reader magazine, summer 2008.[2] *There he had ended by saying that he did not have or believe in any comprehensive theory of human psychology: all he had were sentences, in which one might feel something suddenly opening up, and his uncertain sense of the link between them. Now ten years later, for all his continuing commitment to the openness of possibilities, I say to him I have a much greater sense of the essays in his books being connected chapters in a more urgent endeavour, rather than separate entities as they were, often playfully, in the early volumes. Did he agree that he had committed himself to more of a project now?*

A. Phillips
Department of English, University of York, York, UK

P. Davis (✉)
Centre for Research into Reading, Literature and Society,
University of Liverpool, Liverpool, UK
e-mail: phildav@liverpool.ac.uk

J. Billington (ed.), *Reading and Mental Health*,
https://doi.org/10.1007/978-3-030-21762-4_17

AP: Absolutely yes.

PD: Could you say what that project is? And say how it included both the reading of literature and the practice of psychoanalysis?

AP: I don't think I can say what the project is, and I don't mean that in some mystical or new-age way. Because it partly depends on my not knowing what it is; but that it be worked out through the doing of it. In retrospect, as a younger man I was interested in openness and pluralism. I was brought up to be a hippy—I *am* in a sense still a hippy—so there was an ethos of pluralistic liberalism that I loved, liked and wanted to promote, and was implicit in what I wrote.

Now I think there is a real question about what it is that one wants to be open to and what it is one wants to be closed to. And how one actually works out what is the right and good and best thing to do. We are misleadingly told on the one hand there is a multiplicity, diversity and extraordinary variety of choices and possibilities in our society, but really there is just one game in town—neo-liberal economics, only profiteering. This idea that we have an endlessly plural culture is a complete myth: so working out what could be our real individual choices is more urgent now. When in the early days I was a child psychotherapist I would have said to you, 'I have no interest in helping people, I want to have really interesting and enlivening conversations'—which was at least a better story than being 'saintly'. I would still say that about the conversations, but now I want to help people. I think we should do what we can for each other, and I think really there is no point in anything else other than kindness.

PD: So what are you now more vehemently closed to?

AP: All the projects that are to do with humiliating, diminishing and dominating other people. I don't mean by this I want to promote some pastoral view where everybody is lovely to everybody, because that seems to me inconceivable. But I do want an ethos which is at least educated about the possibility of non-exploitation, non-humiliating relationships. In other words, in psychoanalytic language, I think the basic model which is being given us, if there is an 'us', is that relations between the sexes and within the sexes are fundamentally sado-masochistic: that one person has to be diminished in order for another to feel strong; and there is in this a hatred of dependence and of vulnerability. These so-called dependencies and vulnerabilities are things I want to give an account of, so that we are not phobic about them or need to attack them.

PD: And what deadens or bores you?

AP: There are ways of speaking and ways of reading that make me bored: a monotonous tone in relation to emotionality, a lack of presence, an unwillingness to engage, and a sort of hostility—involving deadening attacks on the relationship.

PD: At the end of an essay on T. S. Eliot, in *In Writing* (2016), you say, 'The soul of man under psychoanalysis is nothing more and nothing less than the relationship between the sexes, about what it is to live with nothing to love and hate but each other'.[3] Nothing but that, but us, now, in the absence of God.

AP: I wouldn't want to limit it to heterosexuality, or to relationships that are actually sexualized. But bafflement is integral to a post-religious life or world: we don't know what we are doing and nobody can tell us. What we do 'know' are quasi-biological facts, and maybe Darwinian facts. We could for example think one of the things we are doing is surviving and if we survive sufficiently, reproducing. But someone could come along and say I don't want to survive, and reproduction is not integral to my relations. The modern question is going to be: where is my real enjoyment, where are the pleasures which are sufficiently sustaining, so that I no longer ask the question what am I doing or what is the point of this.

PD: You are suspicious of survival merely by adaptation, by normalizing. In the T. S. Eliot essay, you re-phrase a warning of his: 'It is human, when we do not understand ourselves, and cannot ignore ourselves, to exert an unconscious pressure on ourselves to turn us into something that we *can* understand'. Then you say this, against that forced understanding, against that pressure to make ourselves too apparently familiar, too literal and too normalized: 'People come for psychoanalysis because there is something about themselves that baffles them and that they cannot ignore' (*In Writing*, p. 246).

AP: Donald Winnicott's word 'compliance' is really useful here, as in contrast to what he calls real 'aliveness'.[4] It has always been a critique of psychoanalysis: what are analysts doing if they are helping people to adapt to a culture that is bad for them. The alternative to adaptation—to a compliance with false social promises, with a false self—is thinking I could create a world that was a better environment to live in. How revisionary can I be?

I would want to talk of a false self—but not of a true self. Winnicott's psychoanalytic model comes from Romanticism: that acorns become oak trees; that we have something in ourselves that we can more or less realize, depending on the quality of the environment. Probably it is better to talk of preferred selves, preferred versions. If there *is* evidence of a true self, the evidence would be a feeling of aliveness and an absence of the feeling of futility and rage. But I prefer the idea there isn't an essential self instead, what John Stuart Mill calls 'experiments in living'.[5] It is like this in my writing or sometimes my speaking: the words occur to me, there is nothing, and then there is something. Words are that kind of thing. Something I am increasingly struck with, is that there is a long period in one's earlier life when one listens to language without understanding it: language comes very late in the day, and that matters.

PD: So many things here about being something other than easily intelligible or compliant … But in these post-religious 'experiments' in attempted freedom, the pragmatic philosophy of William James has become increasingly important to you in this project?

AP: Yes, in the idea of finding enough to be going on with, enough to be going on from. James is by far a greater psychologist even than Freud. To me James is *It*. James has a way of writing that makes psychology seem like something.

PD: He calls it Pragmatism which means: finding thoughts, feelings, ideas that are not absolute truths or complete theories but enough to ride upon, to carry one forward, because of the sudden excitement they arouse, bursting conventional frameworks. One may not know where these thoughts are coming from or leading to, but they make one feel more alive. Like a sudden line of poetry.

That is, I think, why you say psychoanalysis is or should be more to do with inspiration than with set knowledge or conclusive understanding. And that inspiration is also one of the things you read for, reading literature for its experiments in living. It means help towards something that gives you the feel of a possible new future, instead of thoughts going round and round in fixed or addictive circles. You hate all that, don't you, the obsessively repetitive super-ego, the guilt, the depression, the toxic diminishment of being that suffering causes.

AP: Agreed. Guilt, for instance, should be a servant, not a master. And it is a great thing when Ursula says in D. H. Lawrence's *Women in Love*, 'It is an indignity to be unhappy'.[6]

PD: But in the attempt to get away from repeating the past, the future is a funny thing though isn't it? Because by definition the future does not exist, it is always not-yet existent, except as a drive for life that should be more than just hope. In *Side-Effects* (2006) you say, 'We have to make up the future until we get there'.[7] Well, it is as if your best reading is for you about the creation of the future from the past, whereas some authors might only make you regress. And the difference between the future and the past is the difference between light and dark.

AP: It is only worth having a past if you have a future—I can't see the point of it otherwise.

PD: You wrote once in *Side Effects* that the reading of literature is like psychoanalysis in offering a chance to think the strangeness of one's own thoughts: 'a leap into the dark, a place where people can hear what they really think and want, like being told a secret about oneself that someone else has made' (Preface to *Side Effects*). But sometimes, and perhaps more recently now, you seem also to suggest that psychoanalysis may only do precisely what T.S. Eliot warned against: over-rationalise, over-explain, making ourselves too familiar. Could reading be better for you than psychoanalysis then?

AP: It could be, yes. But I think you are describing for me what is a *complementary* difference. Because psychoanalysis does both things: the question about it has always been—is it about insight into yourself or is it about experience? are you learning more about yourself or are you being as it were freed to experience yourself in different ways? They are not incompatible but they can be.

One thing psychoanalysis usefully does is make intelligible things that were previously troubling, puzzling and so on—an intelligibility project; but there is another project which I think I am more interested in, which is one's freedom *not* to be immediately intelligible, in the service of a different kind of evocation or experience. The obvious analogy is listening to music: I don't need to 'get it' but I do need an experience. I don't want to idealise over-literal understanding as the only game in town.

PD: But in reaction, one can over-emphasise the elusive?

AP: That is true. It can become a mystification, a fetish or false lure. That's why you need both sides to work between. And I think literature and psychoanalysis are for me, equally, both incommensurate and overlapping. I move between them, as well as between insight and experience within them. I have never thought there were two things—like art and life, as though they were two realms—but a continuum.

PD: Say more then about what reading literature does for you and your project; what poetry, say, does beyond explanation.

AP: I remember much more the *experience* of reading a book than the book itself, much more what I *felt* than the details of the work. It is like something Wordsworth describes in *The Prelude*:

… but that the soul,
Remembering how she felt, but what she felt
Remembering not, retains an obscure sense
Of possible sublimity, whereto
With growing faculties she doth aspire,
With faculties still growing, feeling still
That whatsoever point they gain, they yet
Have something to pursue[8]

Remembering not *what* exactly, but *how* you felt. It involves what T. S. Eliot says about poetry being 'a form of punctuation',[9] no longer straightforward, in its shifting rhythms and lines of thought. Or like Pater—when he uses a language of celebration which is so under-rated as compared to our more usual language of criticism: 'What is the peculiar sensation, what is the peculiar quality of pleasure, which this work has the property of exciting in us, and which we cannot get elsewhere?'[10] I read *The Winter's Tale* last week: I had read it before but it was *like* reading a new book. I had the experience of thinking: This is the most interesting book I have ever read—which I frequently have. There is enough to think about here for the rest of your life.

PD: But you do then fasten upon startling lines, sudden sentences, and work your essays and thoughts around quotations that are more than just illustrative.

AP: Quotations, yes: you could think they are like seedlings. They are a bit like dreams, they become organizers of experiences, or triggers or provocations. I am reading for the quotations, partly. And why? Because they are like transformative objects, they have an effect on me. Always there is the question anywhere: which bits are they that work for you …

PD: There is something in the writings of the psycho-analyst Marion Milner which we both know: when she speaks of most wanting to read only those books that 'keep her heart up'.[11]

AP: I had a friend at school who used to say that he could only read books that had happy endings. And I would of course reply: Come on, that isn't how life is. But I now think that what he meant was this, at least as I re-describe it for myself. Though life is supposed to be worth living, it is always potentially true that there could be something really unbearable about the whole thing. In the face of that, I want art that is not *only* inspiring but inspiring enough.

PD: But in relation to the dark and unbearable, you write in *Unforbidden Pleasures* (2015) about the paradoxical old Greek saying that the very best thing for us to desire would be never to have been born in the first place: 'And we have been born, and been given this belated knowledge. A knowledge that makes a mockery of our desire; that reveals all our purposes as hiding places and refuges. At least life has taught us this: that life is unbearable'. Or you quote Schopenhauer, the great nineteenth-century pessimist saying 'Dare to know that the world and life can afford us no true satisfaction'.[12]

AP: But how have we been led to have expectations about life that are all too likely to leave us feeling defeated? We must have been educated into wanting the wrong things if our experience is only one of cumulative disappointment. So think of what is *not* like that, amidst the ordinary or neglected pleasures.

It is as though we are leading double lives because at the psycho-biological level we are changing every millisecond of our lives and yet we can have the feeling that nothing changes. So here is a weird parallel life in which it is difficult to discern the changes that are happening. Take rumination, going round and round in circles with the same miserable thought, which is rather like an addiction: involved in this repetitiveness is the wish to stop time, an unconscious attack on one's own development, for fear of where the transformations might take you.

This means being surprised by something new or something you did not know would interest or involve you. One could imagine a spectrum—one end of it is surprise and the other is trauma, but traumas are so surprising that they stop one's experiencing things, so overwhelming are they that one has to close down. Therefore what one's really talking about with surprise is about bearable or fruitful or productive trauma.

PD: This live surprise is what makes you a reader especially of literature, trans-historically, to form a rich and unpredictable miscellany. Is that a refuge against aloneness?

AP: I don't think we are intrinsically alone. I think we are intrinsically related and in something together. But the anxieties attached to that enforce on some of us a developmental project to think of ourselves as separate and isolated and lonely because it saves us from some kind of engulfment. The question is the other way round: why have I needed to isolate myself? what has a certain amount of loneliness been a self-cure for? Because I think the profound experience is embeddedness and intermixture, and the defensive project is separating out.

For people who like reading, the books they care for represent one version of the commonwealth they are living in, all the different conversations they have had. What I love about literature is that there are so many voices—it is incredible, the range of tones and sentences and rhythms and ideas.

PD: It is as though different books might represent different possible moods or modes of being, and they do not simply fit together. You quote Emerson's saying, 'Our moods do not believe in each other'.[13] But isn't there also in your reading now an almost predatory cry for help. 'Help, help' was the cry that William James said lay beneath all religion.

AP: Absolutely, yes, totally right. But help to learn how to live. Not help to be saved or redeemed or rescued. This is the case with all possible truths that we try out: that they are subject to re-description. It seems to me that anything you cannot re-describe is akin to a trauma, and therefore the art—and what education and upbringing are about—is to free one's capacity for re-description.

PD: Reading must help that, when literature itself is a whole series of re-describings of life, enabling us to do or imagine something else?

AP: Yes. We want re-descriptions that are re-enlivening of our selves or what we speak of. A real re-description could not be deliberate: that would be propaganda, and you would be in the realm of the already known.

PD: Could you imagine a world that did not need psychoanalysis or literature?

AP: I could imagine a world that wouldn't need psychoanalysis. It comes out of a symptom, a need for a certain kind of conversation that required psychoanalysis to be invented. A world in which people's conversations and relationships were just better, could do without it. But I think literature is a broader, more diverse thing—I can't imagine a world without literature. You can't get what it offers from elsewhere, though it was once got from religion.

PD: Reading as part of the preparation, then.

AP: What could it be a preparation for?

PD: In your terms, for whatever it turns out it was.

AP: That is right. And for people who have had our sort of education, it is reading that helps. But it does not have to be. I could say I am bored by horse-racing but if someone talks to me about horse-racing, it might be very interesting. There are not *topics* I am bored by, but as I have said there are ways of speaking and ways of reading that make me bored.

The risk is supposing that people who don't read are somehow less. I don't for a moment believe that. It would be to privilege one's own preferences, recruited as a form of your own superiority. Bird-watching could be it instead, have value through the person who cares for it.

PD: And be what we might call, in our terms, a person's poetry. Ruskin says, in his own way, that we are not sent into this world to do anything into which we cannot put our hearts. And that perhaps then, finally, it does not matter *what* exactly it is, except as an exercise for the heart and will—as what you might call the crucial side-effect.

AP: Yes, it is like people talking about whatever it is that mattered to them, in their own way.

PD: And literature is—only, no more, no less than—a version of that?

AP: Exactly. And you tune into what is being said.

PD: Tuning in is most important to you in whatever you do?

AP: Yes I think it is: nothing can happen without tuning in, no relationship. I like the Romantic idea (A) of being able to tune in, and (B) that there is something to be tuned into. What we have been talking about, I think, is all to do with what the philosopher Gilles Deleuze calls 'the capacity to be affected'.[14] To be affected in the encounter between two bodies, two people, a person and a book, and so on; in the passage of emotional energy to and fro that always potentially augments or diminishes the capacity to act and think and live well.

Notes

1. A. Phillips, *Promises, Promises: Essays on Literature and Psychoanalysis* (London: Faber & Faber, 2000).
2. A. Phillips (in conversation with Philip Davis), 'Possibilities', *The Reader*, 30 (2008), 29–36.
3. A. Phillips, *In Writing* (London: Hamish Hamilton, 2017).
4. D. W. Winnicott, *The Maturational Processes and the Facilitating Environment: Studies in the Theory of Emotional Development* (New York: International Universities Press, 1965).
5. J. S. Mill, *On Liberty*, in Collected Works of J. S. Mill, ed. by J. M. Robson (Toronto: Toronto University Press, 1977), vol. 18, pp. 260–67.
6. See: D. H. Lawrence, *Women in Love*, ed. by David Farmer, Lindeth Vasey, and John Worthen (Cambridge: Cambridge University Press, 1987), p. 193.
7. A. Phillips, *Side Effects* (London: Hamish Hamilton, 2006), p. 97.
8. W. Wordsworth, *The Prelude: 1799, 1805, 1850*, ed. by Jonathan Wordsworth, M. H. Abrams and Stephen Gill (New York: W. W. Norton, 1979), 1805, II: 333–41.
9. See *The Poems of T. S. Eliot*, ed. by Christopher Ricks and Jim McCue, vol. 1, p. 409.

10. *Walter Pater: The Critical Heritage*, ed. by R. M. Seiler (London: Routledge, 1980), p. 57.
11. Marion Milner, *A Life of One's Own* (Hove: Routledge, 2011), p. 12.
12. Adam Phillips, *Unforbidden Pleasures* (London: Penguin Books Ltd., 2016), p. 167.
13. R. W. Emerson, 'Circles', in *The Essential Writings of Ralph Waldo Emerson*, ed. by Brooks Atkinson (New York: Random House, 2000), p. 254.
14. Gilles Deleuze and Felix Guattari, *A Thousand Plateaus*, trans. by Brian Massumi (London: Bloomsbury, 2004), p. 288.

Part V

Reading and Health: Implementation—Barriers and Enablers

18

Reading and Mental Health

Ellie Gray, Grace Farrington and Mette Steenberg

Ellie Gray, 'Clinical Implications of Existing Practice and Research in Reading and Mental Health'

The findings from multiple studies on the role of reading in mental health, including my own (see Chapter 9, 'Ellie Gray and Gundi Kiemle, "Interpretative Phenomenological Analysis (Community Mental Health)"'), have a range of implications for clinical practice. As a clinical psychologist, I have a particular interest in how the community reading groups I studied appear to offer therapeutic benefits which in some ways mirror and in other ways are distinct from those occurring in standard psychotherapy or bibliotherapy in clinical mental health contexts. My first task in what follows is to outline some of these similarities and differences.

E. Gray (✉)
Cumbria Partnership NHS Foundation Trust, Cumbria, UK
e-mail: ellie.gray@cumbria.nhs.uk

G. Farrington
The Reader, Liverpool, UK
e-mail: graceframe@thereader.org.uk

M. Steenberg
Aarhus University, Aarhus, Denmark
e-mail: mette.steenberg@cas.au.dk

J. Billington (ed.), *Reading and Mental Health*,
https://doi.org/10.1007/978-3-030-21762-4_18

My second goal is to focus in particular on the value of reading interventions in addressing the 'treatment gap'.[1] Despite the large number of people experiencing mental health problems in the UK, only a proportion receives appropriate treatment.[2] This gap in services is partly attributable not only to limited resources and long waiting lists but also, significantly, to the stigma associated with a person's acknowledging mental health difficulties.[3] How might a reading intervention help to overcome these issues?

Self-Help Bibliotherapy

This term refers to the use of self-help literature which clinically advises on behaviour change.[4] Professionally authored instructional materials guide the reader through self-help programmes with a view to improving self-management.[5] These materials are applied to a variety of populations in a range of formats[6] including written, audio and internet-based materials, delivered individually or in groups, accompanied by varying levels of therapist contact (none/face to face/phone/email).[7] Self-help bibliotherapy has developed into what is now commonly known as 'Books on Prescription'[8] which provides access to self-help literature from local libraries for specific difficulties, including anxiety[9] and depression.[10]

Self-help bibliotherapy schemes, including Books on Prescription, are frequently found in primary care services in the UK[11] as part of an attempt to reduce the treatment gap. In accordance with government drives to improve access to evidence-based mental health interventions,[12] mental health practitioners recommend empirically tested self-help bibliotherapy materials consistent with National Institute for Health and Clinical Excellence (NICE) guidelines.[13] A series of meta-analyses and literature reviews indicate that self-help bibliotherapy is a reasonably effective intervention for a range of mild to moderate mental health problems, including depression, anxiety and assertiveness difficulties.[14] Evidence from clinical practice and randomised controlled trials (RCTs) provides further support for self-help bibliotherapy, particularly in treating depression and anxiety.[15] There are limitations to the interpretation of this evidence owing to a number of factors: the variable strength of effect across presentations (with some problems—anxiety for example—yielding more promising results than others, such as impulse control); inconsistencies in sample size and population (crossing clinical and non-clinical participants); and often a lack of clarity around the term 'bibliotherapy' (see below) such that it is questionable whether studies are comparable. However, the tentative conclusion that self-help bibliotherapy is no less effective than individual psychotherapy[16] has emerged together with some recognised advantages of the former over the latter. Employing self-help bibliotherapy over standard face-to-face therapy may save clinical time (Robertson et al., 2008) and enhance cost-effectiveness (Chamberlain et al., 2008). Clinical evaluations also indicate that Books on Prescription schemes require reduced training and supervision, result in shorter waiting times (Reeves & Stace, 2005) and provide an alternative to medication (Robertson et al., 2008). Self-help bibliotherapy can also be empowering for the client, improves self-management and is less stigmatising than traditional mental health services (Papworth, 2006; Turner, 2008). These benefits, by freeing up resources and increasing access to services, go some way towards reducing the treatment gap.

One drawback of self-help therapy from a clinical perspective, however, is that it is largely reliant upon the aims and principles of Cognitive Behavioural Therapy (CBT). Although self-help bibliotherapy does make use of other psychological models (Cognitive Analytic Therapy, for example),[17] CBT remains the dominant theoretical framework[18] which is not universally suitable (Chamberlain et al., 2008). Even where a range of self-help approaches are available, those prescribing them (general practitioners, for example) do not necessarily possess the clinical skills to select the most appropriate therapeutic model. Furthermore, some individuals may not be ready to engage in therapy to directly address their mental health problems; without a skilled therapist to address these concerns—and to offer interpersonal warmth as part of the therapeutic relationship[19]—people may disengage from services altogether. Self-help bibliotherapy, if overly problem-focused and reliant upon correctly identifying and targeting the 'problem' as a single phenomenon may not be amenable to those with more complex presentations. Its frequent dependence on user literacy and cognitive skill also limits its application to certain presentations and client groups and the focus on symptom change or reduction can overlook other aspects such as quality of life and general well-being.

Creative Bibliotherapy

This term broadly refers to the use of imaginative literature to elicit therapeutic effects.[20] Where self-help bibliotherapy seeks to promote cognitive change by instructing and informing, creative bibliotherapy encourages emotional engagement with the text, evoking real feelings and offering what Joseph Gold terms a 'lived-through quality'.[21] There is limited empirical evidence of the effectiveness of creative bibliotherapy (Pehrsson & McMillen, 2005), often restricted to case studies, anecdotal accounts or bibliographic lists.[22] In part, this is because creative bibliotherapy has a more informal history and evolution within clinical practice. That's to say, it has not sought explicitly to address the treatment gap or respond to overarching concerns, but has grown up piecemeal as an adjunct or enabler of the psychodynamic process within the consulting room. As such, creative bibliotherapy as it is practised in mental health care often has considerable overlap with narrative medicine[23] and psychotherapeutic practices, as outlined below.

The 'life story' has received attention in psychotherapy, both because psychotherapeutic practice involves exploration of life histories, in terms of past events and experiences, to create a contextual understanding of present difficulties,[24] and because narratives are fundamental to making sense of experience.[25] Having a coherent story of experience is considered therapeutic.[26] Hence the clinical application of narrative to psychotherapy[27] and life story work.[28] Imaginative literature can be a vehicle for expressing personal narratives (Pehrsson & McMillen, 2005) and can help supplement or 're-story' one's own narrative, especially where the latter is blocked by difficult events, such as loss. Gold (2001) argues that, by engaging the reader with multiple layers and networks of experience, imaginative fiction enables the reader to select what is relevant to them in organising and understanding their own. This reframing process enables new perspectives, culminating in a cognitive shift which, however small, can have considerable consequences for emotion and behaviour.[29]

In addition to cognitive change, creative bibliotherapy has the potential to facilitate new emotional experiences. Described as a 'symbolic equivalent' of actual experience,[30] fiction, by contrast with traditional psychotherapy, can 'transport the reader to a parallel situation in which they can process their own circumstances from the safety of intellectual and emotional distance' (McNulty, 2008, p. 26). Literature provides a model for discussing painful experiences without explicitly focusing on the individual (Pardeck & Pardeck, 1984). Repressed memories may be elicited, negotiated and tolerated through vicarious involvement in the thoughts and feelings of others (Gold, 2001). Behaviourally, too, creative bibliotherapy may provide a model for new ways of acting. Through identification, the reader may attempt to imitate behaviours or actions,[31] encouraging them to test out adaptive behaviours (Pardeck & Pardeck, 1984) and increase their repertoire of roles (Gold, 2001).

Shrodes (1949/1950 as cited in McCulliss, 2012) proposed a psychodynamic model of creative bibliotherapy. Firstly, the client identifies with experiences/events within the literature and projects their own emotions and drives onto characters, whose intentions and relationships are related to their own difficulties, thereby enhancing self-awareness. The client then expresses their reactions via spontaneous emotional release.[32] Insight and integration follow, whereby the client realises ways of overcoming their struggles by recognising themselves and others in the literature. Bhattacharyya (1997) noted the powerful effects of this process in resolving internal conflicts; as insight comes through identification, the projected unacceptable parts can be owned and integrated, making whole that which was fragmented before (p. 15), thus promoting coherence in identity and narrative. Others highlight the normalising effect of identification (e.g. Gold, 2001), which can help validate attitudes, beliefs and experiences.[33]

There is evidence, then, of the potential impact of creative bibliotherapy within a psychotherapeutic context, upon cognitive, emotional and behavioural processes, both intra- and inter-personally. However, there is limited empirical research, much derived from anecdotal or clinical reports, and it remains unclear whether such processes can occur without the guidance of a therapist (as in self-help), or whether they are suited more to an individual or a group setting.

Group Bibliotherapy

Individual bibliotherapy gradually evolved into group bibliotherapy (McCulliss, 2012), and there is some (albeit limited) empirical evidence of the therapeutic value of group creative bibliotherapy for adult mental health. An Israeli study, for example, compared inpatients' functioning in standard group therapy and group bibliotherapy.[34] Both groups employed an 'affective-support' approach, focusing on emotional expression, group support and cognitive/affective exploration. In group therapy, discussion focused on issues spontaneously raised by members, whereas group bibliotherapy was guided by members' reactions to short stories selected and read aloud by the therapist. Independent ratings of transcriptions of both groups indicated that clients were more active and productive, less resistant and engaged in greater affective exploration and self-disclosure in group bibliotherapy. These findings were attributed to psychodynamic processes similar to those operating in Shrodes' (1949/1950 as cited in McCulliss, 2012) model, occurring between the readers and the text.

As early as 1950, Powell described informal group creative bibliotherapy in psychiatric hospitals, whereby patients met weekly to discuss books (including novels and philosophical works) they read alone prior to the session. Groups emphasised education and recreation, rather than therapy, but, as well as providing enjoyment and satisfaction, Powell reported that such activity 'adds another dimension of thinking and…interpersonal experience'.[35] This is consistent both with the aforementioned facilitation of new perspectives and interpersonal development through individual creative bibliotherapy (e.g. Pardeck & Pardeck, 1984) and with Yalom and Leszcz's (2005) findings in respect of the eleven therapeutic factors of group psychotherapy (including 'interpersonal learning', 'development of socializing techniques', 'recapitulation of the primary family grouping', 'existential factors', 'group cohesiveness').[36] As an everyday non-clinical activity, group reading also helped maintain links between the stigmatised hospital environment and the normality of the 'outside world' (Powell, 1950). Similarly (and again consistent with Yalom & Leszcz, 2005), reading groups provided a 'little society', or microcosm, where attendees were viewed as individuals rather than 'patients'. As this new social context was failure free, attendees were able to test out new ways of being, which may not be possible in their 'patient' role (Powell, 1950), thus enabling the development of socialising techniques (Yalom & Leszcz, 2005). A like finding emerged from a study with stroke inpatients, who felt that participation in a reading group helped re-personalise them, giving identity aside from illness/disability.[37]

Until recently (see Part III), studies of live group bibliotherapy in clinical mental health contexts have been relatively scarce, but there is a small body of literature developing in this area with people with neurological difficulties. Reading literature aloud in groups has been found to promote positive affect, improve engagement and alertness, elicit memory and reduce disruptive behaviour in people with dementia and brain injury.[38] Holm et al. (2005) reported that their storytelling group for people with Alzheimer's disease prompted existential discussions and a sense of fellowship, consistent with Yalom and Leszcz's (2005) existential factors and group cohesiveness. This study also highlighted that, although entertainment and stimulation are valuable benefits of group reading (Higgins et al., 2005), giving structure to such activity is important for moving beyond entertainment merely and reaping deeper psychological gains.

Clearly, both formal and informal group creative bibliotherapy offer some benefit to the reader consistent with processes of individual creative bibliotherapy (enhanced self-expression, interpersonal growth), even without a skilled therapist. However, the cited examples are based on small samples or anecdotal evidence and take place in inpatient/residential settings, focusing primarily on acute mental health or organic difficulties. Such examples do not address the current treatment gap in relation to the functional mental health difficulties that many people experience living in the community.

Community Reading Groups/Live Shared Reading

My own study was concerned with the value of live Shared Reading in the community of literary works (see Chapter 9 'Ellie Gray and Gundi Kiemle, "Interpretative Phenomenological Analysis (Community Mental Health)"'). From a clinical perspective, it was interesting to identify potential areas where Shared Reading groups appeared to be re-enacting aspects of therapy. My primary role as a clinician influenced my interpretation of participants' accounts, but what emerged was that Shared Reading groups seemed to incorporate aspects of both common therapeutic factors (e.g. containment, boundaries, therapeutic relationship), and specific features of individual models (e.g. cognitive behavioural therapy, cognitive analytic therapy). Perhaps this capacity to complement elements of multiple therapeutic orientations reflects the malleability I noticed in Shared Reading in terms of individual tailoring to group members' own needs.

Reading groups could therefore provide alternative access to therapeutic activity without the persons directly engaging in therapy. This may be an important avenue for people for whom traditional services are unsuitable, inaccessible or ineffective. Since traditional psychological therapy does not work for everyone, reading groups may be one way of addressing the aforementioned 'treatment gap' in mental health service provision. It may be that reading groups can be used as an adjunct, as well as an alternative, to psychotherapy, for instance while people are on waiting lists. I often find it difficult informing clients of the length of waiting lists, due to the anxiety, disappointment and frustration this elicits. It is therefore helpful to be able to offer alternative therapeutic activity in the meantime, which may enable clients to develop self-awareness, experience alternative perspectives and explore patterns of relating prior to therapy.

Because Shared Reading is not 'therapy', it could increase provision of therapeutic activity in a way that is currently not available in the NHS, by mixing those living with mental health problems with those without. Not only do Shared Reading groups mix 'well' with 'unwell', but tend to welcome heterogeneity of mental health issues. Again, this contrasts with groups in statutory services, which are usually organised according to presentation or symptom (e.g. hearing voices, alcohol misuse, binge-eating disorder). Reading groups, on the other hand, are relevant to people with a variety of mental health issues, suggesting that they could be delivered simultaneously to people with multiple presentations in mental health services.

The holistic focus on wellness complements the shifting focus of UK mental health services from symptom/problem management to recovery models, which aim to develop personal strengths and resources to enable the service user to lead a meaningful life over which they have control.[39] Participants in our study (Gray et al., 2015) valued being in a non-stigmatising environment where they felt accepted and were seen as 'well', while also having the opportunity to express their 'unwellness'. Importantly, the latter was experienced as a choice because of the group's unpressured nature. The personal agency that this gave to participants is also reflected in the non-obligatory ethos of the reading group, such that people could attend as and when they liked. Again, this is in contrast to DNA ('Did Not Attend') policies often implemented in the NHS following non-attendance, which can result in premature discharge due to difficulties engaging. While such policies may be necessary, community reading groups offer an opportunity to access therapeutic activity which does not require a certain level of commitment (both in terms of attendance, and active participation), thus allowing for potential ambivalence or resistance.

Finally, from a practical perspective, the cost of delivering reading groups is considerably cheaper than traditional psychotherapy, and Shared Reading is widely replicable across educational levels and cognitive skills. Beneficiaries do not have to be literate. I came across group members with varying levels of disability and impaired cognitive function who nonetheless participated by hearing the literature read aloud and being able to participate in the ensuing discussion.

Grace Farrington, 'Reading and Mental Health: The Perspective of Occupational Therapy'

During my placement at Mersey Care NHS Trust (see above Chapter 8), I worked alongside a group of occupational therapists, each of whom had had experience of The Reader's shared group reading model within a mental health setting. Together they produced a rationale for using Shared Reading within mental health service provision, which (with their permission[40]) I summarise below, followed by an interview I conducted with one of the authors.

The rationale took as its starting point the underlying principle of occupational therapy with regard to mental health, as stated by the College of Occupational Therapists: 'health and wellbeing are supported by engagement in a balanced range of occupations that are chosen and valued by the individual'.[41] This placed the reading group within a range of possible activities which, in an inpatient setting, might also include reminiscence, exercise or relaxation sessions. But the therapists involved in Shared Reading suggest that the emphasis on meaningfulness makes reading particularly important:

> Maintaining an acceptable and personally satisfying routine of activities that have meaning and value for the individual gives a structure to time and creates a sense of purpose and direction to life. Such a routine enfolds the individual within a physical and sociocultural context, thus supporting feelings of identity, normality and well-being, even in the presence of disease or disability. (College of Occupational Therapists, 'Recovering Ordinary Lives', p. 3)

The work of occupational therapy in fact tends to take the focus away from disease and disability:

> The centrality of occupation in the thinking of occupational therapists leads to a focus on the strengths of individuals, rather than their problems, and on their contribution to recovery … The service user becomes an active participant in the creation of his or her future, learning hope and building confidence. ('Recovering Ordinary Lives', p. 10)

The authors of the rationale comment on what deeply constitutes recovery thus:

> Modern mental health services are directed to provide opportunities for self-exploration that help to develop interests rather than attempting to cure people back to so-called 'reality'.[42] Reading is one such method that can be utilised to help facilitate this process by providing new ways of expressing feelings and knowledge.

The rationale gives the following summary of this process:

Motivation for Occupation (Reading):
- Provide/develop leisure interest
- Promotion of self-expression, identity and choice

Pattern of Occupation (Reading):
- Structure and routine
- Engagement in a planned structured activity

- Role development: as participant, reader; group interactions, community building
- Responsibility for own leisure time

The rationale tries to strike a balance between the way in which Shared Reading facilitates the development of certain skills (including communication and interaction, process and motor skills, as well as literacy), and the degree to which this might be enjoyed as a valuable 'leisure' activity that is effective precisely by *not* concentrating on skills which are a by-product of involvement in the meaning itself. While there is a recognition that leisure is 'essential to occupational functioning', nonetheless even the words leisure or pleasure are names that are often in reaction against instrumentalism: rather than capturing the deep characteristics of the activity of reading, these descriptors are first of all intended not to scare or deter. But what is really at stake is that deeper meaning of recovery, including the recovery of a sense of self, within the context of redundancy—not only as job loss but as loss of existential purpose in the world. In an article published in a magazine for Occupational Therapy professionals, Susan Yee points out that in contemporary society one's identity is often heavily dependent upon a sense of one's occupation, and yet often what accompanies mental illness is the loss of employment. So-called leisure activities are important in offering 'a safe venue for persons to re-engage in doing', enabling the individual potentially to reassess their own 'life importance'.[43] Anne Louise Humphreys, reporting on the benefits, from an occupational therapy perspective, of a reading group for chronic pain sufferers who are no longer able to work, regards reading as a meaningful activity likely to produce what Csíkszentmihályi called a state of 'flow'.

> Occupational flow describes a point at which someone is presented with a 'just-right challenge' where their skills are balanced harmoniously with the challenge and the person is focused upon a clear task with strong concentration and focused attention. This state is associated with loss of inhibiting self-consciousness, and a heightened awareness of present being.[44]

One group member, who had not been in employment for twenty years, after his pain forced him into early retirement, said of the reading group: 'I feel like I'm in work again; [the group] makes you *think* and I haven't had that for *such* a long time' (Billington et al., 2014). As Humphreys observes, he misses not simply the routine but the whole-self engagement with which work had provided him: this 'flow' experience allows him to recover, if only for a short period of time, what he has been missing.

The rationale collectively produced by the Mersey Care occupational team continues by identifying a set of skills that may be used or developed within the reading group. These are efforts that may be achieved without consciousness of effort (via 'flow') when they are means of enjoyment or excitement not ends in themselves. But the modern framework must still foreground them:

Communication and Interaction Skills:
- Non-verbal: requires being socially appropriate for group setting/can address social skills
- Verbal skills through discussions
- Vocal expression
- Relationships—stimulates constructive conversations between group members
- Promotes constructive dialogue and communication techniques
- Skills and knowledge development

Process Skills:
- Increase concentration
- Seeking and retaining information for discussion
- Decision-making
- Memory recall

Motor Skills:
- Posture
- Energy: channelling a person's energy into positive activity; also requires the maintenance of attention
- Fine motor and dexterity

Other:
- Increase self-confidence
- Reduce anxiety
- Group working
- Relaxation

The authors of the rationale comment further that: 'Reading groups have demonstrated an ability to build community and promote social interaction and social inclusion. Research shows that these areas are fundamentally affected by mental health difficulties'.[45] Although this rationale applies specifically to reading groups in inpatient mental health settings, the use of the language of well-being extends its relevance to reading in community settings.

In an interview with Chris Vaughan, one of the authors of the rationale, Chris remembered 'a certain impression' he had had as a result of his own personal involvement in the groups. I was interested in this language as something distinct from the (necessarily) professional and official language of the framework for the rationale. 'The transformative effect that these groups have is quite remarkable', Chris went on. 'I've seen aspects of people – things they say, how they present – which I wouldn't have had an opportunity to see anywhere else'. Chris assisted in running other kinds of groups as part of his role and recognised that there were similarities with the kinds of interventions offered by members of the city's Philharmonic Orchestra, or by visitors from the local dance school. These too are able to engage the patients on the ward and provide a means of participating in a creative activity. 'I suppose it's about expression', Chris said: 'freedom of expression'. 'And a kind of individualism – or individualised kind of … I don't know, outpourings if you like – that often are contained or forgotten, because so many people are medicalised aren't they?'

Chris gave an account of a woman in her early eighties who had been on the acute psychiatric ward for a relatively long time—months instead of weeks—during a 'very severe bout of depression'. The woman had received help for her depression on previous occasions, but (her husband had commented) 'it had never been this bad before'. She had been undergoing a course of ECT treatment (Electroconvulsive Therapy), but had not responded, so that 'the care staff were finding it difficult to determine how best to treat her'. Chris knew the woman was very well-read, and would be likely to be interested in the reading group, but he had not quite known whether she was ready for it or whether she might feel a little too overwhelmed.

However, a student who was helping out on the ward decided one week to take the woman in to join the group. They were reading a chapter from a Dickens novel, Chris remembers:

> A lot of the people were familiar with Dickens, and were keen to take turns to read. And this lady had just been kind of passively participating in a way: she was listening to others read and following the text. You could tell she was still very much attentive and engaged. And then after a pause, about halfway

through the session, she said 'Can I read now?' She asked that without any prompting at all.

And then she read a passage in the most *beautifully* enunciated way I can ever remember. And everybody was just staggered because that kind of expression, it hadn't been revealed to anyone before. It was almost as though things just stood still when she announced that she'd like to read, and then read perfectly, and then suddenly said, 'Shall I stop now?' When she started reading it was almost as if she'd crossed a threshold, in a way, in her recovery. That's how I'd describe it. And then she went on to become a regular member of the group until she became well again, and then asked if she could attend the group as an outpatient, which we arranged.

There is a moment when this ceases to be an 'intervention' and becomes simply an act of reading. This is what allows the woman voluntarily to engage in a way that is more active than might at first be apparent: it is as though the woman has been attentively waiting for the right moment to speak. Moreover, it appears that what Chris had meant earlier by expressive 'outpourings' was not so much the mental relief that might be afforded by an offloading of personal trouble, but closer to a vocal expression from that person's inner being. As he re-tells the story, he goes back to imagine the kind of position in which the woman would have been finding herself at this time:

Anhedonia [inability to experience pleasure] often accompanies the conditions with which many patients we work with are admitted into hospital. It's that lack of pleasure in most things that would generally gratify us as humans, which also informs a patient's outlook, world view, sense of a future. And she was very flat, very low, and probably the future for her was very bleak, didn't hold an awful lot. I suppose for most of her stay she was confused as to where she was; or she didn't probably see where else she could go from here.

Chris several times referred to the idea that Shared Reading may be particularly important in helping to expand people's options and provide access to certain 'freedoms'. He had noticed this particularly in the high-secure hospital where he had first had experience of observing the effect of Shared Reading (see Chapter 8). The wards were the most extreme version he had encountered of a setting in which 'life was so clearly defined and structured for patients', and the 'freedoms' patients had 'to make some choices linked to their own volition' were very much limited. Even as a staff member, he could sense the effects of that limitation on the ward:

> There are lots of security protocols and things are really slowed down to a snail's pace, and as a consequence things don't happen in a spontaneous way. Whereas in the group there was a kind of fluidity, because no-one knew really where the conversation was going to take us.

This is about freedom in time, in thought, in present existence outside a set programme or an institutional requirement. For Chris, this extended to his own position: normally, he felt, he would be expected as the health professional to demonstrate expertise, and to be able to manage a situation, be in control of what was happening. In the reading group, he felt that this expectation did not lie solely with him; there was a different shared order in operation. This finding on behalf of both staff and patients seems rooted in a principle of relative non-selection—the generous principle of not narrowly focussing or planning or excluding too much in advance. It's important to leave room for choice and improvisation. Of course, group leaders have in mind key places and emphases within any given literary text and work hard to manage these groups carefully; of course, stakeholders and commissioners of the reading group recommend particular participants to the reading group to encourage them in particular areas and conditions of life. But the rich human inclusiveness of the literary material supersedes these goals. The participants, themselves largely *un*selected in fact, voluntarily find in the works what interests them without pressure. The resulting upshots within the texts and the readers alike are largely unexpected and uncontrolled. This is what Chris is calling 'freedom' for human flourishing, not 'contained' by narrowly programmatic or 'medicalised' ends.

Mette Steenberg, '"Time to Read": A Referral Model of Shared Reading for Vulnerable Adults in Central Region Denmark'

Mette Steenberg holds a dual position as researcher at Aarhus University, Interacting Minds Center and as Director of The Danish Reading Society (Laeseforeningen).

Based on the idea of 'culture on prescription', the purpose of Time to Read was to develop and implement Shared Reading as an aesthetic quality-ensured mental health activity within local municipalities in the Central Region, Denmark. In order to meet this goal, the project developed a referral model in which health professionals working with health promotion and prevention referred adults suffering from depression, stress or anxiety to Shared Reading groups delivered by librarians at the local libraries for mental health promotion.

Stakeholders and Roles

The project involved four main stakeholders. The Danish Reading Society (Læseforeningen), Aarhus University, the Central Region, Denmark (a regional government mainly responsible for health care) and five municipalities within the region (municipalities). These agents were brought together in a joint effort to:

1. Implement Shared Reading as a continuous activity within local health promotion schemes (municipalities)
2. Document the mental health benefits both qualitatively and quantitatively (Aarhus University)
3. Train and supervise librarians in order to ensure quality (The Danish Reading Society/Læseforeningen).

Læseforeningen and Shared Reading was selected and financially supported by Central Region Denmark as a regional strategic initiative in the process of developing the field of culture and health within the region. Shared Reading was chosen because of its well-defined method which is not context specific and thus transferrable to various municipalities. This methodological advantage furthermore represented a possibility for documenting quantitatively the mental health effects on a larger population exposed to the same intervention (see Chapter 12).

The Danish Reading Society/Læseforeningen was the project owner and had responsibility for activities, timeline and budget. As the first step, the organisation identified key figures within those municipalities in the region who were already working in some capacity with Shared Reading and who either had experience with, or could see the advantage of, working across sectors.

The result was a 10-person steering committee consisting of two representatives each from five municipalities, including one leader from the library services (most of them leaders of development and learning) and one from the health sector (some with decision-making authority). The committee represented a mix of leaders and preventive medicine consultants working directly with citizens.

Motivations for joining the project were firstly being part of a research project that documented the mental health benefits of Shared Reading (libraries), and secondly being able to offer a new activity for vulnerable adults (health sector). It is interesting to note that representatives from the health sector were less motivated by the aspect of documentation than might have been expected of a sector working within an evidence-based medicine paradigm. This can be explained by the fact that the health professionals involved did not represent the strategic level of health politics, but mainly worked in direct contact with vulnerable citizens and were thus mostly motivated by developing new suitable activities for an increasing number of citizens. The library representatives, on the other hand, represented the level of strategic development within the organisation and were concerned with developing a more active social role for libraries (see Chapter 5), and therefore highly aware of the need to document the mental health effects of literary reading in order to make a case for culture as prescription.

The Referral Model: Literature on Prescription

The original idea of a referral model was based on health professionals, often prevention consultants,[46] referring vulnerable adults (suffering from depression, stress or anxiety, excluding those in acute psychiatric treatment and/or with active drug abuse) to Shared Reading groups delivered by librarians at the local library. However, in the five different municipalities the referral model took on different forms due to local cultures of collaboration.

In two municipalities, referral was carried out within the ordinary process of (secondary) preventive measures for citizens already within the health system, targeting those suffering from both somatic diseases and mental health issues. Time to Read was offered as an activity as part of a health-promotion conversation between the health user and the health professional seeking to clarify the optimal preventive measures for the individual in question. In addition, other sectors and partners within the municipality were informed of the activity and were instructed to direct interested participants to the person responsible for referral.

In one of the three municipalities, the focus was on prevention. The reading group was offered also to citizens outside of the health system, through advertisement in local newspapers and social media, and, as a consequence of the preventive strategy, involved a different set of referral partners including MDs (general practitioners).

In the two remaining municipalities, the referral model wasn't implemented either because of lack of referral or due to local forms of collaboration and models of referral.

One municipality operated referral within the library sector exclusively, based on this library's previous experience with Shared Reading groups. However, as the library had no direct contact with the target group, recruitment failed, and the reading groups were never established. In this respect, it is interesting to notice that this particular municipality differed from the others in having selected a steering committee member who worked strategically on developing health and culture initiatives at the level of health politics. Nevertheless, failure to identify key professionals working directly with health promotion at user level meant that referral from the health area to library was never implemented.

Another city chose their health representative from within the leadership of the World Health Organization's (WHO's) Healthy Cities Network, which strives to promote healthy citizens through local and voluntary engagement. Those referred attended Shared Reading on a voluntary basis, and the referral method was successful. However, as participants' mental health conditions were not identified by health professionals, due to self-referral, this group could not form part of the research design.

Criteria for and Obstacles to Successful Implementation

Analysing the referral method in practice, three essential criteria stand out for successful implementation across the three municipalities in which recruitment and referral worked well, all three reflecting a process of taking ownership:

1. The identification and engagement of one or more key professionals, working in health promotion and prevention, and in direct contact with citizens, who can take responsibility for referral, seems to be the most consistent criterion of success across the three municipalities. These professionals worked strategically to implement referral within existing structures and to spread knowledge about Shared Reading as a mental health activity to other sectors (e.g. jobcentres), for the widest possible recruitment within the target group. In the context of jobcentres, Shared Reading was not an easy referral option as citizens were already assigned to many different training programmes aimed at the labour market. However, because Shared Reading was not aimed directly at developing specific competences for the labour market, the activity was often rejected.
2. Development of a solid, sometimes already existing, working relationship across the library services and the health sector. In all three municipalities, they formed local steering groups, which went even further in developing culture and health initiatives and/or took Shared Reading to new sectors or target groups.

3. Development of a culture of sharing across the municipalities. One municipality discovered a need for 'showcasing' Shared Reading for potential participants, an idea that was formalised in information-events in all three municipalities. Potential participants were invited to a Shared Reading session at the local library in which the person responsible for referral also participated to enable immediate referral.

Obstacles:

1. Lack of understanding of the activity, and who could benefit, by professionals. In the beginning, it was not stressed clearly enough that Shared Reading, based on reading aloud and facilitated dialogue, is for everyone and does not require previous knowledge of literature. Thus, health care and other professionals would only suggest participation in reading groups to those who were already keen readers.

   To overcome this obstacle, Læseforeningen showcased Shared Reading to those professionals in direct contact with the target group for optimal communication of the intervention.
2. The discontinuity of the intervention. Shared Reading was offered as a 10-week intervention once every half year (starting September and January). The discontinuity made it difficult for professionals to integrate it into the ordinary prevention routines.

   One solution was for the person responsible for referral to communicate starting dates well in advance and send reminders a few weeks before start-up. However, quite a few people were still lost as the target group was generally not able to commit to anything in the distant future.

Further Implementation, Obstacles and Solutions

In the phase of implementation and recruitment, health promotion professionals were the key to success. However, in the current phase of the project, the steering committee is struggling to identify ways in which Shared Reading can be implemented at the level of health politics locally in order for the intervention to become a budgeted activity. This seems to be a regular paradox in health promotion: that professionals working directly with users, and consequently having a focus on practice, at times have to carry out their work without strategic support, even in direct opposition to local politics.

The barrier in this case is a lack of understanding on the part of leaders in health of (1) what mental health really is and how it relates to health more generally, and (2) the idea that participation in cultural activities plays an active role in quality of life and thus health.

The solution here is both one of communication, including offering models that people can relate to—'oh, so it's like joining a football club, I get out of the house and secure some fun spare time for myself and exercise my body at the same time?', as one politician said—and continuing the labour of documenting, both qualitatively and quantitatively, the effects of participation in aesthetic processes, so that quality of life can be turned into figures in the health budget.

Another concern in relation to implementation is quality assurance. There is a discrepancy which is not yet solved between the two sectors: health and culture. The health sector depends on documentation and quality assurance and has a direct professional goal of making people healthy, thus requiring a well-defined quality-assured method, an idea which is new to the library services. However, in this particular project, as the library sector wishes to document mental health effects of Shared Reading, both sectors have, at the level of the steering committee, come together in an understanding of the need to develop quality assurance. At the level of reading-group leaders however, quality assurance in terms of supervision has represented a challenge. As described in Chapter 5, in Time to Read, Shared Reading groups are delivered by highly motivated librarians who see their role as Reader Leaders as a way of fulfilling a key interest in and passion for 'sharing their joy of literature with others'. Nevertheless, while they enjoy their work and find it close to their hearts as librarians, some have expressed an insecurity in relation to the personal aspect involved in being a group leader in the context of mental health, as they would normally engage with citizens more indirectly through book recommendations. In this light, supervision became a challenge, as the librarians were not used to being put on the spot in the more social and human aspects of their profession. To overcome this challenge, Læseforeningen makes an effort to build an informal and supportive learning environment through quarterly team meetings.

Summing Up the Time to Read Experience

Each municipality looks different and has different conditions to work in. No matter what the specific contexts some elements are important to make a successful referral model:

- Developing local ownership of the project, identifying health and culture professionals within the community who take an active role.
- Having professionals with direct contact with relevant citizens and working relationships across sectors.
- Communicating what Shared Reading is and for whom it could be relevant.
- Developing a culture among librarians working as reading guides where personal and human skills are at the centre of their professional role.

Notes

1. N. Ridgway and C. Williams, 'Cognitive Behavioural Therapy Self-Help for Depression: An Overview', *Journal of Mental Health*, 20.6 (2011), 593–603.
2. D. M. Clark, R. Layard, R. Smithies, D. A. Richards, R. Suckling, and B. Wright, 'Improving Access to Psychological Therapies: Initial Evaluation of Two UK Demonstration Sites', *Behaviour Research and Therapy*, 47.11 (2009), 910–20.
3. For example: G. Kupshik and C. Fisher, 'Assisted Bibliotherapy: Effective, Efficient Treatment for Moderate Anxiety Problems', *British Journal of General Practice*, 49 (1999), 47–48; N. Mead, W. McDonald, P. Bower, K. Lovell, D. Richards, and C. Roberts, 'The Clinical Effectiveness of Guided Self-Help Versus Waiting List Control in the Management of Anxiety and Depression: A Randomised Controlled Trial', *Psychological Medicine*, 35.11 (2005), 1633–43; T. Reeves and J. M. Stace, 'Improving Patient Access and Choice: Assisted Bibliotherapy for Mild to Moderate Stress/Anxiety in Primary Care', *Journal of Psychiatric and Mental Health Nursing*, 12.3 (2005), 341–46.
4. Consistent with L. Brewster, 'Reader Development and Mental Well-Being: The Accidental Bibliotherapist', *Aplis*, 22.1 (2009), 13–16.
5. W. Songprakun and T. V. McCann, 'Evaluation of a Cognitive Behavioural Self-Help Manual for Reducing Depression: A Randomized Controlled Trial', *Journal of Psychiatric and Mental Health Nursing*, 19.7 (2012), 647–53.
6. D. Fanner and C. Urquhartt, 'Bibliotherapy for Mental Health Service Users Part 1: A Systematic Review', *Health Information and Libraries Journal*, 25.4 (2008), 237–52; D. E. Pehrsson and P. McMillen, 'A Bibliotherapy Evaluation Tool: Grounding Counselors in the Therapeutic Use of Literature', *The Arts in Psychotherapy*, 32.1 (2005), 47–59.
7. For example: E. Kaltenthaler, G. Parry, and C. Beverley, 'Computerized Cognitive Behaviour Therapy: A Systematic Review', *Behavioural and*

Cognitive Psychotherapy, 32.1 (2004), 31–55; D. McCulliss, 'Bibliotherapy', in *Research on Writing Approaches in Mental Health*, ed. by L. L'Abate and L. G. Sweeney (Bingley: Emerald, 2011), pp. 67–83; J. A. Pardeck and J. T. Pardeck, 'An Overview of the Bibliotherapeutic Treatment Approach: Implications for Clinical Social Work Practice', *Family Therapy*, 11.3 (1984), 241–52; and S. P. Thomas, 'Bibliotherapy: New Evidence of Effectiveness', *Issues in Mental Health Nursing*, 32.4 (2011), 191.

8. S. Starker, 'Do-It-Yourself Therapy: The Prescription of Self-Help Books by Psychologists', *Psychotherapy*, 25.1 (1988), 142–46; D. Chamberlain, D. Heaps, and I. Robert, 'Bibliotherapy and Information Prescriptions: A Summary of the Published Evidence-Base and Recommendations from Past and Ongoing Books on Prescription Projects', *Journal of Psychiatric and Mental Health Nursing*, 15.1 (2008), 24–36; M. Gunning, C. Richards, and N. Prescott, 'Reading for Well-Being,' *Community Practitioner*, 84.4 (2011), 40–41; A. Porter, J. Peconi, A. Evans, H. Snooks, K. Lloyd, and I. Russell, 'Equity and Service Innovation: The Implementation of a Bibliotherapy Scheme in Wales', *Journal of Health Services Research and Policy*, 13.2 (2008), 26–31; and R. Robertson, S. J. Wray, M. Maxwell, and R. J. Pratt, 'The Introduction of a Healthy Reading Scheme for People with Mental Health Problems: Usage and Experiences of Health Professionals and Library Staff', *Mental Health in Family Medicine*, 5.4 (2008), 219–28.
9. H. Kennerley, *Overcoming Anxiety: A Self-Help Guide Using Cognitive Behavioural Techniques* (London: Constable & Robinson, 2009).
10. P. Gilbert, *Overcoming Depression: A Self-Help Guide Using Cognitive Behavioural Techniques*, 3rd edn (London: Constable & Robinson, 2009).
11. For example, Gunning et al., 2011; J. Turner, 'Bibliotherapy for Health and Well-Being: An Effective Investment', *Aplis*, 21.2 (2008), 56–61.
12. Department of Health, 'National Service Framework for Mental Health: Modern Standards and Service Models', 1999. Retrieved from http://www.dh.gov.uk/prod_consum_dh/groups/dh_digitalassets/@dh/@en/documents/digitalasset/dh_4077209.pdf; R. Layard, 'Mental Health: Britain's Biggest Social Problem?' (London: Prime Minister's Strategy Unit, 2004).
13. For example, National Institute for Clinical Excellence, 'Depression: The Treatment and Management of Depression in Adults' 2009. Retrieved from http://www.nice.org.uk/nicemedia/live/12329/45888/45888.pdf; National Institute for Clinical Excellence, 'Generalised Anxiety Disorder and Panic Disorder (with or without Agoraphobia) in Adults: Management in Primary, Secondary and Community Care, 2011. Retrieved from http://www.nice.org.uk/nicemedia/live/13314/52599/52599.pdf.
14. For example: T. R. Apodaca and W. R. Miller, 'A Meta-Analysis of the Effectiveness of Bibliotherapy for Alcohol Problems', *Journal of Clinical Psychology*, 59.3 (2003), 289–304; Chamberlain et al., 2008; M. Papworth, 'Issues and Outcomes Associated with Adult Mental Health Self-Help

Materials: A "Second Order" Review or "Qualitative Meta-Review"', *Journal of Mental Health*, 14.4 (2006), 387–409; Ridgway and Williams, 2011; R. W. Marrs, 'A Meta-Analysis of Bibliotherapy Studies', *American Journal of Community Psychology*, 23.6 (1995), 843–70; and P. C. Den Boer, D. Wiersma, and R. J. Van den Bosch, 'Why Is Self-Help Neglected in the Treatment of Emotional Disorders? A Meta-Analysis', *Psychological Medicine*, 34.6 (2004), 949–71.

15. Kupshik and Fisher, 1999; Reeves and Stace, 2005; Songprakun and McCann, 2012; A. Van Straten, P. Cuijpers, and N. Smits, 'Effectiveness of a Web-Based Self-Help Intervention for Symptoms of Depression, Anxiety and Stress: Randomized Controlled Trial', *Journal of Medical Internet Research*, 10.1 (2008), e7.
16. P. Cuijpers, A. van Straten, and F. Smit, 'Psychological Treatment of Late-Life Depression: A Meta-Analysis of Randomized Controlled Trials', *International Journal of Geriatric Psychiatry*, 21.12 (2006), 1139–49.
17. E. Wilde McCormick, *Change for the Better: Self-Help Through Practical Psychotherapy* (London: Sage, 2008).
18. P. Cuijpers, 'Bibliotherapy in Unipolar Depression: A Meta-Analysis', *Journal of Behavior Therapy & Experimental Psychiatry*, 28.2 (1997), 139–47; van Straten et al., 2008.
19. R. Richardson, D. A. Richards, and M. Barkham, 'Self-Help Books for People with Depression: The Role of the Therapeutic Relationship', *Behavioural and Cognitive Psychotherapy*, 38.1 (2010), 67–81.
20. For example: A. J. Gianinni, 'Use of Fiction in Therapy', *Psychiatric Times*, 18.7 (2001), 56–57; W. McNulty, 'Harry Potter and the Prisoner Within: Helping Children with Traumatic Loss', in *Popular Culture in Counselling, Psychotherapy, and Play-Based Interventions*, ed. by Lawrence C. Rubin (New York: Springer, 2008), pp. 25–42; A. Tani, 'Reading to Bond: Enhancing the Attachment Bond Between Incarcerated Mothers and Their Children' (Doctoral dissertation). Retrieved from ProQuest, published by University Microforms International, 2010 (UMI No. 3442856).
21. J. Gold, *Read for Your Life: Literature as a Life Support System* (Markham, ON : Fitzhenry & Whiteside, 2001).
22. A. J. L. Baker, 'The Power of Stories/Stories About Power: Why Therapists and Clients Should Read Stories About the Parental Alienation Syndrome', *The American Journal of Family Therapy*, 34.1 (2006), 191–203; Giannini, 2001; McNulty, 2008; R. J. Riordan, F. Mullis, and L. Nuchow, 'Organizing for Bibliotherapy: The Science in the Art', *Individual Psychology*, 52.2 (1996), 169–80.
23. Semina texts include: Trish Greenhalgh and Brian Hurwitz (eds), *Narrative-Based Medicine* (London: BMJ Books, 1998); Rita Charon, *Narrative Medicine: Honouring the Stories of Illness* (Oxford: Oxford University Press, 2008).

24. A. Carr and M. McNulty, 'Intake Interviews, Testing and Report Writing', in *The Handbook of Adult Clinical Psychology: An Evidence-Based Practice Approach*', ed. by A. Carr and M. McNulty (Hove: Routledge, 2006), pp. 253–88.
25. L. Burns and R. Dallos, 'A Different World? Literary Reading in Family Therapists' Personal and Professional Development', *Journal of Family Therapy*, 30.1 (2008), 222–46.
26. M. Divinsky, 'Stories for Life: Introduction to Narrative Medicine', *Canadian Family Physician*, 53.2 (2007), 203–205.
27. For example, A. Morgan, *What Is Narrative Therapy? An Easy-to-Read Introduction* (Adelaide: Dulwich Centre Publications, 2000).
28. R. Thompson, 'Using Life Story Work to Enhance Care', *Nursing Older People*, 23.8 (2011), 16–21.
29. J. Toner, 'Cognitive Behavioural Therapy', in *The Pocket Guide to Therapy: A 'How To' of the Core Models*, ed. by S. Weatherhead and G. Flaherty-Jones (London: Sage, 2012), pp. 33–57.
30. D. McCulliss, 'Bibliotherapy: Historical and Research Perspectives', *Journal of Poetry Therapy*, 25.1 (2012), 23–38.
31. A. Bhattacharyya, 'Historical Backdrop', in *The Therapeutic Use of Stories*, ed. by K. N. Dwivedi (London: Routledge, 1997) pp. 1–18.
32. S. McArdle and R. Byrt, 'Fiction, Poetry and Mental Health: Expressive and Therapeutic Uses of Literature', *Journal of Psychiatric and Mental Health Nursing*, 8.6 (2001), 517–24.
33. B. Usherwood and J. Toyne, 'The Value and Impact of Reading Imaginative Literature', *Journal of Librarianship and Information Science*, 34.1 (2002), 33–41.
34. Hill and O'Brien, 1999, cited in Z. Shechtman and R. Nir-Shfrir, 'The Effect of Affective Bibliotherapy on Clients' Functioning in Group Therapy', *International Journal of Group Psychotherapy*, 58.1 (2008), 103–17.
35. J. W. Powell, 'Group Reading in Mental Hospitals', *Psychiatry: Interpersonal and Biological Processes*, 13.1 (1950), 213–26.
36. I. D. Yalom and M. Leszcz, *The Theory and Practice of Group Psychotherapy*, 5th edn (New York: Basic Books, 2005).
37. M. Higgins, C. McKevitt, and C. D. A Wolfe, 'Reading to Stroke Unit Patients: Perceived Impact and Potential of an Innovative Arts Based Therapy', *Rehabilitation in Practice*, 27.22 (2005), 1391–98.
38. J. C. Gardiner, M. Furois, D. P. Tansley, and B. Morgan, 'Music Therapy and Reading as Intervention Strategies for Disruptive Behaviour in Dementia', *Clinical Gerontologist*, 22.1 (2002), 31–46; A. Holm, M. Lepp, and K. C. Ringsberg, 'Dementia: Involving Patients in Storytelling—A Caring Intervention. A Pilot Study', *Journal of Clinical Nursing*, 14.2 (2005), 256–63; and M. J. Skrajner and C. J. Camp, 'Resident-Assisted Montessori Programming (RAMP): Use of a Small Group Reading Activity

Run by Persons with Dementia in Adult Day Health Care and Long-Term Care Settings', *American Journal of Alzheimer's Disease and Other Dementias*, 22.1 (2007), 27–36.

39. G. Shepherd, J. Boardman, and M. Slade, *Making Recovery a Reality* (London: Sainsbury Centre for Mental Health, 2008).
40. The following, each of whom at the time was working as a Band 5 OT, were all involved in contributing to the document: Jenny Fleming, Jill Corker, Kelly Johnston, David Cooper, Chris Vaughan, Rachel Albrecht, Hazel Budnarowski, Lisa White, Maria Gleeson, Linsey O'Donnell, Karen Birchall, Georgia Fair, Samantha O'Shea, and Laura Tyndall.
41. 'Recovering Ordinary Lives: The Strategy for Occupational Therapy in Mental Health Services, 2007–2017' (London: College of Occupational Therapists, 2006), p. 3.
42. N. Jacobson and D. Greenley, 'What Is Recovery? A Conceptual Model and Explication', *Psychiatric Services*, 52.4 (2001), 482–85.
43. S. Yee, 'Re-capturing an Important Piece of Self Through Leisure Occupations', *Occupational Therapy Now*, 9.1 (2007), 11–13 (p. 11).
44. J. Billington, A. Jones, A. L. Humphreys, and K. McDonnell, 'A Literature-Based Intervention for People with Chronic Pain', *Arts and Health: An International Journal for Research, Policy and Practice*, 8.1 (2014), 13–31.
45. D. Harrison and A. Sellers, 'Occupation for Mental Health and Social Inclusion', *The British Journal of Occupational Therapy*, 71.5 (2008), 216–19.
46. Prevention consultants, often nurses located at local health centres, see people after they've been to the doctor and possibly also after having gone through treatment, hence 'secondary prevention' (see below).

19

Reading for Dementia

Martin Orrell, Tom Dening, Nusrat Husain,
Sally Rimkeit, Gillian Claridge and Dalice Sim

Martin Orrell and Tom Dening, 'A Provisional Case for the Value of Reading in Relation to People Living with Dementia'

The Context

Currently, there are over 850,000 people with dementia in the UK, with estimated annual service costs of £8.7 billion.[1] The disease causes progressive cognitive deterioration, and in time, the associated loss of functional ability makes living independently impracticable. About 280,000 people with dementia live in care homes[2] and experience high levels of inactivity, boredom and poor quality

M. Orrell (✉) · T. Dening
Institute of Mental Health, University of Nottingham, Nottingham, UK
e-mail: M.Orrell@nottingham.ac.uk

T. Dening
e-mail: Tom.Dening@nottingham.ac.uk

N. Husain
Psychology and Mental Health, University of Manchester, Manchester, UK
e-mail: nusrat.husain@manchester.ac.uk

S. Rimkeit · G. Claridge · D. Sim
University of Otago, Wellington, New Zealand
e-mail: Sally.Rimkeit@ccdhb.org.nz

J. Billington (ed.), *Reading and Mental Health*,
https://doi.org/10.1007/978-3-030-21762-4_19

of life. Those living in care homes have a major impact on NHS resources because of their increased health needs and high risk of hospitalisation. Around 80% of people in residential care homes display Behavioural and Psychological Symptoms of Dementia (BPSD). These symptoms are often treated with antipsychotic drugs which can cause serious adverse events, including stroke and death, and are not clinically effective. It has been estimated by the NHS Institute for Innovation and Improvement that using psychosocial interventions for BPSD could save £54 million per year by avoiding 1348 cases of stroke and 118 falls compared with antipsychotic medication and the related NHS costs.

This has prompted a renewed interest in psychosocial interventions in dementia. Research into non-drug interventions has been identified as a national priority by the Prime Minister's Challenge on Dementia. Sir Mark Walport, Director of the Wellcome Trust, has added, 'The dementia challenge will not be resolved by the natural sciences alone. It will also require progress in social care'.[3]

At present the evidence is variable. However, nonpharmacological treatments (cognitive stimulation therapy, tailored activity programme and occupational therapy) have been found to be more cost-effective than usual care.[4] A recent systematic review showed that psychosocial interventions can help meet the needs of people living with dementia—the need to connect with others, make a meaningful contribution and reminisce—and concluded that further well-designed research was needed to strengthen the evidence base for psychosocial interventions in long-term care.[5]

Why Reading?

Some dementia symptoms are exacerbated because of a lack of suitable activity provision—especially cultural and arts-based activities—both for people

---

D. Sim
e-mail: dalice.sim@otago.ac.nz

S. Rimkeit
Capital and Coast District Health Board, Wellington, New Zealand

G. Claridge
School of Language and Culture, Institute of the Pacific United,
Palmerston North, New Zealand
e-mail: gclaridge@ipu.ac.nz

living in the community and in care homes. This causes boredom, frustration and a lowered sense of well-being and independence, as people with dementia can no longer practice things they used to enjoy (reading novels, for example).[6] Meaningful activity has a positive effect on the health, self-esteem, happiness and life satisfaction of older people. As advocated by the 'Use It or Lose It' theory, participating in activities can postpone cognitive decline and frequent cognitive activity may reduce the risk of dementia. Recent research and practice is paying more attention to psychological and social interventions to help meet the needs of people with dementia and their carers.

The model of Shared Reading pioneered by UK charity The Reader is a widely used, non-threatening and accessible read-aloud activity in which groups, with 2–12 members, meet weekly for 60 minutes (see Chapter 6). The groups are delivered by trained facilitators who read aloud with participants a range of literary texts, usually poetry. Participants are encouraged to reflect on personal memories or matters stimulated by the text and/or to read aloud themselves.

A pilot study of Shared Reading conducted by the Centre for Research into Reading, Literature and Society[7] observed the effect on Behavioural and Psychological Symptoms of Dementia (BPSD) using the Neuropsychiatric Inventory Questionnaire (NPI-Q) (a clinical scale that measures the presence and severity of: delusions, hallucinations, agitation/aggression, anxiety, depression/dysphoria, elation/euphoria, apathy/indifference, disinhibition, irritability/lability and motor disturbance). This preliminary study found significant improvement in BPSD—symptoms closely associated with caregiver burden—and indicated that there were possible immediate benefits for people living with dementia and their carers. As well as helping to improve mood and reduce agitation, the groups were also noted to be 'stimulating and soothing at the same time'. People with dementia said that Shared Reading was very enjoyable and supportive—'elevating'—allowing them to 'connect' with others, providing 'structure to focus on' and creating 'a space in that present moment'. Staff also showed very strong support, highlighting opportunities to 'trigger memories', promote 'active listening' and attention, and enable group members to 'interact in a meaningful context' unrelated to other care tasks, where they could share personal reflections and experiences authentically. Staff also saw benefits to themselves: 'If the service users are happy then we're happy'. A second study[8] found a positive effect on the quality of life, as measured by the DEMQOL-Proxy[9] (an interviewer-administered carer-rated measure which evaluates various aspects of mood, including contentment, energy levels, cheerfulness). Qualitative data also supported the benefits of the groups. It was found that Shared

Reading produced a sense of identity and prompted both relevant past experiences and new ideas through a concentrated mental and emotional 'present-ness' in connection to the literature.

Reading aloud groups offer a cheap and popular intervention which can be replicated in a variety of health and social care settings. In generating quality of life and BPSD improvements, Shared Reading has potential to release additional economic benefits by offering a non-drug intervention which is in line with NICE guidelines in respect of dementia, namely 'offering a range of activities to promote wellbeing that are tailored to the person's preferences'.

What Needs to Happen Next?

Shared Reading now needs more robust scientific and statistically powerful evaluation to determine clinical and cost-effectiveness compared to usual care. Specifically, what is required is a large-scale multi-centre randomised controlled trial involving people with mild to moderate dementia who live in care homes or attend community day centres in the UK. The trial should measure the effectiveness of a reading aloud group intervention, as compared with usual care, in relation to mood and quality of life, behavioural and psychological symptoms (BPSD), costs and service use.

Such a trial would need to work closely with people with dementia, family carers and care home staff to adapt existing materials for group reading to make it possible for care staff to run Shared Reading groups effectively. With appropriate support to ensure adherence to The Reader's model, Shared Reading could be widely delivered by care assistants in residential and community settings so that large numbers of participants could be recruited to the study.

As adaptation of the read-aloud model will be necessary for future routine use, the trial should develop and evaluate a standardised training package for care staff (using interactive seminars, videos, case studies, as well as a training manual—as per cognitive stimulation therapy—and providing a body of reading material). Training care staff to deliver the intervention will further reduce delivery costs and increase the accessibility and spread of the intervention.

The trial should ideally incorporate systematic economic evaluation to determine the cost-effectiveness of the model delivered at scale, and exploration of its wider implementation. There are often problems implementing non-pharmacological interventions in practice even when there is clear evidence of benefit. These benefits cannot be realised unless these barriers can be overcome. The trial will need to produce evidence on how the Shared Reading intervention is introduced and operationalised in routine practice, how it is experienced by different stakeholders, and what contextual factors and causal mechanisms affect outcomes.

Nusrat Husain, 'A Case for the Value of Reading with Older People in the BME Population'

The Context

The two most common mental health issues in old age are dementia and depression and they may develop together. Individuals with dementia commonly suffer from depression[10] resulting in reduced quality of life. Individuals with a history of depression in later life may be associated with an increased risk of developing dementia.[11] A higher prevalence of depression has been indicated in the ethnic minority groups compared to white Europeans,[12] with research indicating depression persists more frequently in Pakistanis over the age of 50 years old.[13] The Alzheimer's Society estimate that almost 25,000 people with dementia are from the Black and Minority Ethnic (BME) groups in England and Wales; the figure is expected to rise to 172,000 by 2051, almost a seven-fold increase. The prevalence of depression and dementia is similar if not higher in the BME community compared to the White British elders,[14] yet to our knowledge there is no intervention currently present to address this. The BME population is more likely to be living in low-income areas, and this inequality is further aggravated by the marked ethnic disparities in access to mental health care often due to cultural differences such as language barriers, family support and different explanatory models.[15] While generally the public understanding of dementia has improved, a stigma remains in relation to the condition,[16] with the levels of stigma being higher in the BME community.[17] The Department of Health's 'key priorities' include recognising and addressing the particular needs of BME populations in respect of dementia and enhancing the mental health and well-being of people living with dementia by improving access to psychology therapies and cultural activities as an alternative to liberal and inappropriate prescribing of medication.[18] Several studies have looked at the impact of alternative therapies in the treatment of dementia.[19] Relatively little is known about this or any other intervention among BME groups.[20]

These circumstances make a pressing case for the discovery and development of non-medical interventions which are readily accessible and can help reduce social and health inequalities.

Why Reading?

Literacy and reading for pleasure are among the strongest indicators of social and educational opportunity and mobility.[21] Poor literacy is aligned with many of the social determinants of health inequalities—poverty, low socio-economic status, poor housing, low well-being and poor mental health. Literacy and reading are thus prime examples of how inequalities in resource and in the capacity to control the direction of one's life (through, e.g., the greater educational opportunity which literacy and wide reading can offer) can impact upon health. It is also an area where the NHS can work systematically with voluntary and third sector organisations, in preventing the unequal consequences of ill health.

Several studies have demonstrated the impact of The Reader's model of Shared Reading on mental health issues, including depression as well as dementia.[22] (See also Chapters 5 and 6). The key elements of the model as identified in these studies are:

- A rich, varied, non-prescriptive diet of serious literature, enhancing the ability of people to think and speak of important emotional thoughts and meanings otherwise difficult to locate and express.
- Making the literature 'live' in the room—as a human presence, not just an object of study or chat—through skilful reading aloud, ensuring everybody can take part regardless of levels of literacy, educational, ethnic or cultural background.
- Creation of small communities, often across widely different backgrounds, with a closer relation of private to public or individual to social than is customary as a result of the human coalescing and emotionally sharing force of the literature.
- Regularity: meeting weekly offers valuable continuity and structure for people whose lives may be chaotic or empty.

The emphasis on a personalised, inclusive, regular activity, which combines a non-pharmacological approach with social connectedness, has strong potential benefits for the especially disadvantaged BME community, in which (the particularly high number of) people living with dementia and depression experience chronic social isolation and low well-being, as well as poor access to mental health care and culturally appropriate services.

What's to Be Done?

The Reader's Shared Reading model is delivered to a wide range of disadvantaged groups and The Reader is already collaborating with NHS England and Wales by bringing reading groups to service users in ways which benefit their health and well-being. What is needed now is a pilot study of how this successful intervention can be extended and culturally adapted to meet the special needs of a specific community within the BME population. I have suggested my own constituency of severely disadvantaged older adults within the British South Asian communities in the North-West—who are particularly isolated and at high risk of developing mental health difficulties—as an obvious place to start since The Reader originated in the North-West region and has already forged strong links with local health and governmental bodies.

The study's purpose would ideally be three-fold.

First, it would need to explore the feasibility of establishing community Shared Reading groups in a British South Asian community. This could be achieved through running separate focus groups (i) with individuals living with dementia and their relatives and carers (ii) with health professionals and organisations who work with individuals experiencing dementia and related mental health issues.

Second, the study should investigate the acceptability of the intervention to individuals from the British South Asian population by (i) a test run of the reading group with a group of participants at a care home with British South Asian residents and (ii) in-depth qualitative interviews with participants, their relatives and the health care providers to understand the experience of participants. The study would be essentially qualitative in nature but might consider trialling with participants the suitability for this population, and for the study, of certain standard assessments/measures: for example, The Geriatric Depression Scale (GDS) (which has been used successfully in the Pakistani elderly population[23]).

Critical to the success of the reading group will be the choice of material. Since Shared Reading began in 2001, The Reader has built up a bank of tried and tested materials—including a published anthology of poems and extracts from the Renaissance to the present day for reading with older people.[24] Crucial for this study, however, will be advice from experts in South Asian literature as to: choices of literature (fiction and poetry especially); whether the latter should be delivered in the original language, or in translation, or both; whether and how South Asian literature might be mixed with other literatures. It is anticipated that the 'test' reading group will have most success if the facilitator is drawn from the BME community (preferably the immediate, local one).

Thirdly, the study will need to evaluate the ability of such groups to become sustainable, by documenting the barriers and enablers to the NHS's working systematically with voluntary and third sector organisations in preventing the unequal consequences of social isolation and ill health—possibly offering a prototype model for such cooperation.

I am well-versed in such issues because I have collaborated with The Reader and the University of Liverpool on designing just such a project and in successfully securing funding for this valuable project. We have been unable to carry out the study to date for want of suitably qualified research personnel who can speak, read and understand one or more British South Asian languages (Urdu, Gujarati, Hindi, Bengali, Punjabi). This is the first known barrier to overcome. We now plan to start the project in the North-West later this year and if we find this feasible and acceptable we will explore the possibility of testing this intervention in South Asia.

Sally Rimkeit, Gillian Claridge, Dalice Sim, 'Reading for Dementia: A Pilot RCT'

Reading and Older Adults

The elderly are known to spend more time reading than any other age group. A UK-based study of 4000 adults found that more than four-fifths of them enjoy reading, rating it more important than watching television.[25] Reading has been demonstrated to have a positive effect on life expectancy, contributing to the retarding of the deleterious effects of ageing by supporting the brain's resilience to pathological damage.[26] This 'cognitive reserve',[27] produced by habitual reading, was most famously demonstrated in the 'Nun Study'[28] which analysed data from convent archives, annual examinations and posthumous brain specimens of 678 Catholic sisters. The study showed a strong association between higher linguistic ability in early life and better cognitive ability and protection against clinical symptoms of Alzheimer's disease, despite pathological brain changes, decades later. The first linguistic assessments were based on the idea density and grammatical complexity displayed in hand-written autobiographies by the nuns in their youth. This association between literacy skills in young adult life and protection against dementia held after education and occupation were controlled for. Within this model of cognitive reserve, there is increasing evidence that some people can tolerate age-related brain changes and Alzheimer's pathology and still maintain cognitive function without dementia.[29] It is possible that reading and literacy can play a part.

The link between book reading, cognitive reserve and protection from dementia risk is supported by a recent prospective cohort study in the USA which suggests that limited literacy correlates to dementia risk. 25.5% of those with limited literacy (less than 9th-grade reading level) developed dementia (as tested by study criteria for 'likely' dementia) over the 8 years follow up of the study, as compared to 17% with adequate literacy.[30] A 2016 estimate of the proportion of dementia cases attributable to illiteracy, using the population attributable fraction (PAF) from United Nations prevalence data from South Korea, Latin America, South Asia/Middle East and Africa, concludes that public policy efforts to improve literacy rates will have a significant impact on protection against later life dementia and will potentially save many billions in health dollars.[31] In the Rush Memory and Aging Project (Chicago, USA), early and late life cognitive activity, including reading books, visiting the library and writing letters, together accounted for 15% of the residual variability in cognitive function after adjusting for neuropathology in the brain. The authors hypothesise that cognitive activity, such as book reading, can support cognitive reserve to counterbalance cognitive loss associated with neuropathologic burden.[32] In a study of people living beyond aged 90, the lifestyle factors of going to church or synagogue and reading or having stories read aloud during the nonagenarian years were the most significant lifestyle factors to lower risk of developing dementia over the next five years.[33] This is interesting because both church and synagogue services largely consist of the repetition of well-known 'stories' in the form of bible and torah readings.

Reading and Mental Health in Older People

The Recovery and Discovery Model

The recovery model in mental health care uses an approach that supports people to live as meaningful a life as possible despite persistent symptoms of illness. Recovery-oriented practice broadens the person-centred approach by promoting hope and eschewing therapeutic nihilism. This model is particularly salient for use in dementia care, as it acknowledges that recovery does not represent cure, but instead offers the opportunity for persons to regain confidence and identity within their communities and to exercise their choice to do things and develop relationships that give their lives meaning.[34] The most rigorously studied of the psychosocial interventions which aim to help people with dementia live as well as they can with the condition is cognitive stimulation therapy (CST). CST has been shown to compare favourably with cognitive enhancing medications in improving quality of life in community-dwelling people with dementia[35] and is now recommended by the National Institute for Health and Care Excellence (NICE Guideline, 2018). A twice-weekly, seven-week, manualised step-by-step intervention, CST provides activities which are not necessarily those which the person living with dementia would choose for himself or herself. Arguably, facilitating access to community-based arts activities that the person once loved, or now chooses to take interest in, promotes recovery-(and discovery-) oriented practice more fully than CST.[36] Currently, studies in the UK, USA or globally on the effect of reading for people living with dementia fall short of the 'gold standard' for robust experimental design set by research into CST.[37] Pilot evidence suggests, however, that the value of reading short items of poetry aloud for people with dementia, because of the rhythm and rhyme, seems to maintain concentration and interest. The content of the poetry may also trigger relevant past experience and fresh acts of thought (Longden, et al., 2016). Enjoyment, enhancement of social interaction and relationship, and the sense of engaging in an authentic experience that can be sustained by family members are also key themes (Billington et al., 2013).

Dementia-Friendly Reading Materials

With 47 million people worldwide now experiencing dementia, many of whom have been avid readers throughout their lives, enhancing access to and enjoyment of literary fiction seems both valid and effective. However, there appear to have been few strategic efforts to engage the elderly, especially those living with dementia, in reading. The only formal guidelines on providing library services to people with dementia, for example, are those from the International Federation of Library Associations and Institutions (IFLA).

In their guidelines, the IFLA emphasise the obligation of public library services to provide access to 'culture, literature and information to all, including persons with disabilities'. They enjoin library services to 'lead the way in tailoring collections' for this population.

However, problematically, these guidelines recommend that for adults with dementia 'children's picture books with big and clear illustrations are appropriate'. It is true that people living with dementia may find lone and group reading difficult to access and enjoy because of specific cognitive impairments.[38] Support persons frequently offer individuals living with dementia children's books to read in the belief that their reading ability diminishes along with their memory loss, in a 'de-developmental model' of regressed linguistic functioning, and this diminished ability might be on a par with that of a child learning to read.

But linguistic studies have suggested that for common dementia types, such as Alzheimer's disease or vascular dementia, language comprehension might be compromised by 'attenuated span capacity, difficulty focusing attention, encoding and activation of long-term knowledge, rather than from the loss of linguistic knowledge'.[39] People with mild to moderate Alzheimer's disease generally retain the linguistic knowledge they previously gained in their reading life and their literacy is not significantly worse than adult controls, but is significantly better than children's scores.[40] People with mild to moderate Alzheimer's disease retain the ability to recognise the meaning of words that are not commonly used (such as 'sew', 'soot' 'dough or 'height', as tested in the Addenbrookes-III), especially if they are encountered in a familiar context such as a well-known story.[41]

Hence, ludic readers who have now developed dementia may not need to have the vocabulary of once-loved literary classics dumbed down, as they are likely to have retained understanding of irregular syntax and low-frequency lexis. Children's books or books written for the adult learner reading English as a second language, both of which rely on high frequency words and simple syntax, may lack sophistication and be infantilising for the skilled English reader with dementia.[42] This is especially concerning, given the findings of recent neuroscientific research which indicates that it is the complex syntax of literary (as opposed to expository) texts which evoke recruitment of a wide range of brain networks. In doing so, classic literature has the power to excite the mind with discovery and creativity.[43] While several researchers have provided practical recommendations for making text more 'dementia-friendly' (see below), there is no advice on adapting classic fiction for this audience.

Our Research Programme on Shared Reading Groups for Dementia

We are in the process of undertaking a robust, three-step programme of research to fill the gap in current understanding and provision of Shared Reading groups for people living with dementia. Step 1, a feasibility study, and Step 2, a pilot randomised control trial (RCT), have been completed and study findings have informed the design of Step 3, a fully powered RCT which is now underway. Our primary research question is: Can participation in a book group, appropriately facilitated, improve the quality of life of persons living with dementia? Secondary measures test for improvements in cognition, mood, theory of mind and thriving at the care home. The NZ Health and Disability Ethics Committee has provided important consultation and approval throughout the programme.

Step One: The Feasibility Study

In 2015–2016, we completed a feasibility study to discover the attitudes and opinions of people living with dementia towards reading targeted adaptations of classic literature and discussing them in book groups.

Protocol

The participants were 7 people (4 male), aged from 66 to 84 years, diagnosed with dementia. Four lived in community with family and three in a secure dementia unit at the care home where the focus groups took place. Their avowed reading preferences were for fiction over non-fiction, and they liked action stories best, then crime, romance and mystery. Biography was most popular in non-fiction.

We created and published a version of Charles Dickens' classic tale *A Christmas Carol* for the book groups as (1) the story is widely familiar to readers and written in Dickens' inimitable style; (2) the book groups were held during the festive Christmas season (November 2015). As there was no peer-reviewed information available on how to adapt literary fiction for improved access and enjoyment for people with dementia, our adaptation utilised evidence-based recommendations available at the time, from peer-reviewed publications of studies on 'aphasia-friendly' educational materials, including minimum font size 14, plenty of white space, 1.5 line spacing, san serif font, reducing of information to bite-sized chunks, repeating the referent newly on each page, and simplified language and syntax.[44] The illustrations were carefully chosen from adult classic editions of *A Christmas Carol* found at the Alexander Turnbull Library in Wellington, New Zealand, for the 64-page book. The adaptation was given to the participants at an initial individual interview, together with the original text in a large print non-illustrated edition, and a commercially produced illustrated children's adaptation. It was important that the three books were perceived as printed books, rather than just A4 hand-outs, for an authentic experience of book reading.

Two focus groups were held, one involving day care participants with mild to moderate dementia, the other with participants in residential care with more severe dementia. The focus groups were audio recorded, transcribed and analysed using IPA (see Chapter 9 above). Both focus groups provided equally lively discussion, with striking levels of engagement by those with advanced dementia.

Results

Three key themes emerged:

1. **The participant as a lively reader**. All participants were keen readers and entered into a spirited discussion of their relationship to reading in childhood and adulthood. 'Books always took me to another adventure, another part of the world, a new topic to understand'. Participants enjoyed talking about excerpts even if they could not recall reading them previously. The idea of a book group was enthusiastically welcomed: 'That's a great idea. We could descend on them with our ideas'.
2. **The participant as guardian of the voice of Dickens and a preference for Dickens' language**. The children's adaptation was regarded as 'too simple. It lost Dickens. It tells the story, the guts of the story, but you lose the voice of Dickens. You don't have access to his imagination'. The pleasure participants took in the language was demonstrated through the generation of their own, often humorous wordplay.
3. **The participant as a discerning book reviewer**. While they wished to experience the style and rhythm of the original language, participants offered many helpful suggestions for making the adaptations more 'dementia-friendly', including use of a list of characters, strong contrast of

print and paper, judicious shortening of the story, and lively illustrations that capture the spirit of the text and avoid childish pictures.

The feasibility study successfully tested the practicality of creating and trialling an adapted book appropriate to the tastes and needs of people living with dementia. What was most striking and salient was their command and appreciation of the 'wonderful words' of the original classic writer, even if the context was not always grasped. This vindicated our choice of classic, well-known and time-honoured, texts. It was keeping track of the characters and plot that was at issue. Simplification was not always appreciated and was sometimes seen as infantilising.

From the feasibility findings, we conclude that adaptations of literary fiction for readers with dementia should re-tell classic stories in episodic form, preserving as much as possible of the original language. Too much reading makes too many memory and attention span demands on the reader with Alzheimer's disease. The adaptations should give each double-page spread a sense of unity in itself, as a stand-alone reading experience as well as a step in the overall narrative. They should provide a cast list at the beginning of the story and repeat the referents on each new page (e.g. repeat 'Scrooge' rather than using the pronoun 'he'). The older eye requires large font with clear print on contrasting white paper. Illustrations should enliven the story, without being childlike. Classic tales are valued for their familiarity and inimitable quality.

On the basis of these findings, we have now published five further dementia-friendly adaptations of classic tales and poetry. The use of the same five books throughout the study enhances the fidelity of the book group intervention for the pilot and full RCT.

G. Claridge, B. S. Rimkeit, A Dovetale Press Adaptation, A Christmas Carol, Charles Dickens, Second Edition ISBN 978-0-473-37294-1.
G. Claridge, B. S. Rimkeit, A Dovetale Press Adaptation, Little Women, Louisa May Alcott ISBN 978-0-473-37295-8.
G. Claridge, B. S. Rimkeit, A Dovetale Press Adaptation, Sherlock Holmes, The Adventure of the Blue Carbuncle ISBN 978-0-473-37293-4.
G. Claridge, B. S. Rimkeit, A Dovetale Press Adaptation, The Garden Party & The Doll's House, Katherine Mansfield ISBN 978-0-473-37291-0.
B. S. Rimkeit, G. Claridge, A Dovetale Press Selection, Poetry for the Restless Heart ISBN 978-0-473-37292-7.

Step 2: The Pilot RCT

Protocol

The main purpose of the pilot RCT was to test the practicability of conducting a twice-weekly, 7-week book group intervention and RCT in a population of people living with dementia in a care home. The study design was modelled on Spector's CST protocol (Spector, 2010). Primary goals were to assess the feasibility of the recruitment and consenting process, the pre- and post-assessment process, and the scheduling and facilitating of the book group intervention. We carefully evaluated the resourcing of time and energy for care home nursing staff, clinical assessors, and care home activity staff, for each of these processes. Bupa NZ provided a grant for the publication of the dementia-friendly books and resource-in-kind in recruiting, consenting and facilitating the book groups in their care homes. After the completion of data collection, we met with Bupa staff to gain comprehensive feedback on staffing resourcing and burden.[45]

The primary assessment measure was the Resident QoL-AD (Quality of Life in Alzheimer's Disease) self-report, a 15-item questionnaire.[46] Secondary measures were Addenbrooke's-III cognitive assessment,[47] Thriving of Older Persons Assessment Scale (TOPAS),[48] The Geriatric Depression Scale Short Form (GDS–SF),[49] and The FACES Test of Theory of Mind.[50] To assess behavioural changes in participants, the Neuropsychiatric Inventory (NPI)[51] was completed by family support persons. QoL-AD-Proxy and TOPAS-Proxy were asked to be completed by family support persons from the participant-dyad.

20 dyads of people with living with dementia and their family support persons were selected from two Bupa care homes in the lower North Island of New Zealand. A poster in each care home invited residents to express an interest in the study. Senior nursing staff assisted in selecting and consenting residents who they thought might meet study criteria in respect of dementia diagnosis, communication, vision and non-disruptive behaviour, as measured by the InterRAI.[52] Each care home had 10 participants living with dementia: 5 randomised to the book group and 5 randomised to 'usual activities'. Our design recommended that one care home enrol participants with mild to moderate dementia (in rest home or hospital level care) and the other care home enrol participants with moderate to severe dementia (in secure dementia level care).

Each book group consisted of five participants living with dementia. Family support participants in the dyad did not join the book groups. The groups lasted about 45 minutes and were facilitated by diversional or activity therapists from the Bupa care home. All sessions were audio recorded with the participants' permission. Before the start of the study, we ran a training session on how to facilitate the dementia-friendly book groups. We also provided a written facilitation manual with step-by-step instructions, to enhance study fidelity. The training manual gave advice on how to encourage the participants to share personal views and opinions, talk about any memories that the readings evoked and link characters or events to anything that was going on in their lives. The book groups were designed to be strengths-based for people with dementia, many of whom, we anticipated, could still enjoy sharing a 'good read', with all its psychosocial and cognitive benefits. Facilitators were asked to avoid the use of closed, factual questions which might cause discomfort or stress to the participant. The programme allowed a week each for *A Christmas Carol*, *Sherlock Holmes* and *Little Women*, two weeks for the *Katherine Mansfield* short stories, and two weeks for selections from *Poetry for the Restless Heart*.

Results

The pilot study allowed the opportunity for review from our sponsor, Bupa NZ. Feedback from Bupa Care was that, with good management, recruitment and consenting of potential participants by nursing staff could be a rewarding endeavour, which allowed staff to engage with interest in the study design and purpose. The book group intervention could be carried out as an adjunct to the normal activities of the care home without undue stress on staff. Facilitation of twice weekly book groups for 7 weeks by activity staff was found to be inherently feasible, if incorporated into the care home's activity schedule. Facilitators found that setting up audio recording of the sessions was one of the most onerous tasks.

In the case of one of the care homes, the facilitators could not attend the pre-intervention training session. It became clear from the transcripts of the book group sessions that the quality of the facilitation was inferior to that of the care home whose activity staff did attend. This lowered the fidelity of the intervention, introducing potential bias into the results.

Care homes found it too cumbersome to recruit participants with stratified levels of dementia severity, and in the end, both care home book groups contained a mixture of participants with all stages of dementia. Several participants with mild to moderate dementia complained that some of the more impaired participants were distracting for them.

Each pre- and post-assessment by a clinician from the research team took approximately one hour to complete for each participant with dementia and appeared to be well-tolerated and even enjoyed. Several participants expressed disappointment when the assessment session was over. The total assessment was conducted over two shorter sessions for participants with more impaired concentration and processing speed.

On evaluating whether the assessors could practically remain blinded at post-assessment, we found that blinded assessment was generally practical and achievable. In all but one case (where the participant described the book group activity after the primary post-assessment measure was completed), the assessors did not know which treatment the participant had received.

The response rate for completing the proxy QoL-AD and TOPAS assessments by the support persons was disappointing. This was also true for the completion of the NPI by family support persons. Furthermore, assessments (requested pre- and post-intervention) could not be kept blinded.

The pilot data shows differences in all outcome variables when the intervention participants are compared to the control participants. The participants living with dementia allocated to the book group intervention show mean improvements in QoL-AD, TOPAS, ACE-III, and GDS, and FACES tests. The small numbers of participants preclude our finding a statistically significant difference between the groups, but analysis of this sample indicates what size of differences we might expect between intervention and control in the full RCT. We have calculated that to fully power a robust RCT, we will need a total of 260 participants from care homes, with 130 participants in each study arm. Based on the differences seen in the pilot study, we have calculated this sample size provides a power of at least 85%. Standard power requirements for RCTs are 80%, and so our sample size will allow for up to 20% attrition. In this older population with dementia, the extra buffering in sample size is important; in our pilot study, two of the 20 participants died during the course of the study.

We are currently analysing the qualitative data from the pilot study, and we anticipate that results will be published in 2020.

Step 3: An International RCT

The findings from the feasibility study and pilot RCT have informed the design of the full RCT. In the full RCT, we are limiting participants to those people living with mild to moderate dementia and excluding those with more severe disease. Potential participants will not be required to have a formal diagnosis of dementia (which we found was often missing in care home records), but care home staff will have a strong suspicion that the potential participant is living with dementia. Participants will be eligible if they score above 35 and below 86 on the Addenbrooke's-III cognitive assessment (ACE-III) (Noone, 2015) at pre-assessment. This will reduce frustration for participants within the book groups who might be distracted by participants with more severe dementia and also increase efficiency of the assessment process. The disadvantage is that this ACE-III assessment occurs after the initial selection process through the InterRAI information. This may mean that some persons who have already consented to being in the study may then not be eligible to participate.

We have simplified the protocol in eliminating the support person-participant and the participant-dyad. In the full RCT, the only participants are those residents at the care home with dementia. Hence, we have eliminated the QoL-AD-proxy and TOPAS-proxy assessments. The Health and Disability Ethics Committee acknowledge and commend the new study design, which they emphasise better focuses on the 'voice' of the person with dementia, rather than proxy evaluation. However, we continue with the NPI assessments through formal carers at the care homes, to assess for changes in behaviour.

To enhance study fidelity, we are extending the facilitators' manual, providing videos of Dr Claridge facilitating book groups and offering more intense in-house training. In contrast to the pilot study, the full RCT sessions are not being audio recorded.

International collaboration has been established for completion of the full RCT. Data collection has commenced in New Zealand through Drs Rimkeit, Claridge and Sim at the University of Otago, supported by a NZ Lotteries Grant. Josie Billington and Philip Davis of the University of Liverpool will be completing data collection in the UK, supported by funds from their host university. Professor David Edvardsson and Jen Austerberry of La Trobe University, Melbourne, will be running the RCT in Australia. Bupa Care continues to provide resource-in-kind by recruiting and consenting participants and facilitating the book groups in their care homes in New Zealand and Australia. HC-One care homes are providing resource-in-kind with support from Professor Graham Stokes in the UK.

This is the largest and most strongly powered RCT into dementia and Shared Reading to date, and results are anticipated to be available in 2020.

Our hypothesis is that for persons living with dementia Shared Reading can, by promoting recovery and even discovery, actually enhance the quality of life.

Notes

1. See Department of Health (2018), 'Dementia: Applying All Our Health', https://www.gov.uk/government/publications/dementia-applying-all-our-health/dementia-applying-all-our-health#facts-about-dementia and The Alzheimer's Society (2019), 'Key facts and Statistics on Dementia', https://www.alzheimers.org.uk/about-us/news-and-media/facts-media.
2. Alzhiemer's Society, 'Fix Dementia Care: NHS and Care Homes', 2016.
3. Quoted in *The Guardian*, 26 March 2012.
4. M. Knapp, V. Iemmi, and R. Romeo, 'Dementia Care Costs and Outcomes: A Systematic Review', *International Journal of Geriatric Psychiatry* 28.6 (2013), 551–61.
5. V. Lawrence, J. Fossey, C. Ballard, E. Moniz-Cook, and J. Murray, 'Improving Quality of Life for People with Dementia in Care Homes: Making Psychosocial Interventions Work', *British Journal of Psychiatry*, 201.5 (2012), 344–51.
6. V. H. Menec, 'The Relation Between Everyday Activities and Successful Aging: A 6-Year Longitudinal Study', *Journal of Gerontology*, 58B.2 (2003), S74–S82.
7. J. Billington, J. Carroll, P. Davis, C. Healey, and P. Kinderman, 'A Literature-Based Intervention for Older People Living with Dementia', *Perspectives in Public Health*, 133.3 (2013), 165–73.
8. E. Longden, P. Davis, J. Carroll, and Josie Billington, 'An Evaluation of Shared Reading Groups for Adults Living with Dementia: Preliminary Findings', *Journal of Public Health*, 15.2 (2016), 75–82.
9. S. C. Smith, D. L. Lamping, S. Banerjee, R. Harwood, B. Foley, P. Smith, J. C. Cook, J. Murray, M. Prince, E. Levin, A. Mann, and M. Knapp, 'Measurement of Health-Related Quality of Life for People with Dementia: Development of a New Instrument (DEMQOL) and an Evaluation of Current Methodology', *Health Technology Assessment*, 9.10 (2005), 1–93, iii–iv.
10. Y. E. Geda, R. O. Roberts, D. S. Knopman, R. C. Petersen, T. J. Christianson, V. S. Pankratz, G. E. Smith, B. F. Boeve, R. J. Ivnik, E.G. Tangalos, and W. A. Rocca, 'Prevalence of Neuropsychiatric Symptoms in Mild Cognitive Impairment and Normal Cognitive Aging: Population-Based Study', *Archives of General Psychiatry*, 65.10 (2008), 1193–98; and E. Teng, J. M. Ringman, L. K. Ross, R. A. Mulnard, M. B. Dick,

G. Bartzokis, et al., 'Diagnosing Depression in Alzheimer Disease with National Institute of Mental Health Provisional Criteria', *American Journal of Geriatric Psychiatry*, 16.6 (2008), 469–77.

11. M. A. Butters, E. M. Whyte, R. D. Nebes, A. E. Begley, M. A. Dew, B. H. Mulsant, et al., 'The Nature and Determinants of Neuropsychological Functioning in Late-Life Depression', *Archives of General Psychiatry*, 61.6 (2004), 587–95; and A. F. Jorm, 'History of Depression as a Risk Factor for Dementia: An Updated Review', *Australian and New Zealand Journal of Psychiatry*, 35.6 (2001), 776–81.
12. L. Bayard-Burfield, J. Sundquist, and S. E. Johansson, 'Ethnicity, Self-Reported Psychiatric Illness, and Intake of Psychotropic Drugs in Five Ethnic Groups in Sweden', *Journal of Epidemiology and Community Health*, 55.9 (2001), 657–64; K. Bhui, D. Bhugra, D. Goldberg, J. Sauer, and A. Tylee, 'Assessing the Prevalence of Depression in Punjabi and English Primary Care Attenders: The Role of Culture, Physical Illness and Somatic Symptoms', *Transcultural Psychiatry*, 41.3 (2004), 307–22; S. B. Thapa and E. Hauff, 'Gender Differences in Factors Associated with Psychological Distress Among Immigrants from Low- and Middle-Income Countries—Findings from the Oslo Health Study', *Social Psychiatry and Psychiatric Epidemiology*, 40.1 (2005), 78–84; F. B. van der Wurff, A. T. Beekman, H. Dijkshoorn, J. A. Spijker, C. H. Smits, M. L. Stek, and A. Verhoeff, 'Prevalence and Risk-Factors for Depression in Elderly Turkish and Moroccan Migrants in the Netherlands', *Journal of Affective Disorders*, 83.1 (2004), 33–41; S. Weich, J. Nazroo, K. Sproston, S. McManus, M. Blanchard, B. Erens, S. Karlsen, M. King, K. Lloyd, S. Stansfeld, and P. Tyrer, 'Common Mental Disorders and Ethnicity in England: The EMPIRIC Study', *Psychological Medicine*, 34.8 (2004), 1543–51; and R. Williams and K. Hunt, 'Psychological Distress Among British South Asians: The Contribution of Stressful Situations and Subcultural Differences in the West of Scotland Twenty-07 Study', *Psychological Medicine*, 27.5 (1997), 1173–81.
13. R. Gater, T. Tomenson, C. Percival, N. Chaudhry, W. Waheed, G. Dunn, G. Macfarlane, and F. Creed, 'Persistent Depressive Disorders and Social Stress in People of Pakistani Origin and White Europeans', *Social Psychiatry and Psychiatric Epidemiology*. 44.3 (2009), 198–207.
14. A. Shah, 'Estimating the Absolute Number of Cases of Dementia and Depression in the Black and Minority Ethnic Elderly Population in the UK', *International Journal of Migration and Health and Social Care*, 4.2 (2008), 4–15.
15. A. G. Bhikha, S. Farooq, N. Chaudhry, and N. Husain, 'A Systematic Review of Explanatory Models of Illness for Psychosis in Developing Countries', *International Review of Psychiatry*, 24.5 (2012), 450–62.

16. A Beattie, G. Daker-White, and J. Gillard, '"How Can They Tell?" A Qualitative Study of the Views of Younger People About Their Dementia and Dementia Care Services', *Health and Social Care in the Community*, 12.4 (2004), 359–68.
17. V. Seabrooke and A. Milne, 'Early Intervention in Dementia Care in an Asian Community: Lessons from a Dementia Collaborative Project', *Quality in Ageing*, 10.4 (2009), 29–36; J. La Fontaine, J. Ahuja, N. M. Bradbury, S. Phillips, and J. R. Oyebode, 'Understanding Dementia Amongst People in Minority Ethnic and Cultural Groups', *Journal Advance Nursing*, 60.6 (2007), 605–14; N. Azam, *Evaluation Report of the Meri Yaadain Dementia Project* (Bradford: Bradford District Health and Social Care Communications Team, 2007); J. Mackenzie, 'Stigma and Dementia—East European and South Asian Family Carers Negotiating Stigma in the UK', *Dementia: The International Journal of Social Research and Practice*, 5.2 (2006), 233–48; and J. Mackenzie, D. Coates, F. Ashraf, T. Gallagher, and L. Ismail, *Understanding and Supporting South Asian and Eastern European Family Carers of People with Dementia* (Bradford: University of Bradford, Bradford Dementia Group, 2003).
18. Department of Health and Social Care, 'Prime Minister's Challenge on Dementia 2020: Implementation Plan' and 'Implementation Plan, Annex 2: Roadmaps to Delivery 2020'.
19. A. King, R. F. Oman, G. S. Brassington, D. L. Bliwise, and W. L. Haskell, 'Moderate Intensity Exercise and Self-Rated Quality of Sleep in Older Adults—A Randomised Controlled Trial', *Journal of the American Medical Association*, 277.1 (1997), 32–37; A. Bowes and H. Wilkinson '"We Didn't Know It Would Get That Bad": South Asian Experiences of Dementia and the Service Response', *Health and Social Care in the Community*, 11.5 (2003), 387–96; A. Wiles and D. Booker, 'Complementary Therapies in Dementia Care', *Journal of Dementia Care*, 11.3 (2003), 31–35; G. D. Cohen, S. Perlstein, J. Chapline, J. Kelly, K. M. Firth, and S. Simmens, 'The Impact of Professionally Conducted Cultural Programs on the Physical Health, Mental Health and Social Functioning of Older Adults', *The Gerontologist*, 46.6 (2006), 726–34; Billington et al., 2013; and Longden et al., 2016.
20. Brownfoot Associates, *The Needs of People with Dementia and Their Carers Within Three Ethnic Minority Groups in Haringey*. A Report Commissioned by Haringey Housing and Social Services and the London Regional Office of the Alzheimer's Disease Society, Haringey (Social Services Department/Alzheimer's Disease Society, 1998); and D. Jolley, 'The "Twice a Child" Projects: Learning About Dementia and Related Disorders Within the Black and Minority Ethnic Population of an English City and Improving Relevant Services', *Ethnicity and Inequalities in Health and Social Care*, 2.4 (2009), 5–9.

21. 'Reading for Change', Organisation for Economic Co-operation and Development (OECD), 2002. https://www.oecd.org/edu/school/.../33690904.pdf (accessed 9 March 2019).
22. J. Billington, P. Davis, and G. Farrington, 'Reading as Participatory Art: An Alternative Mental Health Therapy', *Journal of Arts and Community*, 5.1 (2014) 25–40; J. Davis, 'Enjoying and Enduring: Groups Reading Aloud for Wellbeing', *The Lancet*, 373.9665 (2009), 714–15; C. Dowrick, J. Billington, J. Robinson, A. Hamer, and C. Williams, 'Get into Reading as an Intervention for Common Mental Health Problems: Exploring Catalysts for Change', *Medical Humanities*, 38.1 (2012), 15–20; E. Gray, G. Kiemle, J. Billington, and P. Davis, 'An Interpretative Phenomenological Analysis of the Experience of Being in a Reader Group', *Arts & Health: An International Journal for Research, Policy and Practice*, 8.3 (2016), 248–61; S. Hodge, J. Robinson, and P. Davis, 'Reading Between the Lines: The Experiences of Taking Part in a Community Reading Project', *Journal of Medical Humanities*, 33.2 (2007), 100–04; E. Longden, P. Davis, J. Billington, and R. Corcoran, 'Shared Reading: Assessing the Intrinsic Value of a Literature-Based Intervention', *Journal of Medical Humanities*, 41.2 (2015), 113–20.
23. A. M. Taqui, A. Itrat, W. Qidwai, and Z. Qadri, 'Depression in the Elderly: Does Family System Play a Role? A Cross-Sectional Study', *BMC Psychiatry*, 7.1 (2007), 57; H. A. Ganatra, S. N. Zafar, W. Qidwai, and S. Rozi (2008) 'Prevalence and Predictors of Depression Among an Elderly Population of Pakistan', *Aging and Mental Health*, 12.3 (2008), 349–56.
24. A. Macmillan, *A Little Aloud* (London: Random House, 2010).
25. K. Rumbold and C. Clark, *Reading for Pleasure: A Research Overview* (London: The National Literacy Trust, 2006).
26. K. E. Stanovich, R. F. West, and M. R. Harrison, 'Knowledge Growth and Maintenance Across the Life Span: The Role of Print Exposure', *Developmental Psychology*, 31.5 (1995), 811.
27. Y. Stern, 'Cognitive Reserve in Ageing and Alzheimer's Disease, *Lancet Neurology*, 11.11 (2012), 1006–12.
28. D. A. Snowdon, S. J. Kemper, J. A. Mortimer, L. H. Greiner, D. R. Weikstein, and W. R. Markesbery, 'Linguistic Ability in Early Life and Cognitive Function and Alzheimer's Disease in Late Life: Findings from the Nun Study', *Journal of the American Medical Association*, 275.7 (1996), 528–32.
29. D. A. Snowdon, 'Healthy Aging and Dementia Findings from the Nun Study', *Annals of Internal Medicine*, 139.5 (2003), 450–45.
30. A. R. Kaup, 'Older Adults with Limited Literacy are an Increased Risk for Likely Dementia', *Journals of Gerontology Series A Biological Sciences and Medical Sciences*, 69.7 (2014), 900–06.
31. S. W. Suh, 'Impacts of Illiteracy on the Risk of Dementia: A Global Health Perspective', *Journal of Alzheimer's Disease*, 53.2 (2016), 731–41.

32. R. Wilson, P. A. Boyle, L. Yu, L. L. Barnes, J. A. Schneider, and D. A. Bennett, 'Life-Span Cognitive Activity, Neuropathologic Burden and Cognitive Aging', *Neurology*, 81.4 (2013), 314–21.
33. A. Paganini-Hill, C. H. Kawas, and M. M. Corrada, 'Lifestyle Factors and Dementia in the Oldest-Old: The 90+ Study', *Alzheimer Disease & Associated Disorders*, 30.1 (2016), 21–26.
34. K. S. Jacob, 'Recovery Model of Mental Illness: A Complementary Approach to Psychiatric Care', *Indian Journal of Psychological Medicine*, 37.2 (2015), 117–19.
35. A. Spector, M. Orrell, and B. Woods, 'Cognitive Stimulation Therapy (CST): Effects on Different Areas of Cognitive Function for People with Dementia'. *International Journal of Geriatric Psychiatry*, 25.12 (2010), 1253–58.
36. A. Holm, M. Lepp, and K. C. Ringsberg, 'Dementia: Involving Patients in Storytelling—A Caring Intervention: A Pilot Study', *Journal of Clinical Nursing*, 14.2 (2004), 256–63; L. Phillips, S. A. Reid-Arndt, and Y. Pak, 'Effects of a Creative Expression Intervention on Emotions, Communication and Quality of Life in Persons with Dementia', *Nursing Research*, 59.6 (2010), 417–25; J. Billington, J. Carroll, P. Davis, C. Healey, and P. Kinderman, 'A Literature-Based Intervention for Older People Living with Dementia'. *Perspective in Public Health*, 133.3 (2013), 165–73.
37. Y. Young, P. Camic, and V. Tischler, 'The Impact of Community-Based Arts and Health Interventions on Cognition in People with Dementia: A Systematic Literature Review', *Aging and Mental Health*, 20.4 (2016), 337–51; US National Endowment for the Arts, *The Arts and Aging: Building the Science* (Washington, DC: US National Endowment for the Arts, 2013).
38. I. Papathanasiou and P. Coppens, *Aphasia and Related Neurogenic Communication Disorders* (Burlington, MA: Jones & Bartlett Learning, 2017), pp 473–74.
39. K. A. Bayles, 'Effects of Working Memory Deficits on the Communicative Functioning of Alzheimer's Dementia Patients', *Journal of Communication Disorders*, 36.3 (2003), 209–19.
40. J. L. Cummings, J. P. Houlihan, and Mary Ann Hill, 'The Pattern of Reading Deterioration in Dementia of the Alzheimer Type: Observations and Implications', *Brain and Language*, 29.2 (1986), 315–23; and A. Leff and R. Starrfelt, *Alexia: Diagnosis, Treatment and Theory* (London: Springer Verlag, 2014).
41. D. A. Bolata, G. C. Burgess, M. J. Cortese, and D. R. Adams, 'The Word-Frequency Mirror Effect in Young, Old and Early-Stage Alzheimer's Disease: Evidence for Two Processes in Episodic Recognition Performance', *Journal of Memory and Language*, 46.1 (2002), 199–226.

42. S. Rimkeit and G. Claridge, 'Literary Alzheimer's: A Qualitative Feasibility Study of Dementia-Friendly Book Groups', *New Zealand Library & Information Management Journal*, 56.2 (2017), 14–22.
43. J. L. Keidel, P. M. Davis, V. Gonzalez-Diaz, C. D. Martin, and G. Thierry, 'How Shakespeare Tempests the Brain, *Cortex*, 49.4 (2013), 913–19; and A. M. Jacobs, 'Neurocognitive Poetics: Methods and Models for Investigating the Neuronal and Cognitive-Affective Bases of Literature Reception', *Frontiers in Human Neuroscience*, 16.9 (2015), 186.
44. Bayles, 2003; G. C. Gilmore, K. E. Groth, and C. W. Thomas, 'Stimulus Contrast and Word Reading Speed in Alzheimer's Disease', *Experimental Aging Research*, 31.1 (2005), 15–33; and T. Rose, L. Worrall, and K. McKenna, 'The Effectiveness of Aphasia-Friendly Principles for Printed Health Education Materials for People with Aphasia Following Stroke', *Aphasiology*, 17.10 (2003), 947–63.
45. D. Sim, S. Rimkeit, and G. Claridge, *Report of the Study: Reading for Pleasure: The Benefits of Participating in a Dementia-Friendly Book Group at the Care Home—A Pilot Study of a Randomised Controlled Trial* (Wellington: University of Otago, 2018).
46. R. G. Logsdon, L. E. Gibbons, S. M. McCurry, and L. Teri, 'Quality of Life in Alzheimer's Disease: Patient and Caregiver Reports', *Journal of Mental Health and Aging*, 5.1 (1999), 21–32.
47. P. Noone, 'Addenbrooke's Cognitive Examination-III', *Occupational Medicine*, 65.5 (2015), 418–20.
48. A. Bergland, M. Kirkevold, P.-O. Sandman, D. Hofoss, and D. Edvardsson, 'The Thriving of Older People Assessment Scale: Validity and Reliability Assessments', *Journal of Advanced Nursing*, 71.4 (2014), 942–50.
49. J. A. Yesavage, 'Geriatric Depression Scale', *Psychopharmacology Bulletin*, 24.4 (1988), 709–11.
50. S. Baron Cohen, A. M. Leslie, and U. Frith, 'Does the Autistic Child Have a "Theory of Mind"?', *Cognition*, 21.1 (1985), 37–46.
51. J. L. Cummings, M. Mega, K. Gray, S. Rosenberg-Thompson, and D. A. Carusi, 'The Neuropsychiatric Inventory: Comprehensive Assessment of Psychopathology in Dementia', *Neurology*, 44.12 (1994), 2308–14.
52. J. P. Hirdes, G. Ljunggren, J. N. Morris, D. H. M. Frijters, H. F. Soveri, L. Gray, M. Bjorkgren, and R. Gilgen, 'Reliability of the interRAI Suite of Assessment Instruments: A 12-Country Study of an Integrated Health Information System', *BMC Health Services Research* 8.227 (2008).

20

Reading in Secure Settings
Nick Benefield and Kathryn Naylor interviewed by Fiona Magee

Nick Benefield, Kathryn Naylor and Fiona Magee

Nick Benefield in Interview with Fiona Magee,[1] 'Whilst Not Falling Apart'

A psychotherapist and policy-maker, Nick Benefield, recently retired, was Advisor to the Department of Health Personality Disorder and Offender Personality Disorder Programme and Head of the Department of the Health/National Offender Management Service. Along with colleagues, he is responsible for establishing in criminal justice settings the environmental model of living, management and care known as PIPES—Psychologically Informed Planned Environments.

FM: What's the thinking behind PIPES?

NB: PIPES are established in both prisons and in criminal justice settings in the community. They are part of a pathway approach to the longer term care and management of high risk offenders. It is not sufficient to lock a person up and get them fed and watered; we need to create environments that support psychosocial life and character development, to further

N. Benefield (✉)
Advisor to Offender Personality Disorder Pathway, NHS England, Leeds, UK
e-mail: nick.benefield@icloud.com

K. Naylor · F. Magee
Mersey Care NHS Mental Health Trust, Liverpool, UK
e-mail: Kathryn.Naylor@merseycare.nhs.uk

J. Billington (ed.), *Reading and Mental Health*,
https://doi.org/10.1007/978-3-030-21762-4_20

day-to-day stability and long-term hope. I think it is one of the most optimistic things happening in prisons at present.

It is a life programme and a long business. We track improvements in prisoners' social and psychological behaviours, their general psychological health, as well as ultimately a reduction in their risk of offending. Already we have some evidence that people are doing a lot better. We've only been at this now for seven years, so only a few have come out so far, but of the ones who do come out, the indicators are that they feel more stable and equipped to be back out in the world when they come to leave prison.

FM: How did you develop your ideas about what is the way to look after people?

NB: After social work training, I began working at a place near Cirencester called The Cotswolds Community, which was in the process of changing from being a children's prison into a therapeutic unit. I was a residential social worker and social therapist there for twelve years.

I was responsible for a lot of very difficult kids, in a place that had no locked doors, no punishments, eight staff, and we ran a small farm-holding, milked cows, kept sheep, baked bread. It was hands-on working with people and I learnt all about therapeutic social work and about what Donald Winnicott (paediatrician and psychoanalyst) called 'good enough'[2] upbringing. I still see some of those children—they're men with families of their own now. Most appear to have done well.

I started my own analysis and trained as a psychotherapist. After developing social group work and Family Service Units in London, I took on the Directorship of Hammersmith Mind. After eight years, I took on NHS commissioning—eventually commissioning forensic services in the North West for Ashworth Hospital and all the medium and low secure services. I started a multidisciplinary team there which included a prison governor, a psychiatrist, a nurse, a psychologist, a social worker, a probation officer, so you had a more integrated team commissioning all of those services.

FM: And the fact that it is a 'mixed team' is important?

NB: Yes. The health service, in my view, lost the core task for psychology some years back when psychology services became more specialist and access more limited. In the context of the Offender Personality Disorder Programme, I wanted psychologists to go and work on the floor in prisons with the officers, so they are fully present as the psychological mind in the present setting. I wanted them freed up from doing just assessments and offender treatment programmes, to being able to make a difference to the day-to-day lives of people—spotting and getting people early, working with them, seeing it as a life-long plan and thinking about them all the way throughout into the community; so it's more than just a psychological intervention.

FM: How did you first come to commission reading groups?

NB: I first found out about the UK charity The Reader in 2006, when I met Jane Davis (founder and director) and we talked about how Shared Reading might fit into the idea of how you engage people through methods other than traditional therapy. Reading groups were the first of what we call the 'enrichment projects' as part of this. I funded an initial piece of work with The Reader back in 2010 and they now run reading groups in every PIPE in the UK.

FM: Why did you think Shared Reading would be a good fit?

NB: My feeling is that people in these settings can get a new start in this area of experience by being read to. Reading is a very rewarding experience. If we think about what happens for children when they are being read to: they make sense of their environment and how they fit into it. In some way it builds a picture for them about how the world is and then they can actually marry it with the reality. We learn about good and bad, right and wrong, kindness and unkindness—the whole range of emotions and many life scenarios. These ideas can be rehearsed and worked out—better understood without too much anxiety. Children (and later, adults) hear stories and they build up *internal narratives about how life is both for themselves and others.*

FM: Internal narratives? Can you tell me more about that idea?

NB: A man or a woman in a prison has done something very wrong that got them there and they have a story, an internal narrative, about their life—how they got to where they got to. Often it's things like, 'It's all because of my ex' or 'This happened to me when I was young' or sometimes, 'It wasn't me, it didn't really happen'. Those narratives are there, fundamentally, to preserve their sanity. If you've harmed someone you've got to have a narrative that makes it possible in some way to live with it. The alternative is that you become very defensive and bury it so it's untouched and you drop it away from consciousness.

What we need is men and women in this position to be able to gradually face that difficulty, to change the narrative about it, because their existing narrative is incorrect—it doesn't give them any responsibility ('my dad beat the living daylights out of me') or blames the victim. What you need is for them to have a more complex narrative that gives them an understanding that they both own a responsibility and aren't solely responsible. In other words, some choices and decisions were driven by all sorts of other factors in their lives.

FM: What sort of factors?

NB: Most of the men and women in the offender personality disorder programme have chronically deprived, often traumatised and broken early years. I don't mean that's the *reason* they commit bad acts but I would say there's a direct relationship between early deprivations and traumas and later anti-social behaviour. If a child has a positive environment that is socially and relationally rich, that supports the neuropsychological development of the individual brain to some degree. If the *opposite* happens, we now know that this tends to lead to poorer quality of relating later, a poorer containment in the individual and poorer emotional management.

FM: What do you mean by containment?

NB: I mean holding onto yourself, being yourself, being able to relate to others whilst not falling apart yourself; I mean not being disruptive and being collaborative—so you can have friends and relationships, which of course go up and down but you can generally *manage*. I'm talking about what we might call an internalised moral capacity and things like being assertive but at the same time still considering others. All of these things are subtle but very important latent social skills and a significant number of the prison population have not been given the experience to develop these skills. Around 34,000, at the last estimation, fit the criteria for having a severe personality disorder likely to be related to their criminal offending and are probably a risk to themselves and particularly to other people. There's a lot of people we don't help; prison provision might work as a deterrent for individuals who are relatively normal psychologically, but actually most of these men and women *aren't* as robust.

FM: But there is help that can be given? Can you tell me more about what form that takes?

NB: My work is about trying to understand; if children get most of this ability to learn early by the way they're reared and attached and safe, what might we do with a man or woman in their early thirties who's committed a serious crime and is in prison? We can't regrow brains, but we *can* provide an experience which they can internalise—give them a good experience that they enjoy, feel valued in and respected by, that is social and in some way equated to early childhood experience of attachment and safe relationship.

Over the years I've been to so many prisons and secure hospitals and I was disheartened by the poverty of these environments—low levels of support for improving relating, no art, no creative workshops—so little through which you might learn something new and fresh, that might feed you in some way and give you a sense of something other than the basic day-to-day provision. The Reader seemed to be ready-made for bringing a new level of ongoing psychosocial enrichment into those environments.

FM: You're not talking here, are you, about teaching literacy, but something else?

NB: If people want to learn to read and write, that's great but that must not be the purpose of why, in the context of the Reader groups, we are 'reading to' people in prison. To me, what the reading groups should be about is giving special time to these men and women without laying any expectation on them.

If you just stick with the idea of trying to teach people to read, it can become bound up with shame and failure—you can get to the literacy issues, but not until you've first overcome the discomfort, the anxiety, the inhibition, the early failure, all that sense of 'I stutter over words and I can't get them right, and yet I'm a 30-year-old man who was tough on the street'. These are things we know are very hard for people to overcome. To be read to is to be given a reading plus experience.

FM: What is the value of this 'special time' they are getting in the reading group? What does it do?

NB: I think there are a few things going on. Firstly, getting these men and women to read together in a group gives them a richer experience of *social* life and allows them to test out how to be orderly with one another too. Can I be relatively normal in a group of other people? Can I have my views challenged? Can I be listened to or listen and wait for other people to speak? All very simple social skills these people often have missed out on.

And secondly, it gives them a richer *interior* life. It allows people to rework experiences, to rework aspects of themselves, taking on other references and viewpoints. If I'm a man who has done harm, and I'm in a high secure prison my place in the world in one sense is a very rigid fixed point—this is who and what I am, I am a serious offender in prison—doing my time. The approach we take to running a PIPE setting, including the reading groups, allows for some *re-triangulation*: it allows the identity of the person to become a little more fluid and able to incorporate something else other than their fixed narrative—does that make sense?

FM: Back to the idea of changing narrative?

NB: Yes, because when you read, and particularly in a group, all the time you're hearing other people's views. What happens is you don't have to keep your old narrative going—you become less defensive and you can test out a new narrative, and the thing is you're doing it with the story—the story removes it slightly from you, so you don't have to expose yourself too far, you can put something out there and see what people make of it. You're growing your capacity to explore varying views on how life is, to test out various ideas and perspectives.

What you're essentially asking the people in the reading group to do, is to put themselves in somebody else's place. There is a brilliant book, *This is Water*, by the philosopher David Foster-Wallace—we bought it for all the PIPE teams—and it's about how you've got to keep at the job of thinking, 'So what's happening on the other side, what's it like to be the other person?' Because if you don't, the danger is you only get to the division that says, 'They are different than me and I don't like their difference' and that's that. Life is then only one-dimensional, my view alone.

FM: I visited one of the reading groups in HMP Frankland recently, and the clinical lead there said to me: 'The men see the reading group as a break away from their treatment, but in fact it is part of their treatment'. Do you agree?

NB: Yes! But we don't need them to see it as part of their treatment. However, we do need the prison or hostel to understand that it has a therapeutic potential. The other concern is that this is early days in a long-term initiative and we have to be careful about how this sort of provision is perceived. It's only several years ago, remember, that there was a ban on books in prison. All these enrichment activities—reading, singing and drama—they can be seen as in some way too pleasurable for offenders and so we might receive a negative press.

FM: Because … not punitive enough?

NB: Look, none of this is a science, but it's my feeling that when we put someone into prison, we need to maximise it as an opportunity—with reading, with singing, with any enrichment projects and good relating and good 'parenting'—if we want to help people to become better citizens. We pay maybe £50,000 a year to put one man into prison. Why waste that? It must be seen as an investment.

We should treat our prisons as better places, as part of our world, and then *our* world would be better. I was recently visiting a prison in an Overseas Territory and it was a place where we would all agree conditions were shameful. And, OK, compared to that, in our prisons we generally follow good human rights; the prisons themselves are generally clean and tidy, but actually the experience of being a human in a prison? If we were to go and live in a prison for a month or two, I think we would have a new perspective on how much the setting supports good human relating. We've no right under criminal law to deprive prisoners of anything other than their liberty. What an institutional environment such as a prison does a lot of the time is it quashes the capacity for human interaction. I understand that, to some extent, it has to, for lots of very good reasons about safety and risk, but my principle is, if you treat people badly you get bad people (from babyhood onwards) and if you treat them as well and respectfully as possible, then you're generally going to get better, more responsive people. The trouble is that, like a lot of things, prisons are an industrial model for a human problem—and trying to change that is a hard balancing act. A good many prison Governors and staff work to reduce the worst impact but it's often an uphill struggle because the conditions work against it.

FM: I'm interested in your emphasis on the 'human'. That's about, is it, compassion? But also imperfection?

NB: The men and women we work with, they're real people with real difficulties and we can make a difference in the time we've got where we deprive them of their liberty—we can maximise the opportunity, in PIPE settings at least, for supporting the improvement of human relating. We want people to be better related and better relaters. If you can't get on being in the presence of other people, you are more likely to be in trouble. Many of these men and women are deeply troubled by their relationship to others: personality disorder, which is what most of them have, is fundamentally a difficulty in the relationship between the person themselves and the world—'this doesn't look right', 'that person's not behaving properly', 'he shouldn't have said that': relating, for them, is troubled and it's persistent, pervasive and problematic.

FM: But not hopeless?

NB: Donald Winnicott said, 'The delinquent act is an act of hope';[3] in other words if I take, I take because I think I might one day have. Many people act that hope out through acts of physical taking, so stealing for example—many years ago we looked after a boy who used to steal and every time he stole he threw the money down the toilet, just flushed it all away, never kept or used it. It was the act of taking that was the thing. I'm very moved by people in prisons sometimes—I'm quite hard-nosed in other ways because I know how harsh the world can be for people—but I've met people in prison for whom, I realise, their resilience and their still holding something means … there is a hope for them, you know?

FM: What about the prison officers—how do they fit into this thinking?

NB: I once said to two prison officers who complained that each day started so badly with angry exchanges as men were unlocked at breakfast, 'When you go to unlock a prison door and take your key out of your fob, just for thirty seconds think about the man, the individual, behind that door. *Then* open the door'. I was back there a few weeks later and they said, 'You know you told us to do that thing about the keys, well we've started doing that and mornings are a lot better here now'.

It's a different way of working. I've met a lot of officers who've told me that they were miserable, they didn't want to come to work, but since they've been working in the PIPE setting that's all changed. They can't imagine why nobody ever told them this is what it could be like in prison. They've started to feel they can treat prisoners thoughtfully, with more respect and as individuals—I hear prison officers talk to me about individual prisoners in a way that they never would have done years ago; they speak as though they're talking about real human beings whom they understand have done bad things, they must look after them safely, but they have expectations and hope for them. That is a great gain. And it leads to more steady and stable prisoners because they feel cared about by the staff and related to.

If we could just get people to understand that prisons are depersonalised worlds in which humans are organised into institutional living that tends to replicate their life experiences in a negative fashion. We want prisons to be the opportunity to provide them with emotionally reparative experiences. To make time in prison more live and human because these people don't get much experience of that and if they're going to come out and live in the world again here they will need to be more emotionally and socially literate.

FM: It's a big ask of everyone involved—the men and the officers—isn't it?

NB: Yes, I suppose it is. The men in particular perhaps. We are asking them to trust: they have to trust and that can be hard. They come to the reading group and they have to watch the reader and the others in the group in order to think, 'Is this safe?'. Just the listening, speaking and tolerating other people's responses is so big an issue if you have had few opportunities to develop safe experiences of being with others. They're not asking a conscious question about safety but that's what's going on.

A lot of the men couldn't engage, they wouldn't start therapy and so we had to try and work out what happens when you are confronted with something unexpected in relating terms—like the reading group for example. Why might they find it hard to take up something that is offered and which, over time, might help. We wanted to understand and learn *what makes engagement safe*, what are the rules? What happens in this fearful, uncertain space of the first engagement with an unknown 'other'. It is surprising how little we are able to maintain that sort of attention, and for people who have had poor early experiences of sufficient attention to their emotional states it is very important.

Kathryn Naylor in Interview with Fiona Magee, 'The Things That We Have'

Dr Kathryn Naylor is an associate specialist in forensic psychiatry at Ashworth Hospital, one of the three high-security psychiatric hospitals in England, alongside Rampton and Broadmoor, providing services for patients who, presenting a grave danger to themselves or other people, require treatment and care in conditions of high security. The majority come from prison, or through the court system, or from a secure unit. Rehabilitative and creative activity includes Shared Reading groups involving both staff and patients. Dr Naylor has been leading one such group, as part of a research study, undertaken by Centre for Research into Reading Literature and Society, University of Liverpool.[4] *The interviewer, Fiona Magee (a member of the CRILS research team) based the conversation on selected transcripts from the recorded reading group sessions and began with one session which focused on Robert Browning's poem, 'Along the Road'.*

I walked a mile with Pleasure;
She chattered all the way,
But left me none the wiser
For all she had to say.

I walked a mile with Sorrow
And ne'er a word said she;
But oh, the things I learned from her
When Sorrow walked with me![5]

KN: Participants may often find it so hard to articulate their feelings and actually know what their feelings are. So if you say 'What's sorrow?', they may really struggle. They've all experienced sorrow so much, that I think it would be good for them to recognise that bit.

FM: One man in the group who was asked what he might 'learn' from Sorrow, as the poem suggests, said, first, 'Regret', then after a long pause, changed it to 'Remorse'.

KN: For the men that we look after, 'remorse' is a word that may be bandied around a lot. And they don't always know what it is, though they know they're supposed to feel it. But if you can't feel for yourself what's happened because you don't understand those feelings, it's very hard to feel for somebody else. It's all mediated through the same bit of your brain—physical pain, emotional pain and pain for others—empathy.

FM: About not understanding your own feelings—I am wondering if the value of stories and poems lies in trying to shift that a bit?

KN: When we made the poster, advertising the voluntary reading group, we said it's 'therapeutic not therapy'. What we think is going on is that it becomes more abstract and less concrete. So at first it's very concrete and literal to participants—'We don't understand this' or 'It must be about this, because that's what it says in the poem'—and gradually more abstract thought comes out.

FM: You often ask them, 'Can you imagine what this is like?' Can you tell me a bit more about what you mean by 'abstract'?

KN: The things that are not in the words. So when we are reading, there are the words and the narrative, but there's all the other stuff that's going on in your head that brings the story to life. You're imagining it—your imagination, your past experience, and something might just strike you. Group-members often haven't had an experience of being read to, they often have very poor literacy, and their illness makes it difficult for them to take or change a perspective, and think about what can be taken away—abstracted—from the poem, about what other meanings things might have beyond the concrete words. It means taking a leap from the word on the page to what that's like.

FM: Some of the poems, such as William Stafford's 'A Ritual to Read to Each Other' speak of the need for human connection:

> I call it cruel and maybe the root of all cruelty
> to know what occurs but not recognize the fact[6]

One of your group-members talks of people being scared to show their real emotions in prison. Another—the same man who had said 'Remorse' in the previous session—just says, 'Missed friendship'—like a brief message in one or two words, with years beneath it.

KN: He is talking about all the things he misses. Something gone beyond your control isn't it: 'missed'. It's not 'I miss a friendship' it's … it's gone.

This is really important for them because friendships in Ashworth … you don't have friends really. So, you arrive, you know that people have done things like you've done, or worse than you've done and you have to tolerate them, and you're told where you're going to be, on what ward. They find friendships really difficult and they talk about not wanting to be friends with anybody in the whole hospital, and for many of them, they haven't even really got friends outside, so they don't even get visitors. I think that one of the few things that they do find different here, in the Shared Reading group, is some sort of comradeship.

FM: There are blocks and resistances too in these groups: stuff that people do not want to feel.

KN: Yes. A group member might describe a feeling but not actually put himself in it emotionally, because that would be too difficult to tolerate. Not connecting: it's protective. I know how difficult they can find any feedback that's personal, because they feel unlovable and unlikeable and other people are untrustworthy. So anything that you feedback to them that's personal, they dismiss, or ignore. If they were reading in the group and I said 'Oh that was well read', that would be very difficult for them to accept because it's personal and it's about 'you' and they'd think I was lying or fobbing them off or being patronising. But I *could* say 'The way that you read that made me feel really sad' because it's about me, not about them. It's still praising their reading and they can accept that because it's not about them.

FM: You are describing the lack of an emotional vocabulary. But there are also breakthroughs.

KN: Yes. When one of the group says, 'My soul had gone'—that is one moment.

FM: Even without the vocabulary, you can see that everyone in the group can feel it.

KN: Or saying 'I just didn't know what to do' when he has been so scared of the scaredness, of the fear.

FM: What does the reading group do for them?

KN: I think instead of thinking about what does a reading group do for the people who are in it, start thinking more about what are the needs of the people that we are looking after, and then what would meet those needs. So, they lack connection with other people. They lack connection with their own emotions. They find it really hard to take other people's perspectives. They find it hard to think outwardly instead of just inwardly. Hard to develop friendships. Hard to sit and sustain concentration and attention. And then the side-things of literacy and numeracy and medication. And the abstract thought—starting to recognise what that is, in a safe way.

And then you think, well actually reading does all that. That's what reading does. And you can see it happening. You only have to get people in a room together for a sustained period and you can see something different is happening.

FM: Can you describe it?

KN: Well, one thing I wanted to say before is about this emptiness they've got, and wanting to fill this emptiness. A lot of what they are trying to do as well is check that they are still here and fill that emptiness.

FM: Check they are still here?

KN: Well, one of the features of borderline personality disorder is chronic feelings of emptiness. I think about it as like having a gnawing stomach because you're hungry, but imagine that all the time. Only it's not food. You might put food in because you think that's what it is, but actually it's all that love and attention that's missing. So you are constantly seeking to feed it in, to try and fill this emptiness, but you can't.

And so by starting to think instead of, 'What's this hole inside *me*?', thinking 'What are other people feeling? Can I fill that hole in a different way?', by beginning to stop focusing on this hole, you can start thinking about the things that we have that fill that hole.

FM: That 'we' have?

KN: The rest of people that don't have borderline traits. So, you know, your love, and what you feel for yourself, is not just about you is it? It's about the relationships you have with the people that are close to you. So if you're feeling a bit down, you might choose to phone somebody up? Because you know that you love them and they're going to be nice and it's going to make you feel better because you love them. Or you might go and watch nature. Or go for that swim. It's something else that's filling that hole but it's not about you having to fill it inside. You know that other things will make you better.

FM: So they often *don't* know other things will do that for them?

KN: No. So they harm themselves. In an attempt to feel better and fill the hole. Or take drugs to fill the emptiness inside. Or eat.

A lot of them have this emptiness inside and nothing to fill it, so the group helps them start finding something else.

Notes

1. A version of this interview first appeared in *The Reader*, 63 (2016), 19–30.
2. D. W. Winnicott, *Playing and Reality* (London: Tavistock Publications, 1971).
3. D. W. Winnicott, *Deprivation and Delinquency*, ed. by C. Winnicott, R. Shepherd, and M. Davis (London: Routledge, 1984).
4. See Chapter 9; see also M. Weston and E. McCann, 'Get into Reading with Mersey Care NHS Trust', *Mental Health and Social Inclusion*, 1.15 (2010), 12–16; and L. Dyer, 'Setting Up a Reading Group', *Mental Health Practice*, 13.8 (2010), 21–23.
5. R. Browning, *Poems*, 2 vols (London: Chapman and Hall, 1849).
6. W. Stafford, *The Way It Is: New and Selected Poems* (Minneapolis: Graywolf Press, 1999).

21

Reading in a Clinical Context
Andrew Jones and James Ledson in interview with Kate McDonnell

Andrew Jones, James Ledson and Kate McDonnell

KM: What drew you to pain medicine in particular because I guess it's not necessarily the most glamorous part of medicine?

AJ: I became interested in it in my first house job in a small North London district general hospital. There was a very keen palliative care nurse there; this was the time when palliative care was changing from hospice being the place where you went into to die to trying to manage people's pain and to keep them out in the community. The mainstay of that approach is something that is considered completely obvious now, which is to give regular doses of long-acting opiates but this was very new then. When I started Anaesthetics, I was interested in pain medicine so whenever I went anywhere, a training post, I let it be known and I was put in the pain clinic. I built up a reasonable training by doing that.

A version of this interview first appeared in *The Reader*, 65 (2017), 17–27.

A. Jones (✉) · J. Ledson
Royal Liverpool and Broadgreen University Hospitals
NHS Trust, Liverpool, UK
e-mail: Andrew.Jones@rlbuht.nhs.uk

J. Ledson
e-mail: James.Ledson@rlbuht.nhs.uk

K. McDonnell
The Reader Organisation (TRO), Liverpool, UK
e-mail: katemcdonnell@thereader.org.uk

J. Billington (ed.), *Reading and Mental Health*,
https://doi.org/10.1007/978-3-030-21762-4_21

JL: For me it was a slow burn. I first became interested when I was a House Officer. The hospital where I worked had an acute pain nurse, which was pretty much unheard-of at the time. I was working, amongst other things, in orthopaedics and this nurse and I would go round the ward and we'd make changes to people's medications to try and help them get over their operations. I'd also worked as an auxiliary nurse in a hospice before I went to medical school, so palliative care was something that I'd been exposed to before I knew any medicine. I went into Anaesthetics and I was most interested in pharmacology and physiology. After I'd been in Intensive Care for a while I started again with acute pain on the wards. From there, I became interested in the psychological side too and that drew me further into the chronic pain service. For people with acute pain, after an operation for example, you can treat the pain or help with the symptoms; they get better and the pain goes.

KM: What would you say are the particular challenges of pain medicine?

AJ: You have to be realistic about what you may achieve. You're not going to cure anybody, so you need to have the mindset that you are doing the best for the patient and that the patient will appreciate you're doing the best you can—it's important they feel better than they would do if you weren't doing what you are doing.

JL: It's very much a switch from a therapeutic cure, which you know does not exist, to providing support over a long period of time and trying to help people get through their setbacks and flare-ups. Sometimes it's great. You see someone in the clinic and they say 'I'm doing fine. I don't want you to make any changes'. But where people say 'I'm really quite terrible at the moment', that's probably where we do the most good; where we're the most useful. Don't forget, these are people who have been coming a long time to pain clinic; they've been around hospital doctors and have been around primary care an awful lot. They know that there's no point going to Accident & Emergency. There's no point going to see the GP. So their point of contact with any support is very often us and only us.

KM: So the doctor/patient relationship is critical in treating pain?

JL: A lot of our patients say that the simple greeting 'How are you?' fills them with dread because they don't know what to say to that person socially. They understand that the person probably isn't that interested that they're in pain, and they're worried that they will bore them so they keep it to themselves. Being able to come to the clinic and to express how they're feeling is an important part of the therapeutic relationship. Sometimes I feel like we're almost treated as a GP because people will come and they'll present us with problems that aren't related to pain in the clinic.

AJ: I think we fulfil that role more than GPs do now, the GP role has been changed so much. I did toy with the idea of becoming a GP when I first qualified and it was the day-to-day care that appealed to me, which I now get from the pain clinic, and which I wouldn't get if I was in General Practice in its present form. The relationship with the patients is very important. A lot of medicine is protocol and algorithm driven whereas in the clinic people are coming to see you because with your experience and knowledge you're not just following the protocol. I find that quite—I don't know what the word is really—satisfying.

KM: At the same time, it must be hard to be exposed to a lot of hopelessness.

AJ: Some of the negative feelings get channelled into anger on our patients' behalf. Many of them are from an inner city environment and most of them—the vast majority—are living on benefits, and they've had a constant assault on their living standards for many years. They're constantly having to go to assessments.

JL: That adds an extra layer of complexity to the condition, and to your therapeutic relationship; sometimes people are frightened to report an improvement because it might have a financial consequence. Those assessments do not allow for good days and bad days, good weeks and bad weeks. I've had patients who've been videoed round the supermarket and someone saying 'You carried a watermelon to the checkout, there's nothing wrong with you'. It just so happened it was a good day and he wanted a watermelon.

KM: It sounds quite holistic, as if the life of somebody coping with pain becomes bigger than if you were treating somebody you could fix.

JL: There are the things that we can do medically—injections and blocks, writing prescriptions. At the same time we're involved in the social and the psychological side. It's not uncommon for me to say 'I'm sorry we're not very good at treating this but we can perhaps help you to live with it better'.

AJ: I think we should drop the use of the word 'pain' in terms of the patients we look after because pain is only an aspect of the suffering and disability they're going through. The label of Chronic Pain is out there and people use it so we have to stick with it but it's not a very accurate description of what's happening to these patients. It probably simplifies the condition in the view of many people. I'm pretty sure a lot of doctors and a big part of the general public think 'Well, you're in pain, why don't you take a pain killer?' It's not a very helpful stance. What they really have is suffering. They do not have a localized symptom. Their whole life is awful.

JL: Often treatment is not so much a case of trying a new intervention but of reverting to something that worked previously and then stopped working. Pain is a dynamic thing and the treatments that help are also dynamic. In the same way that you have setbacks and flare-ups of your pain, there is a dynamic alteration in things that can be useful over time.

AJ: That's why we irritate and upset hospital management—patients keep coming back for years and years, whereas in theory, once we get someone stabilised on treatment we should discharge them but it isn't as simple as that. Jim and I both have backgrounds as anaesthetists where quality control is dead simple. The patient wakes up at the end; they're still alive; they can't recall anything about the operation; job done. Pain is much more complex. It's hard to have valid end points to demonstrate that you've done anything good in pain.

JL: Yes, the measures of success are all financially driven—things like patients not attending A&E, not needing to go to primary care.

AJ: How many people have you got back to work? Those measures are foisted on us sometimes and they are foisted on us to reduce our funding. The syndrome of chronic pain doesn't fit these models.

KM: Is there a pattern in the way people react to pain?

AJ: There is with all of them a sense of loss of the person they were before they had chronic pain. I'm at the stage of life where I can't do things that I used to be able to do but I've taken nearly sixty years to get to this stage. With chronic pain the loss happens very quickly and intensely.

JL: It's like a bereavement, particularly with people who have been active beforehand. When physical activity is no longer part of their life it leaves a huge void.

KM: When I started off with my condition I used to be really annoyed with my body, very angry and frustrated.

AJ: That's massive. Some of the work we explore in CBT classes is the idea of accepting that this is how you are now without that acceptance meaning that it's beaten you.

JL: You can be accepting of the situation without being hopeless and those two things are very easily confused. It's a fine line to tread. People can't really move on until they've accepted the chronicity because they will be searching for that magic bullet, that thing that will cure them.

KM: Do you find people who have extreme reactions?

AJ: Every single patient we've met has been different. They have similarities and themes but everyone reacts in their own way. You see despairing people. Occasionally you see somebody who puts on a front of stoicism, though I suppose if people really are stoic, we won't meet them.

KM: You were saying people, including many doctors, often don't understand pain. Do you feel attitudes or treatment are getting better?

AJ: The public awareness of chronic pain has probably greatly improved. The idea that we should have pain clinics and that they should be funded by the NHS has improved. In terms of medical students and junior doctors understanding chronic pain, I don't think it's any better. Do you know how much chronic pain is taught in medical schools? None at all! When medical students come to us, it's not just a revelation in terms of pain: it's a revelation that there's a whole world out there that they're not being taught about.

KM: What about your understanding of it?

JL: It changed over time for me. Starting out as a junior doctor, and probably as a consultant as well, at the beginning, I would have expected there to be a pharmacological solution or an intervention that would work, and interestingly that's often the point most of our patients start out from too. Over time, I've begun to be able to scratch the surface of how insidiously pain affects every part of your life.

AJ: That makes us very old-fashioned doctors in that we have improved our practice by learning from our patients over time. That is unusual in the modern medical context, where training is thought to be the key thing, not learning. What we think of as the marvels of modern medicine—surgery, anaesthesia, antibiotics, effective treatments for a whole gamut of ailments and conditions—is comparatively modern. Anaesthesia was first described in 1846 and all the modern marvels, imaging, antibiotics, they've all happened since then. Yet for about three millennia humanity has had doctors and virtually no therapeutic weapons. I think that what we're doing with pain medicine is to go back to that time. We're using fairly primitive techniques but there's still a need for us. And in some ways we have to compensate for the limited armamentarium by being more empathetic and by concentrating on the holistic stuff.

KM: What was it about Shared Reading that made you think it might help?

AJ: A professor in anaesthetics at University of Liverpool put us onto CRILS' study on the benefits of Shared Reading for people with depression (see Chapter 4) as he thought the findings were highly relevant to the needs of our own patients. There is a strong association between chronic pain and depression. People with chronic pain have three times the average risk of developing psychiatric symptoms such as mood or anxiety disorders, and depressed patients have three times the average risk of developing chronic pain. We, too, felt this might prove a useful intervention for patients with pain so we contacted The Reader and CRILS.

JL: My thoughts about Shared Reading and chronic pain have changed as I've become more involved. Initially I thought, yes, that would be a great benefit to people who are socially isolated and who will be able through it to have some sort of group dynamic and shared experience with others who have chronic pain. I realised quite quickly that there was an awful lot more going on. I suppose I undervalued at first the ability of Shared Reading to improve people's emotional literacy, which enabled them to articulate their condition better. There's one patient in particular whose treatment plan has radically changed because she became more emotionally aware and she was able to articulate a side of her distress.

AJ: The striking thing in the reading group is that everyone is so animated and engaged, and that's an unusual reaction for people with chronic pain. When we start the CBT groups, people are usually very inward looking and challenging you to get them engaged but the reading group wasn't like that, right from the early days. Of course some talk more than others and some say very little but they all seem to get the same benefit. They have the group thing but I'm sure the actual reading, as Jim said, has changed them.

KM: How would you describe emotional literacy?

JL: It's being more aware of your own emotions and your own feelings and also being able to use that awareness as a doorway to examine your behaviours. If you imagine somebody who is really cross and is railing and ranting that's very different to somebody who says—to themselves—I'm actually very angry at the moment. The person who says I'm angry is likely to be able to do something more effective about it than the person who is ranting and raving.

KM: Is it to do with being able to step outside the emotion?

JL: A little bit, yes. That probably comes with being able to vicariously examine characters' behaviours and emotions rather than it being personal straight away. There is no expectation on people who come to the Shared Reading group to talk about themselves but they can nevertheless explore how they feel through the characters in the literature.

KM: How does that help them living with pain?

AJ: We've demonstrated decreases in pain after the group but I think they're better able to deal with it as just pain rather than as global suffering because of the reading group. The rest of the week, even though the pain is bad, they're less distressed by it. Some of the patients I know through the clinic seem much more well after two years of Shared Reading than they were before. There's fluctuation of course but that's against a background of lesser suffering.

JL: It would be interesting to try functional brain scans. Perhaps reading exercises parts of the brain you wouldn't normally exercise.

KM: What do you think is going on in that space of pain still being there but some other thing happening?

AJ: Pain comes about because the central nervous system reordered itself. Neural plasticity. When we do nerve blocks or trigger point injections, that peripheral stimulus seems to change the wiring again and I would be very surprised if it wasn't the case that Shared Reading is doing the same thing, just with a different peripheral stimulus. It's been demonstrated that people do feel improvements in wellness when they listen to music and literature seems to be coming at it in the same way. That's been one of the revelations to me since getting involved in this work, how much arts for health work is going on, which the medical profession knows absolutely nothing about. Fortunately, the arts for health people know very little about what the medical profession is doing too!

KM: How would you compare Shared Reading and CBT in terms of what's going on with thinking?

AJ: CBT is an intellectual understanding of concepts—we're tapping into one part of their thinking but we're not tackling the emotional side of it. CBT gives pain sufferers a new way of looking at their pain, and that's something that Shared Reading can build on.

Some of the things we're trying to achieve in CBT—things we plant the seed of there—come out in a different way, an emotionally realised way in Shared Reading. You might think it's lost because the CBT course is over, but Shared Reading can bring things back or make them more individually 'have-able'.

JL: When people take part in CBT for pain, the model is usually that they have an assessment to decide whether or not it's likely to be useful for them. There is kind of an unwritten contract that you have to engage in a particular way. So for example, you would feel pressure to talk about and examine thoughts that you've had around pain whereas with Shared Reading it's completely voluntary. You can choose whether or not and to what extent you wish to engage with the emotional content of the literature.

AJ: A lot of patients with chronic pain define themselves more by their pain and what they *can't* do or no longer have. Successful therapy, by whatever means, is allowing them to start defining themselves by what they can do and still have. It is well known that you can cause damage by dredging things up from people's past but clearly Shared Reading is a very gentle, safe way of doing that.

JL: One similarity with CBT is that people who have unshakeable beliefs can be challenged by others in the group but, in the case of Shared Reading, because it's often removed from the individual—it's a character in a book—the climb-down is easier. It's easier to change your mind or to take a different perspective. And then on a layer slightly deeper than that, you can choose whether or not you wish to think about the emotions that those characters in the literature have evoked in you and why that might be, again, using it perhaps as a doorway to effect change and changes in cognition principally.

KM: What's holding the door open in that way?

AJ: It's voluntary and it's non-judgemental and non-selective, which we tried to be in the early days with the CBT classes but we have had to screen a bit.

KM: What do you screen for?

JL: I suppose one of the biggest things is if somebody is expecting to come to a course of CBT and have less pain at the end. If people expect that and you can't budge them from that expectation then they're going to be disappointed. With Shared Reading I suspect that people don't have any expectation that it's going to help their pain. So they're pleasantly surprised when it helps their distress. It's wonderfully open-ended. It doesn't claim to do anything or expect anything of anybody. It's not saying the book will do this or that for you. It just says, let's see what happens. That's why I would be worried about people perceiving it as a prescribed treatment.

AJ: When people are in CBT, they are people with pain. When they're in the reading group, they're people with lives. What Shared Reading tends to do is to find other bits of people that are not to do with pain. It doesn't target anything in particular—that's its strength. And we know that pain is essentially an emotional thing which us why it is important that Shared Reading is operating on a much more emotional level than CBT. It looks as though CBT will be of most help if it precedes Shared Reading. You'll get benefit from SR whichever way round you do it, but CBT is most effective as a preliminary or primer.

KM: How do you think it impacts on people's thought processes?

JL: There are ingrained patterns of thinking that are common to everyone with chronic pain and that have an adverse affect on quality of life. This probably applies to depression as well. The two obvious ones are the catastrophising and mindreading. By mindreading I mean you assume that someone has (usually negative) thoughts about you without actually having any evidence for it. Catastrophising is Oh God, it's always going to be like this. This is never going to get better. What we try to do, for example, with flare-ups is to get people to recognise that pattern of thinking and to rationalise it: I've been here before; it's always got better before; there's no reason why it won't do so again. Shared Reading can help with that again through the immersed exploration of the characters—it's recognising self, recognising yourself, sometimes in a good way and sometimes in a more challenging way.

AJ: There are ways of conforming brains so that certain emotions are more to the forefront or background. The frontal lobes are changed in people with chronic pain: there's less density and less connectivity. If you think how much this brain area controls personality, it obviously is an element controlling pain. I dare say Shared Reading is having an effect at that level, allowing the frontal lobes more control of the situation.

KM: Is the implication that chronic pain can change personality?

AJ: It does. Possibly people are reinventing themselves. Not as they were before but as someone they feel more comfortable with.

JL: Could it be that we all have various selves? We've got our perceived self, our hoped-for self, and it seems intuitively true to say that the further apart your hoped-for self and your perceived self are then the more trouble you're in. Could it be that by exploring characters and emotions in books, you're able to redefine your identity to something that fits better, perhaps bringing them closer together, your hoped-for self and your perceived self, the how-others-see-you self? It might be that that's one of the things the Shared Reading addresses. It's a reformulation.

Correction to: Quantitative Methods

Josie Billington, Rhiannon Corcoran,
Megan Watkins, Mette Steenberg, Charlotte Christiansen,
Nicolai Ladegaard and Don Kuiken

Correction to:
Chapter 12 in: J. Billington (ed.), *Reading and Mental Health*,
https://doi.org/10.1007/978-3-030-21762-4_12

The original version of the book was inadvertently published with an incorrect spelling of the author name "Nikolai Ladegaard" in chapter 12 and front matter. The correction to the chapter has been updated with the change.

The updated version of this chapter can be found at
https://doi.org/10.1007/978-3-030-21762-4_12

J. Billington (ed.), *Reading and Mental Health*,
https://doi.org/10.1007/978-3-030-21762-4_22

Index

J. Billington (ed.), *Reading and Mental Health*,
https://doi.org/10.1007/978-3-030-21762-4

M

N

S

W

Y

The manufacturer's authorised representative in the EU is Springer Nature Customer Service Centre GmbH, Europaplatz 3, 69115 Heidelberg, Germany. If you have any concerns regarding our products, please contact ProductSafety@springernature.com

Printed and bound by CPI Group (UK) Ltd, Croydon, CR0 4YY
05/10/2026
02228123-0014